NUTRACEUTICALS AND HEALTH

NUTRACEUTICALS AND HEALTH

Editor

Tai Hu Guan

scitus academics

Nutraceuticals and Health

Edited by **Tai Hu Guan**

ISBN: 978-1-68117-723-6
Library of Congress Control Number: 2016958849

SCITUS Academics LLC,
616, Corporate Way, Suite 2, 4766,
Valley Cottage, NY 10989

www.scitusacademics.com

Notice

Printed in United States of America on Acid Free Paper

PREFACE

In recent years, a new diet health paradigm is changing which places more emphasis on the positive facets of diet. The new lifestyle embraced by people today has altered the basic food habits of the latter. Consumption of the junk food has augmented manifold leading to a number of diseases caused due to improper nutrition. Nutraceutical is the hybrid of 'nutrition' and 'pharmaceutical'. Nutraceuticals, in broad, are food or part of food playing a significant role in modifying and maintaining normal physiological function that maintains healthy human beings. The principal reasons for the growth of the nutraceutical market worldwide are the current population and the health trends. The food products used as nutraceuticals can be categorized as dietary fibre, prebiotics, probiotics, polyunsaturated fatty acids, antioxidants and other different types of herbal/ natural foods. These nutraceuticals help in combating some of the major health problems of the century such as obesity, cardiovascular diseases, cancer, osteoporosis, arthritis, diabetes, cholesterol etc. In whole, 'nutraceutical' has lead to the new era of medicine and health, in which the food industry has become a research oriented sector.

Nutraceuticals and Health explores the role of nutraceuticals in human health, disease prevention, health promotion, and as an adjunct to disease treatment. The book opens with a general background of nutraceuticals and human health, then covers health and disease areas such as cancer, lipidemia and cardiovascular disease, metabolic syndrome with obesity, diabetes and hypertension, respiratory health, the gut microbiome, and cognitive decline. Furthermore, it concludes by addressing the methodological issues that must be addressed in the conduct of epidemiological research on nutraceuticals in health and disease. Contributors are recognized experts in their respective fields.

Nutraceuticals are the emerging class of natural products that makes the line between food and drugs to fade. Although the use of nutraceuticals by people has a long history, only recently scientifically supported nutritional and medical evidence has allowed nutraceuticals to emerge as being potentially effective. The nutraceuticals of both plant and animal origin holds exciting opportunities for the food industries to create novel food products in future. So, it is vital for students, product developers, nutritionists, dietitians, researchers and practitioners, and regulatory organizations.

TABLE OF CONTENTS

1

NUTRACEUTICALS: AN IMPERATIVE TO WELLNESS

Pravin Shende[1,2*], Drashti Desai[1] and Gaud RS[1]

Department of Chemistry IFM, University of Torino, Italy

ABSTRACT

Nutraceuticals have received considerable attention due to their speculative safety, potential nutritive and therapeutic effects. They are alternative to modern medicines and also provide healthy living. To avoid side effects associated with medicines, live longer expectancy and increase the health value of our diet, nutraceuticals are being preferred. They possess numerous therapeutic benefits like anti-obesity, immune enhancement, natural antioxidant, cardiovascular effects, anti-diabetic, anti-inflammatory effects, etc. Major constituents of nutraceuticals are nutrients, herbals and dietary supplements which help to maintain health, function against various diseases and ensure better quality of life. The aim of this article is to provide the current knowledge about the application of various nutraceuticals in different diseases.

Keywords: *Nutraceutical, cancer, anti-oxidant, proliferation, apoptosis, tumour*

ABBREVIATIONS

EPA: Eicosapentaenoic acid

DHA: Docosahexaenoic acid

CSC: Cancer stem cells

EMT: Epithelial mesenchymal transition

EGF-R: Epidermal growth factor receptor

AHCC: Active hexose correlated compound

PEITC: Phenethyl isothiocyanate

NK cells: Natural killer cells

CoQ10: Coenzyme Q10

ROS: Reactive oxidative species

RNS: Reactive nitrogen species

LDL: Low density lipoprotein

COX-2: Cyclo-oxygenase 2

VEGF: Vascular endothelial growth factor

IL: Interleukin

LPO: Lipid peroxidation

INTRODUCTION

Nutraceuticals have been received considerable attention due to their speculative safety, potential nutritional and therapeutic effects. Present day, exploration and exploitation of disease fighting properties of phytochemicals are found in both food and non-food plants which has created a renaissance in human health and nutrition research. However, it has become a social issue as food composition has been scientifically proven to avoid lifestyle-related diseases. Based on assumptions like, to avoid side effects associated with medicines, live longer and increase the health value of our diet, Nutraceuticals are being preferred [1].

Nutraceutical was derived from the words "nutrition" and "pharmaceutical", by Stephen DeFelice L in 1989. They are sometimes also termed as "functional foods". This term is applicable to the products that range from isolated nutrients, herbal products and dietary supplements, specific diets and processed foods such as beverages, soups and cereals. Functional foods or nutrients are foods that have one or more compounds with biochemical and physiological functions beneficial to individual's health. When functional food consumed regularly they provide specific health-beneficial effects (i.e. healthier status or lowering the risk of diseases-beyond their nutritional properties). The definition for Nutraceuticals and functional foods are not yet clear. Functional food is defined as "any food or food ingredients that may provide a health benefit beyond the traditional nutrients it contains", by the US Institute of Medicine's Food and Nutrition Board [2,3].

Nutraceuticals are new generation of food or supplements which is a link between drug and food. In addition, Father of medicine, Hippocrates emphasized on the relation between the use of appropriate food for health and their therapeutic benefits about 2000 years ago [4].

Nutraceuticals can be classified [5] as follows:

A) On the basis of natural source:

Products can be obtained from-

1. Plants- e.g. Indole-3-carbinol(cabbage), lycopene (tomatoes)

2. Animals- e.g. EPA and DHA (fish oil)

3. Minerals- e.g. selenium, iodine

4. Microbes- e.g. Phycocyanobilin (Spirulina), lactobacillus (yogurt)

B) On the basis of pharmacological conditions, or as per chemical constituents of the products

C) Nutraceuticals on basis of below properties:

1. Potential Nutraceuticals (plant-foods polyphenols for diabetes)

2. Established Nutraceuticals (polyvitamins, omega-3 fatty acids)

Most widely used food sources as Nutraceuticals are of natural sources and can be categorized as follows:

1. Dietary fibre- e.g. beans, fruits

2. Probiotics- e.g. yogurt, dark chocolate

3. Prebiotics- e.g. Asparagus, almonds, apples

4. Polyunsaturated fatty acids- e.g. olive oil, walnuts

5. Antioxidants vitamins- e.g. vitamin C, vitamin E

6. Polyphenols- e.g. tea, coffee, spinach

1. Spices- e.g. garlic, turmeric

Nutraceuticals in cancer treatment

Among adults, the leading cause of death is cancer. Treatment of cancer involves expensive and traumatic use of drugs, surgery and irradiation. By change in lifestyle, reduction in the rates of cancer has been observed in recent times. Nutrition and foods are related to 30% of cancers. A deficiency of any of the 40 nutrients essential for life increases the risk of cancer has been proven in animal study [6].

A large subset of organ-specific subtypes are often too unique, histologically and genomically is represented in human cancers. One of the biggest challenges is the absence of validated therapeutic target(s), especially when evaluating the activity of natural agents (Nutraceuticals) for effective clinical management of human cancers [7].

Nutraceuticals have the ability to control and regulate the DNA damaging factors in cancer cells and DNA transcription in tumours. They possess numerous therapeutic benefits like anti-obesity, immunity enhancement, natural antioxidant, cardiovascular, Antidiabetic, and anti-inflammatory effects [8].

The possibility always exists for herbal-based dietary supplements (or Nutraceuticals) to antagonize therapy. The recent research has revealed that certain natural compounds of phytochemical origin has the potential to interfere with the late-stage cancer and altering the metastatic spread of cancer [9]. Certain foods or supplements has shown direct effect on cancer causing genes and make it harder for them to trigger cancer growth while others work to suppress cancer from developing by directly strengthening those genes [10].

A wide-range of phytochemicals has been acquired by plants to protect themselves for their own defence mechanism and from highly reactive oxygen species. In recent years, the demand for food products or supplements containing bioactive compounds and non-food products (i.e. dietetics and pharmaceuticals) has increased. There has been vast growth in the Nutraceutical industries to yield large number of phytochemicals containing Nutraceuticals with diverse composition and health claim due to increased application of phytochemicals in cancer care. Now to develop dietary supplements that can help to prevent or delay the onset of nutrition-related diseases in a specific population groups is a big challenge. This will be possible when effective understanding of the molecular basis for the ways in which these components affect human health is studied [11].

Numerous Nutraceuticals have shown to regulate specific tumour suppressor genes and cancer driving genes. By utilizing a daily diet of Nutraceuticals specific to the entire possible gene combinations found in your particular form of cancer we can inhibit the over-expressed oncogenes unique to that form of cancer [10]. There are many cellular mediators involved to be manipulated from initial development of a single cell, to invasion, angiogenesis, proliferation and metastasis [12].

Promises of Nutraceuticals in cancer research:

1) Pleiotropic activity

2) Target Classical signaling Pathways (NF-kappa B, EGFR, AKT, etc.)

3) Target CSCs, miRNAs, EMT and deregulate epigenetic programing

4) Sensitize tumour cells to chemo/radio- therapy

5) Generally well tolerated

6) Parent structure usable for design of novel synthetic analogues for improving efficacy Challenges of Nutraceuticals in cancer research:

1) Bioavailability: metabolized effectively, high systemic concentrations difficult to achieve

2) Insufficient pre-clinical data to advance combinational multi-agent therapy in clinical setting

3) Lower priority by pharmaceutical industry as they may not be patented (**Table 1**).

Nutraceuticals as anti-inflammatory

Nutraceuticals possessing anti-inflammatory activity are widely used as a complementary therapy for rheumatoid arthritis. Rheumatoid arthritis is a chronic inflammatory disease in which oxidative stress and inflammatory biomarkers are elevated. Synthetic drugs recommended for its treatment has severe side effects due to which new and safer approaches are being adopted for its treatment. Phenolic compounds, polyunsaturated fatty acids, phytosterols, tocopherols and carotenoids are rice sources of food containing anti-inflammatory activity. Examples of food containing those constituents are fish oil, fenugreek, coriander, tomato, carrot, green tea, walnut, etc [17].

Table 1. Nutraceuticals which as widely used in cancer therapy.

Sr.no	Bioactive compound	Source	Mechanism	Ref. no.
	Eugenol	Cloves, basil, cinnamon	Inhibition of cell proliferation and suppression of NFκβ	9
	6-gingerol	Ginger	Acts as anti-inflammatory and as 5-HT3 receptor antagonist	9
	Diosgenin	Fenugreek	Supresses proliferation of cancerous cells and inhibits NFκβ activity	9
	Piperine	Pepper	Inhibition of cell proliferation	9
	AHCC	Mushroom	Immunomodulation and antitumor effects, strengthens and optimizes the capacity of the immune system, stimulates the immune surveillance system, inhibits the immune-suppressive factors produced by the cancer cells, stimulating the activity of the killer cells and increasing production of the cells that attack cancer.	13
	Astaxanthin	Salmon	Induces apoptosis and inhibits tumour invasion by decreasing extracellular matrix production.	14
	Caffeine Theophylline	Cacao, tea, coffee	It has the ability of offsetting the immunosuppressive activity of tumour-produced adenosine	13
	Limonene	Citrus oils from orange, lemon, mandarin, lime, and grapefruit	Has inhibitory effect on cell migration on cancerous cell, acts by inhibiting the activity of ornithine decarboxylase and causes anti-proliferation activity	15
	Allicin	Garlic	Induces apoptosis	15
	Indole-3-carbinol	Cabbage	It helps detox estrogen into favourable metabolite for some period of time. It induces apoptosis and cancer cell death at doses >400 μm and repress cancer cell growth at lower doses of about <200 μm.	14, 15,16
	Isothiocyanates Sulforaphane	Broccoli	It constitutes of PEITC that helps to prevent cancer.	15
	Beta-carotene, lycopene	Tomatoes	Induces apoptosis	15
	Epigallocatechin-3-gallate	Green tea	Inhibits proliferation of tumour cells, inhibits NFκβ , inhibits EGFR, inhibiting Her-2 receptor phosphorylation in breast carcinoma cells, induces apoptosis in estrogen receptor-(ER-) independent breast cancer cells, inhibits proteasome formation and glucose-regulated protein (GRP78) activity and insulin-like growth factor-I receptor (IGF-IR) and preventing invasion of tumours by inducing HMG-box transcription factor 1 (HBP1) transcriptional repressor.	9,15
	Quercetin	Black tea	Induces apoptosis	15
	Curcumin	Turmeric	It inhibits neurotensin-mediated interleukin-8 production and migration of HCT116 and affects cox-2 and IL-1, IL-6	9,14
	Capsaicin	Chilli peppers	Induces apoptosis by mediating TRPV6 by KB cells pathway	15
	Ellagic acid	Black berries, raspberry	It acts on NPC-BM1 cells and inhibits NF- kappB activation	15
	Gallic acid	Promegranate, nuts	It reduces cell proliferation and act on HTB-35 cells	15
	Pterostilbene	Blueberries and grapes	Helpful in breast cancer by inducing apoptosis.	15
	Resveratrol	Almonds, blueberries, grapes	It induces apoptosis and also reduces cell proliferation, supresses the growth of new blood vessels which leads to tumour growth	14,15
	Daidzein Genistein	Soy	Possess weak estrogen like activity and bind to ER- β receptors	9,15
	EPA (eicosapnetaenoic acid) and DHA (docosahexaenoic acid)	Fish Oil/ Omega 3	Tends to slow growth of tumour and shows a suppressive effect of fish oil on angiogenesis and decreases the expression of a key receptor in endothelial cells that makes them responsive to VEGF and also the potential to antagonize the role of Cox-2 by decreasing the production of Cox-2-derived prostanoids in cancer cells in angiogenic process. Fish oil has the ability to prevent cachexia.	13
	Boswellic acids	Salai Guggul	Inhibitors of the enzyme 5-LPO-and act on cancer growth factors by suppressing the production of leukotrienes	13
	Proteases (proteolytic enzymes), a digestive enzymes papain bromelain	Found in the stomach juices, pancreatic juices, and intestinal juices Papayas pineapples	They digest proteins and aiding digestion, proteolytic enzymes have analgesic, anti-inflammatory, antithrombotic, fibrinolytic, immune-modulating, and edema-reducing properties.	13
	Silymarin Silibinin	Milk thistle	Silymarin is a strong antioxidant, inhibits proliferation and causes apoptosis. Silibinin has the ability to suppress the NF-kappa B signalling pathway and reduces function of the epidermal growth factor receptor (EGF-R)	13

	Phycocyanobilin	Spirulina	It is a potent inhibitor of specific enzyme complex and acts by reducing oxidative stress and contains cell wall polysaccharides that stimulate immune-supportive dendritic cells. It also interferes with the angiogenic process.	13
	Cimetidine	antiulcer	It acts as immuno-supportive agent. It can reduce the risk of metastasis in many cancers. It also has immuno-stimulant activity for natural killer cells and cytotoxic T-cells.	13
	Coenzyme Q10	Meat, fish, eggs	It is a fat-soluble substance that possesses vitamin-like properties. It acts as an antioxidant by scavenging free radicals. CoQ10 defends against the onset of cancer and destroys existing cancer.	13
	Melatonin	Pineapples, bananas, oranges	It is an immuno-supportive agent and also stimulates the immune surveillance system. Its immuno-stimulant effect boosts the activity of natural killer cells and cytotoxic T-cells, they amplify their capacity to stimulate natural killer cells and cytotoxic T-cells. Melatonin boosts the ability of dendritic cells to produce interleukin-2, which helps cancer-attacking immune cells reach maturity.	13
	Salsalate	salicylic acid	It acts by supressing the signalling pathways activated by either NK-kappaB or Cox-2. High-dose salicylic acid are more likely to reflect inhibition of NF-kappB activation. Salicylic acid binds to and inhibits an enzyme that is usually required for NF-kappaB activation.	13
	Selenium	Oysters, Tuna fish	It is an immuno-supportive agent. It acts by increasing the capacity of stimulated NK cells and cytotoxic T-cells to express receptors for interleukin-2.	13
	Probiotics	Lactobacilli Bifidobacteria	They are immuno-supportive agents. These are enterically-coated capsules which introduce live healthy bacteria into the gastrointestinal tract. The bacteria that are chosen for this supplement include special strains of Lactobacilli and Bifidobacteria. They stimulate the immune system and activate NK cells and cytotoxic T-cells.	13

Nutraceuticals acts as anti-inflammatory by numerous mechanisms like inhibiting the activation of NK-kappa B, down regulation of the overexpression of CAMs and enzymes like COX-2, phospholipase A2, etc, it also blocks the cover expression of pro-inflammatory cytokines such as IL-1, IL-6, and had the ability to scavenging ROS. The mechanism of as anti-inflammatory nutraceuticals and non-steroidal anti-inflammatory drugs shares a common molecular targets. Both has the ability to inhibit the metastatic processes which lead to inflammation by activation of NK-kappa B, induction and up regulation of pro-inflammatory cytokines, production of ROS [18].

Nutraceuticals as antioxidants

Antioxidants are the substances that act on free radicals or their actions. It has been proven that higher intake of foods/ compounds with antioxidant can reduce various human mortalities. Some compounds that possess antioxidant activities are onion, garlic, turmeric, basil, etc [19].

Antioxidants (nutraceuticals) play a major role in neurodegenerative diseases like Parkinson's disease, Alzheimer's disease, etc. Major components that possess antioxidant activities are flavonoid polyphenols - green tea, apples, non-flavonoid polyphenols- turmeric, grapes, phenolic acids or phenolic diterpenes- rosemary, organ sulfur compounds- broccoli, garlic, etc. They act by directly scavenging free radicals or increasing endogenous cellular antioxidant defenses. They act on ROS and RNS. It also prevents the formation of oxidized LDL [20].

Newer approaches include gene therapy that will produce more antioxidant in body and use of functional foods and novel biomolecules.

Nutraceuticals as anti-aging

In current scenario, there are increased cases of age related degenerative diseases and people are keener to shift towards better quality of life. Hence, the combination of cosmetics and food supplements is a new approach used to provide skin care treatment. It was assumed by Denham Harman in 1th 1950s that aging is a consequence of excessive production of free radicals. This results to cause damage to human body and even oxidative damage to DNA. Nutraceuticals useful as anti-aging acts similar as antioxidants. They also affect the processes that stimulate the production of reactive species; ROS, RON, etc.

Right selection of nutrients plays a vital role in the treatment of various diseases which can be achieved by proper diet containing intake of food supplements rich in vitamin E, folic acid, vitamin B12, iron, etc. main food sources includes egg yolk, green leafed vegetables, beans, nuts, etc [21].

Nutraceuticals as anti-obesity

Obesity is a common chronic disease and a major underline reason for metabolic syndrome which arises when there is an imbalance between energy intake and energy expenditure. Some components widely used as nutraceuticals in obesity are curcumin, bottle guard, black gram, green tea, etc. They secrete leptin and other cytokines like IL-1, IL-6 that are critically involved in obesity and chronic inflammation. They also help in reducing LDL and total cholesterol. Some act by limiting overall food daily intake. Nutraceuticals have ability to affect weight loss and have huge potential to reverse the development of overweight and obesity-related comorbidities [22,23].

Nutraceuticals as anti-diabetic

Diabetes is a metabolic syndrome where a person suffers from high blood glucose. It is caused due to lack of insulin production or the body cells do not respond properly to insulin or both. Some nutraceuticals used to treat and prevent diabetes are Emblica officinalis, fenugreek, green tea, etc. It also includes anti-oxidant vitamins like vitamin C and E and minerals like magnesium and chromium. They generally act by affecting insulin sensitivity and also prevent insulin resistance. Some act by increasing hepatic glycogen concentration and decreasing the concentration of glycogen phosphorylase and glyconeogenic enzymes [22-24] (**Table 2**).

Table 2. Various nutraceuticals used against different diseases.

Sr.no.	Disease	Examples	Ref. no.
1	Alzheimer	Vitamin E and C, alpha- lipoic acid	1
2	Cardiovascular	Flavonoids (onion, black grapes)	1
3	Parkinson	Vitamin E	1
4	Obesity	Chitosan, fenugreek, vitamin C	1
5	Diabetes	Calcium, vitamin D, Emblica officinalis	1
6	Osteoarthritis	Glucosamine, chondroitin sulfate	1
7	Constipation	Buck wheat	3
8	Vision improving	Carrot, mangoes, spinach, kiwi, egg yolk	3
9	Antioxidant	Oats, fruits, carrots	3
10	Anti-inflammatory	Turmeric	3
11	Hypertension	Curry leaf, green tea	22
12	Hyperlipidemia	*Emblica officinalis*	22

CONCLUSION

Nutraceuticals have been emerged as an alternative to modern medicines and have proven health benefits. Most dietary supplements are derived from plants and some from animals. Nutraceuticals has disease prevention capability with good nutritional value and food ingredients with additional health benefits. They are widely accepted by all age groups due to their higher quality, purity, safety and efficacy, promoting health and help to cure diseases. The latest trend is moved towards nutragenomics and nutraceuticals has led to new era of medicine and health.

REFERENCES

1. Chintale AG, et al. Role of Nutraceuticals in various diseases: A Comprehensive Review. IJRPC. 2013;3:290-299.
2. Brower V. A Nutraceutical a day may keep the doctor away. EMBO reports. 2005;6:708-711.
3. Khan RA, et al. Nutraceuticals: In the treatment and prevention of diseases- an overview. Tha Pharma Innovation Journal. 2014;3:147-150.

4. Angel NM, et al. Role of Nutraceuticals in Cancer. International Journal of Pharmacy and Pharmaceutical Sciences. 2012;4:415-420.

5. Chauhan B, et al. Current concepts and prospects of herbal Nutraceutical: A review. 2013;4:4-8.

6. Watson RR. Functional Foods & Nutraceuticals in Cancer Prevention. (1stedn), Iowa State Press. 2003.

7. Ahmad A, et al. Molecular Targets of Naturopathy in Cancer Research: Bridge to Modern Medicine. Nutrients. 2015;7:321-334.

8. Kuppusamy P, et al. Nutraceuticals as potential therapeutic agents for colon cancer: a review. Acta Pharmaceutica Sinica B. 2014;4:173-181.

9. Wargovich MJ, et al. Nutraceutical use in late-stage cancer. NIH Public Access. 2010;29:503-510.http://www.ctoam.com/

10. Ranzato E, et al. Role of Nutraceuticals in Cancer Therapy. Journal of Food Research. 2014;3:18-25.

11. Burns, KM. Therapeutic Foods and Nutraceuticals in Cancer Therapy. Veterinary Technician. 2010; E1-E7.

12. Brower V. Nutraceuticals: poised for a healthy slice of the healthcare market, Nat Biotechnol 1998;16:728-731.

13. Saldanha SN and Tollefsbol TO. The Role of Nutraceuticals in Chemoprevention and Chemotherapy and Their Clinical Outcomes. Journal of Oncology. 2012;1-23.

14. Zeisel SH. Regulation of Nutraceuticals Science. 1999;285:185-186

15. Benkouider C. Functional Foods and Nutraceuticals. 2005;44: 8-11

16. Alokbi SY. Nutraceuticals of anti-inflammatory activity as complementary therapy for rheumatoid arthritis. Pub/med.gov. 2014;30:734-749.

17. Huang MT, et al. Inflammatory Process and molecular targets for anti-inflammatory Nutraceuticals. Comprehensive Reviews in Food Science and Food Safety. 2006;3:127-139.

18. Kaur S, et al. Free radicals and antioxidants (Nutraceuticals): Boom to human health. International Journal of Natural Product Science. 2012;1:175.

19. Kelsey NA, et al. Nutraceutical Antioxidants as novel Neuroprotective agents. Molecules, 2010;15:7792-7814.

20. Dariji VB. The role of nutraceuticals in anti-aging medicine. Acta Clin Croat. 2010;49:537-544.

21. Kaur G, et al. Nutraceuticals in the Management and Prevention of Metabolic Syndrome. Austin Journal of Pharmacology and Therapeutics. 2015;3:1-6.

22. Conroy KP, et al. Pathogenic obesity and nutraceuticals. PubMed. 2011;70:426-436.

23. Davi G, et al. Nutraceuticals in diabetes and m etabolic syndrome. PubMed. 2010;28:216-226.

2

CREATING BENEFITS FROM OMEGA-3 FUNCTIONAL FOODS AND NUTRACEUTICALS

Catharine Clark[1], Bill Lands[2]

[1]Clark Consulting and Coaching, Frederick, USA

[2]American Society for Nutrition, College Park, USA

ABSTRACT

Foods currently eaten by Americans have abundant amounts of essential omega-6 (n-6) nutrients and relatively few omega-3 (n-3) nutrients. The average omega 3 - 6 balance score of typical US foods is about −6. This imbalance causes the average American to accumulate tissue proportions of n-3 and n-6 highly unsaturated fatty acids (HUFA) with about 77% n-6 in HUFA. This HUFA balance links to many chronic health conditions that are made worse by overabundant actions of food-based omega-6 HUFA. Americans currently spend more on treating food-based health conditions than they spend on food. Less medication is needed to treat signs and symptoms when a key dietary cause of the signs and symptoms is prevented. Informed food producers can readily prepare and market new food products with more n-3 and less n-6 nutrients to reverse the current national nutrient imbalance and help people attain and maintain a healthy HUFA balance. New functional foods and nutraceuticals will help consumers shift their financial resources from treating signs and symptoms caused by HUFA imbalance to preventing the nutrient imbalance that causes the need to treat.

Keywords: Eicosanoids, Highly Unsaturated Fatty Acids (HUFA), Inflammation, Omega-3 (n-3) Fatty Acid, Omega-6 (n-6) Fatty Acid

1. INTRODUCTION

Essential fatty acids (EFA) are vitamin-like nutrients needed for healthy human physiology. The 18-carbon polyunsaturated omega-3 (n-3) α-linolenic acid and omega-6 (n-6) linoleic acid are abundant in foliage and leafy vegetables, such as spinach, broccoli and cauliflower. When eaten, the n-3 nutrients compete with n-6 nutrients for metabolism to longer more highly unsaturated fatty acids (HUFA) which accumulate in the phospholipids of tissue membranes. A competitive hyperbolic equation [1] describes the diet-tissue relationship by which the EFA in foods maintain proportions of n-3 and n-6 HUFA in human tissues. The current average EFA intakes in US foods have an omega 3 - 6 balance score near-6, whereas traditional Mediterranean foods averaged near −3 and traditional Japanese foods averaged near +2 [2] . These average scores maintain tissue HUFA balances near 75%, 60%, and 40% n-6 in HUFA, respectively. Measurements obtained from apparently healthy people with different traditional food habits range from 25% to 85% n-6 in HUFA. The %n-6 in HUFA is an objective measure of n-3 and n-6 nutrient intakes [2] .

The HUFA balance predictably linked to average EFA intakes is also associated with a risk for chronic inflammatory disorders [3] . People with more than 50% n-6 in HUFA have a greater risk of death from cardiovascular disease (CVD) than people with less than 50% n-6 in HUFA. Mechanisms for the CVD pathophysiology include conversion of the n-6 HUFA, arachidonic acid, into powerful inflammatory hormone-like eicosanoids that amplify events in vascular inflammatory atherosclerosis and fatal thrombosis [4] [5] . In the absence of dietary n-3 nutrients, intakes of n-6 linoleic acid as low as 0.4 percent of food energy (0.4 en%) can give 50% n-6 in HUFA. Eating less may lead to EFA deficiency, and eating more may increase the risk for excessive n-6 HUFA actions. Thus, dietary n-6 linoleate has a very narrow therapeutic window [4] . An important action of dietary n-3 nutrients is to raise the proportion of n-3 in tissue HUFA and to widen the range of n-6 intake that has a low risk of excessive n-6 HUFA action.

Plant foods common in tropical Africa during early human evolution likely had omega 3 - 6 balance scores near 0, like leafy foliage (0), cassava (−0.1), sweet potato (−0.5), yam (−0.4), plantain (−0.1) and taro (−3) [6] . Over time, people in central and western Africa selectively acquired a genetic haplotype which has faster Δ6 and Δ5 desaturation activity [7] . That gave faster conversion of dietary n-3 and n-6 PUFA to tissue HUFA and ensured supplies of n-3 and n-6 HUFA adequate for human brain and retinal function during rapid infant development. However, it now makes many African-Americans more responsive than Caucasians or Asians to the very high amounts of n-6 linoleate from food oils in the current American diet (7 en%, rather than the 0.4 en% that prevents EFA deficiency). The consequence is a greater tendency for a higher % n-6 in HUFA and for more unwanted chronic inflammatory disorders. African-Americans have higher prevalence of chronic disease including: cardiovascular disease, hypertension, colorectal cancer, obesity, asthma, and periodontitis [8] . In fact, the prevalence of type 2 diabetes (insulin resistance) is nearly twice as high among African-American adults compared to white adults [8] .

2. MULTIPLE CHRONIC CONDITIONS ARE BECOMING FINANCIALLY UNSUSTAINABLE

The general status of health and wellness (or its counterpart, sickness and death) can be described in many ways. For example, the US economy currently allocates more financial resources to healthcare than to food, and food- based imbalances cause the high need for healthcare [9] . The Centers for Disease Control and Prevention (CDC) estimated that chronic health conditions—such as heart disease, stroke, cancer, diabetes, obesity, and arthritis—are among the most common, costly, and preventable of all health problems [10] . Eighty six percent (86%) of healthcare spending is for chronic medical conditions [10] [11] . The US will likely spend $2.7 trillion treating chronic diseases in 2015 (Table 1)—much of which is considered preventable. This is more than total healthcare spending in 2010. The US needs to change its foods.

The US healthcare system is focused on discovering treatments rather than preventing chronic disease [16] . While medications are profitable (and sometimes a useful interim step), they can have undesired side effects, and their continued use is needed when the food-based cause remains unaddressed. Translating knowledge of risk factor mechanisms into effective informed preventive nutrition actions is an important step toward preventing costly, chronic conditions resulting from food-based mediators [9] .

Table 1. Cost of chronic health conditions.

Year	Healthcare Spending($)	% of GDP	Healthcare (Avg $/person)	Chronic Disease Prevalence	Chronic Disease Spending ($)	Chronic Disease (Avg $/person)
2000	1.4T [12]	13.8 [14]	4,878 [14]	70% [15]	1.0T	3.415
2005	2.0T [12]	16.1 [14]	6,868 [14]	75% [16]	1.5T	5.151
2010	2.6T [12]	17.9 [14]	8.402 [14]	86% [11]	2.2T	7.226
2015	3.1T [13]	18.0 [13]	10.125 [13]	86% [11]	2.7T	8.708

Heart disease, obesity, and type-2 diabetes are at epidemic levels in the US, and they have well-documented food-based n-6 mediators [4] [5] . Depression is another epidemic condition not yet recognized by the public to associate with HUFA balance [17] . Chronic disease and depression are mutually reinforcing: chronic disease can exacerbate depression, while depression can lead to chronic disease [16] . Pharmaceutical companies know imbalanced actions of n-6 mediators for which they produce and market many medications to mitigate food-based pathophysiology. Food producers and manufacturers are becoming aware of their opportunity to significantly alter food-based pathophysiology. Their actions in making better-balanced foods available can shift current health conditions toward increased wellness for the public.

Understanding the causal links between foods and food-based health conditions allows deliberate, explicit implementation of effective preventive nutrition programs [9] . When people increase their intake of n-3 nutrients while decreasing excess n-6 nutrients, they lower the health risk assessment (HRA) biomarker, the %n-6 in HUFA. Effective preventive nutrition addressing the root causes of chronic diseases can benefit the US economy. In 2015, the US will spend 86% of its $3.1 trillion healthcare resources treating chronic diseases. Among the most prevalent chronic conditions, allergies rank #3 and asthma ranks #8 for adults, whereas for children, asthma and allergies rank #1 and #2, respectively [11] . Allergies are a major trigger for asthma. In addition, chronic obstructive lung disease and bronchiectasis are ranked #11 in prevalence for adults, and chronic obstructive pulmonary disease (COPD) is the third leading cause of death in the US [18] . A common aspect of all these immune-inflammatory disorders is excessive action of n-6 eicosanoids derived from an over-abundant intake of n-6 nutrients.

The eicosanoids are potent signaling molecules, and n-3 and n-6 eicosanoids act at selective receptor sites in nearly every tissue of the human body [5] . The cysteinyl leukotriene eicosanoids are potent bronchoconstrictors formed by 5-lipoxygenase and leukotriene C synthase after phospholipase releases the n-3 and n-6 HUFA precursors from tissue membrane phospholipids [19] . Both n-3 and n-6 leukotrienes can increase bronchopulmonary distress in asthma and COPD, however formation of n-6 LTC_4 is more intense than n-3 LTC_5 [20] [21] . A major contributor to recruiting leukocytes that amplify inflammatory conditions is the vigorous chemotactic response of the BLT1 receptor with n-6 LTB_4. It is 100-fold greater than the response with n-3 LTB_5 [22] . Inflammation is amplified as food-based n-6 LTB_4 attracts more leukocytes to an area and signals for release of chemokines (a protein activating additional white blood cells).

Macrophages play a key role in the pathophysiology of obesity-induced insulin resistance. These inflammatory cells accumulate in crown-like structures around adipocytes [23] , and become a significant portion (up to 40% [24]) of the cells in obese adipose tissue. Macrophages release cytokines and LTB_4 that recruit more inflammatory cells as adipose tissue develops systemic inflammatory characteristics [23] . LTB_4 acting through the BLT1 receptor directly induces inflammation and insulin resistance [24] . Genetically altered mice missing the BLT1 receptor were protected from glucose intolerance and insulin resistance [24] [25] . Inhibition of LTB_4 could be a future goal for pharmaceutical treatment of insulin-resistance. Conversely, with n-6 LTB_4 actions on BLT1 being 100-fold greater than n-3 LTB_5 [22] , a promising form of primary prevention is reducing dietary n-6 and increasing the intake of n-3 functional foods. Informed food choices can likely decrease obesity, inflammation, and insulin resistance and have fewer side effects than medications or surgical procedures.

The obesity epidemic in the US has not been resolved by the multi-billion dollar weight-loss industry. Now categorized as a disease, obesity and its associated inflammatory processes play key roles in a complex chain of events linked to n-6 nutrients. The endocannabinoid system regulates food intake mediated by products of n-6 linoleic acid (LA) [26] [27] . Elevated endocannabinoids increase weight gain while adipocytes become larger and adipose tissue more inflamed with macrophage infiltration [27] [28] . Balancing weight-promoting n-6 nutrients with n-3 nutrients normalized endocannabinoid tone and body mass. That approach merits careful attention in preventing undesired appetitive behaviors and in maintaining food energy balance.

The large multi-year Look AHEAD clinical trial hypothesized that obesity is a valid surrogate for cardiovascular disease (CVD) [29] , the #1 cause of death in the US for many decades. The trial lowered the average body mass of 5145 overweight or obese participants with intent to reduce non-fatal myocardial infarction, hospitalized angina, and non-fatal stroke [29] . However, following successful weight reduction and increased physical activity, the trial was stopped after nearly 10 years because the hypothesis was not supported [29] . Obesity is an associative, predictive risk factor of CVD; it is not a valid surrogate. The health risk assessment factor, %n-6 in HUFA, has a high correlation with CVD and a causal mechanistic basis [4] [30] . When people examine blood samples from the Look AHEAD participants, they may find an association between %n-6 in HUFA and CVD mortality and morbidity. This would redirect attention toward a more effective preventive nutrition strategy of lowering n-6 intakes and raising n-3 intakes.

As populations shifted from their traditional dietary patterns toward modern Western food habits, they experienced increased prevalence of deaths from chronic disease. One example is the increased deaths from prostate cancer in Japan and Italy [31] . Japanese historically had seafood as a dietary staple, a low %n-6 in HUFA as an objective biochemical outcome, and one of the lowest rates of prostate cancer deaths in the world. As the average %n-6 in HUFA increased from ~35% to 50%, prostate cancer deaths of elderly Japanese rose from 40 to 400 per 100,000 population. In Italy, where a traditional Mediterranean diet was typical in 1970, deaths from prostate cancer were near 250 per 100,000. However, over the next 30 years, as dietary habits became Westernized, the death rate doubled to 500 [31] . During this period prostate cancer deaths of elderly men in UK, France, and US remained near 500 to 600 per 100,000. In the US, it is the 5th leading cause of cancer death [32] . In 2015, there will likely be 220,000 new cases and 27,000 prostate cancers deaths in the US, with higher prevalence and deaths among African Americans [32] . Reducing the dietary intake of n-6 nutrients enables increased n-3 intakes to competitively attenuate actions of the n-6 thromboxane, TXA_2, in facilitating cancer growth [33] .

There is no shortage of peer-reviewed studies listed by PubMed detailing mechanisms by which the innate immune system is amplified by n-6 actions. Thousands of these studies specify the eicosanoids involved (e.g., LTB_4, TXA_2, PGE_2, $PGF_{2\alpha}$, PGI_2). However, there is a shortage of information about which foods cause major imbalances in n-3 and n-6 nutrient intakes. Useful for this purpose are the omega 3-6 balance scores derived from eleven different n-3 and n-6 fatty acids based on information in the USDA Nutrient Database [2] . The scores predict the impact of a food item on the HRA biomarker, %n-6 in HUFA. Balance scores have dimensions of milligrams per Calorie (mg/kcal), and the negative and positive values combine together to give a predicted biomedical outcome for the %n-6 in HUFA. As consumers combine current food items with functional foods that have more positive (less negative) scores, the incremental differences add together, and can significantly shift the %n-6 in HUFA and clinically relevant outcomes in as little as 3 months [34] . This is important as food producers and marketers begin to resolve the current preventable epidemics.

3. ADDRESS THE CAUSE NOT JUST THE SYMPTOMS

Many medications relieve signs and symptoms of food-based chronic conditions. For example, low-dose aspirin decreases the actions of excessive n-6 thromboxane, TXA_2, in blood platelets [5] . However, when the dietary imbalance causing their food-based condition has not been prevented, consumers need continual medication. This fits a profitable business model for pharmaceutical companies and manufacturers of over-the-counter medications. However, some question the benefit of treating signs and symptoms while leaving the food-based imbalance to cause additional harm [3] . Significant increases in chronic disease spending per person are likely to continue in the absence of effective preventive nutrition (Table 1).

Creating functional foods and promoting new food choices is not in business plans of pharmaceutical companies or manufacturers of over the counter drugs. Moreover, if the CDC is correct that the US healthcare system "is not designed to prevent chronic diseases" and "has primarily focused on discovering [new] treatments" [16] , then the healthcare system is financially unsustainable and needs redesigning. Re-allocating $2.7T/year toward preventive nutrition may be sufficient financial incentive to motivate action [9] . Tools and apps are now available [35] to use the known competitive, hyperbolic diet-tissue relationship among EFA [1] and design new functional foods and nutraceuticals for better nutrient balance and health outcomes for consumers. The empirical equation quantitatively describes how lowering n-6 nutrient intake makes n-3 nutrients more effective in creating balanced HRA biomarker values. The concept of Omega Balance [36] addresses the current nutritional cause for many signs and symptoms, and new functional foods with high positive scores will not have adverse side effects seen with current medications. Informed preventive nutrition offers positive outcomes with lower cost.

To examine the benefit of a better HUFA balance, a recent randomized clinical trial on severe chronic headache pain designed two diets quite different from typical American diets in having much lower amounts of n-6 LA [34] . The low-n-6 diet (L6) replaced high-LA foods with low-LA foods. Adding n-3 nutrients to that diet gave a high n-3, low n-6 diet

(H3-L6). During the 3-month clinical trial, the L6 diet gave a significant reduction

of pain in three objective clinical measures as patients' HRA values went from 78% n-6 in HUFA to 75%n-6 in HUFA. More importantly, the H3-L6 group changed their average %n-6 in HUFA from 77% to 61% and experienced progressive reduction in pain during 3 months, a 40% lower need for medications, and an increased quality of life [34] [37] .

This clinical trial demonstrated how rapidly an informed selection of foods can change the HUFA balance and its physiological consequences. The authors noted that more improvement in psychological distress may occur if the intervention was longer [37] . Also, individuals with an aversion to seafood were not fully compliant, and use of n-3 supplements may further improve outcomes [38] . Supplemental nutraceutical n-3 is a constructive alternative to improve HRA biomarkers in an open free-living population setting. In all scenarios with added n-3 nutrients, reducing dietary n-6 intake ensures more positive outcomes on objective and subjective measures of health, and a decreased need for medication in chronic conditions [34] [37] .

4. CREATING FUNCTIONAL FOODS

Investigators developing diets to give a better tissue HUFA balance replaced high-LA oils with macadamia-oil- vinaigrette salad dressing, and used fat-free mayonnaise [38] [39] . Including fatty seafood rich in n-3 HUFA (e.g. wild salmon, trout, tuna, and sardines) plus functional foods created with flax meal (i.e., ground flax seeds) can provide more n-3 nutrients. Easily arranged recipes for muffins, granola, and bean dip create new functional foods by adding flax meal [38] . In considering a better tissue HUFA balance, the Department of Defense (DoD) noted a substantially increased cognitive load on the warfighter produced a need for better protection and recovery from wounds [40] . However, the current diet for active duty military personnel is imbalanced in n-3 and n-6 nutrients, as it resembles the standard American diet [2] [40] [41] . Assessment of 287 active-duty soldiers showed an average 81% n-6 in HUFA [42] . The DoD concluded that restoring omega-3 fatty acids to optimal levels may improve performance and restore impaired personnel to healthy fit status. To sustain US leadership, DoD established goals for 2030 as shown in Figure 1 [40] .

Sample garrison foods were analyzed using the empirical equation noted in the Introduction [1] . They predicted an average value of 78% n-6 in HUFA [41] . Substituting n-3 rich foods, increasing low n-6 variants, and replacing high-LA with low-LA oils resulted in a substantial observed change in the %n-6 in HUFA, thus shifting

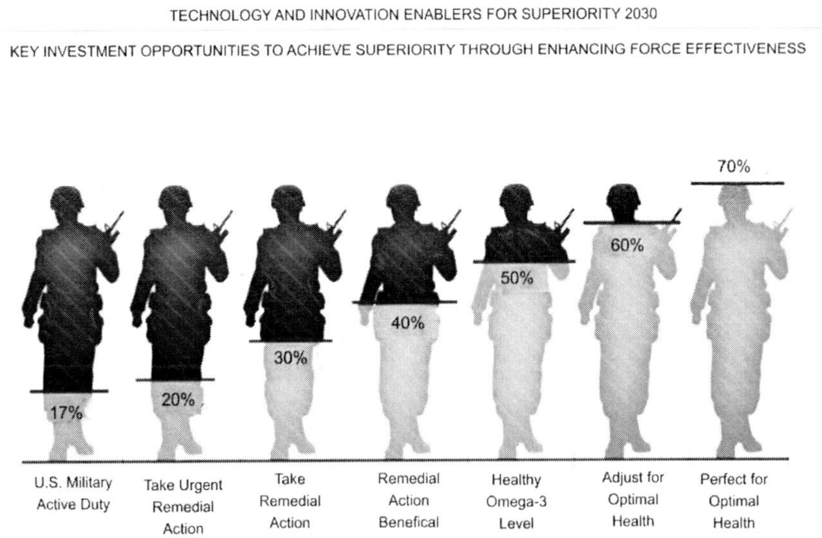

Figure 1. Balance of n-3 in HUFA related to optimal health and force effectiveness. Omega Balance is expressed as %n-3 in HUFA. U.S. Military Active Duty is shown as 17% n-3 in HUFA (i.e., 83% n-6 in HUFA) and optimal health is considered 60% - 70% n-3 in HUFA. Reprinted from Defense Science Board ([40] , p. 57).

dietary patterns of active duty warfighters away from traditional nutrition guidelines [41] and current public advice from the Food and Nutrition Board [4] . The DoD implemented their decision by engaging food producers to assemble functional foods for garrison menus. Results presented in March 2015 during a public lecture showcased functional foods that DoD cooperatively developed with several food companies: Vital Choice, Smartfish, Omega Foods, DuPont, Belovo, and Aidells Sausage Company. New food items included salad dressings using low n-6 soybean oil [43] plus n-3 enriched chicken, eggs and fruit beverages. Researchers noted that lowering dietary n-6 in combination with elevating n-3 acts more potently to lower tissue n-6 HUFA balance than either approach alone [41] . Food producers play a positive role in helping the DoD move toward its goal of resilient warfighters with 40% - 50% n-6 in HUFA. There is much more they can do to expand markets to the broader public.

The Department of Agriculture (USDA) supported development of new peanut cultivars that can be useful as functional foods. Researchers in Florida, Georgia, North Carolina, Oklahoma, Texas and the UK [44] -[47] described new varieties that can replace staples in the American diet. Currently, peanuts, peanut butter, and peanut oil contain large amounts of n-6 have omega 3 - 6 balance scores of −26, −24, and −36, respectively [35] . Variants with less n-6 and much more monounsaturated oleic acid can be effective functional foods. In addition to having improved Omega Balance scores, low-linoleate products have greater shelf life. For many years the fats and oils industry handled low n-6 food oils from coconut or macadamia or from selected cultivars of sunflower, soybean, safflower, and canola which are not yet widely marketed to the public. These oils can be excellent starting points for developing new functional foods to improve the HUFA balance in consumers.

Many nutrition advisors recommend using foods rather than supplements to achieve dietary goals, yet few give consumers explicit data on the amounts of n-3 and n-6 nutrients in foods. Individuals can find information on how to create their own balance of n-3 and n-6 nutrients by downloading the Omega Meals tool onto their personal computer [35] . A simple example is converting snack pretzels (1 ounce (oz), 103 kcal, score = −2.1) into a functional food by combining it with flax oil (3 teaspoons (tsp), 120 kcal, score = +46). The Omega Meals tool combines the data and shows the resulting 223 kcal snack has an omega 3 - 6 balance score of +24.2 which has a very good impact on a person's HRA biomarker, %n-6 in HUFA [35] . To prepare this snack: break up the pretzels in a small bowl, drizzle the flax oil, and stir to coat. This snack is an alternative to a 1.25oz serving of tree nuts which provide 206 - 231 kcal and much more negative balance scores (Table 2). Another functional food combines 4oz low-fat cottage cheese (81 kcal, score = −0.2) with 1 tsp flax oil (40 kcal, score =+46) to give a 121 kcal snack (score = +15). Recipes and meal plans made with Omega Meals can be saved for future use, modified as desired, and printed to share with friends. Every recipe and meal plan displays a chart indicating the likely impact on the predictive HRA biomedical value, the %n-6 in HUFA [35] .

The top 100 Key Foods for Americans [48] have an average Omega Balance Score near −6 [2] , related to a HRA value of 78% n-6 in HUFA (like common American diets). Removing ten foods with the most negative scores leaves 90 Key Foods with an average Score of -3 and an HRA value of 63% n-6 in HUFA (like traditional Mediterranean diets). Possible alternatives to the removed items are in Table 3.

Table 2. Balance of n-3 and n-6 fats in tree nuts. The milligrams of n-3 and n-6 essential polyunsaturated acids (PUFA) per ounce of tree nuts. The color code for Balance Scores reflects the likely impact food items will have on the HRA value, % n-6 in HUFA.

Tree Nuts (1 oz)	PUFA n-3	PUFA n-6	BALANCE SCORE
Walnuts	2574	10,799	−44
Brazil nuts	15	6769	−40
Peanuts	3	4675	−28
Pecans	280	5848	−28
Pistachio	73	3823	−23
Almonds	1	3494	−21
Cashew nuts	18	2206	−14
Hazelnuts	25	2221	−12
Chestnut	[illegible]	[illegible]	[illegible]
Macadamia	58	367	−1.5

very good effect
good effect
OK effect
not very good effect
bad effect
awful effect

Table 3. Possible Alternatives for Widely Consumed US Foods. Ten foods from the top 100 Key Food for Americans [48] are shown with their corresponding Balance Scores and possible alternatives. All Scores are based on milligrams of n-3 and n-6 essential polyunsaturated acids (PUFA) per Calorie.

Food with a Very Negative Score	Balance Score (per kcal)	Possible Alternatives	Balance Score (per kcal)
Soybean oil	−50	Olive oil	−8
		Canola oil	−12
		High-oleic sunflower oil	−4
Mayonnaise	−46	Fat free mayonnaise	0
		Mayonnaise with canola or olive oil	−10
Tub margarine	−39	Butter	−1
		Coconut oil	−2
Microwave popcorn	−37	Low-fat microwave popcorn	−7
"Italian" dressing	−35	Fat free "Italian"	0
		Lemon and olive oil	−8
		Flax & olive oil vinaigrette	+19
Potato chips	−29	Baked potato chips	−8
		Pretzels with flax oil	+24
Stick margarine	−28	Butter	−1
Vegetable shortening	−28	Lard	−10
		Coconut oil	−2
Peanut butter	−24	High oleic peanut butter	−4
		Flax-peanut butter	+4
		Gouda Cheese	+0.4
Tortilla chip snacks	−22	Taco-flavor tortillas	−6
		Flour tortillas	−5

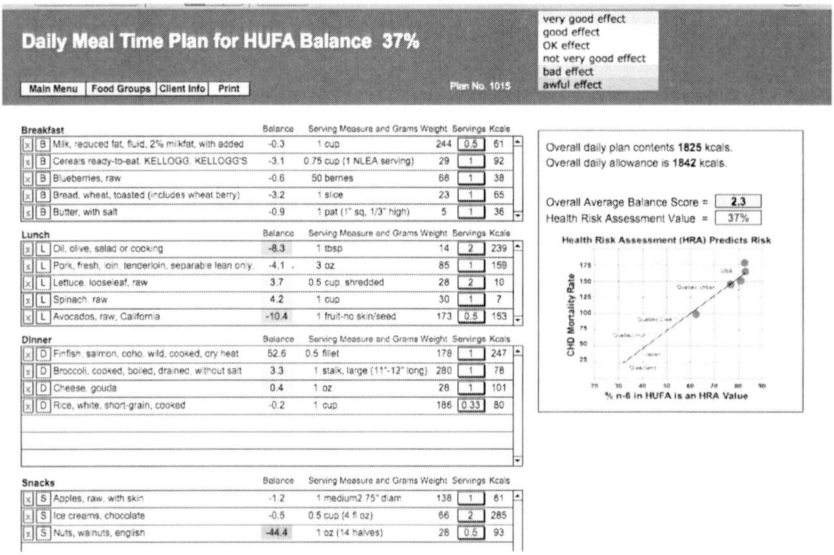

Figure 2. Daily Meal Plan with a Balance Score of +2.3. The meal plan using the Omega Meals tool [35] shows foods eaten at different mealtimes. Highlighting scores by color visually indicates the impact of each food item on the biomedical HRA value, %n-6 in HUFA.

The top 100 foods do not include seafood which has positive Balance Scores: scallops, +15; shrimp, +29; crab, +30; flounder, +30; mussels, +32; white tuna, +46; sea bass, +49; sardines, +53; striped bass, +55; Coho salmon, +57; Eastern oysters, +57; kippered herring, +70; and canned pink salmon, +83. Also, marine plants are becoming more available to US consumers: kelp, −2; laver, +14; and wakame, +26. The American Heart Association and the American Psychiatric Association recommend eating seafood twice a week. Consumers need help in finding more functional foods with positive scores that lower their %n-6 in HUFA [36] , improve health and quality of life [34] and shift personal finances from treatments to other desired uses [9] .

Figure 2 illustrates an Omega Meals plan that initially had an overall Balance Score of −6.9 with an estimated HRA value of 82% n-6 in HUFA (near typical American values of −6 to −7 and 75% - 80%, respectively). It was altered by replacing turkey (−15.9) with salmon (+52.6) to give an overall Score of +2.3 and a predicted HRA value of 37% n-6 in HUFA (near traditional Japanese levels). This plan can be changed further by replacing walnuts (−44.4) with the pretzel/flax oil snack described above (+24); olive oil (−8.3) with coconut oil (−2.1); and avocado (−10.4) with a glass of wine (0). The overall Balance Score would then be +9.5 with an estimated HRA biochemical outcome of 19% n-6 in HUFA (near traditional Greenland Inuit levels). Existing food items already allow people to make food choices that lower their HUFA balance, and new functional foods and nutraceuticals certainly will make that task much easier. Such new consumer items can positively shift US financial outlays from healthcare treatments to economic development [9] .

5. CONCLUSION

A quantitative empirical relationship describes how dietary n-3 and n-6 essential fatty acids maintain the proportions of n-3 and n-6 in tissue HUFA. Traditional food habits of different populations maintain HUFA balances

that range from 25% to 85% n-6 in HUFA and associate with the incidence and severity of many different chronic disorders made worse by n-6 eicosanoids. The combined impact of multiple food choices creates HUFA imbalances in Americans. New food choices with more positive omega 3 - 6 balance scores can reverse imbalances. Consumers need new functional foods and nutraceuticals to help them avoid the need to medicate preventable health conditions and to maintain better a quality of life. Tools and apps for making explicit food choices allow individual consumers to arrange balanced food combinations in their homes. In addition, the tools guide food producers and marketers to make balanced combinations available to the many consumers who do not have time to prepare foods at home. The US spends more on treatment of food-based chronic conditions than it does on food. Prevention costs less than treatment. Informed actions using more functional foods and nutraceuticals can shift some of the $2.7T the US spends annually treating chronic conditions toward preventing the need to treat.

ACKNOWLEDGEMENTS

Dr. N. Schoene gave helpful advice on this manuscript.

AUTHOR CONTRIBUTIONS

Both authors shared in the preparation of the manuscript.

CONFLICTS OF INTEREST

The authors declare no financial arrangements related to this manuscript. CC is a clinical nutrition consultant and BL is a retired professor of biochemistry.

REFERENCES

1. EFAeducation.org (2015) Relating Diets to Tissue HUFA. http://efaeducation.org/?p=188
2. 2. Lands, B. and Lamoreaux, E. (2012) Using 3-6 Differences in Essential Fatty Acids Rather than 3/6 Ratios Gives Useful Food Balance Scores. Nutrition & Metabolism, 9, No. 46. http://www.ncbi.nlm.nih.gov/pmc/articles/PMC3533819/pdf/1743-7075-9-46.pdf
3. Lands, B. (2011) Prevent the Cause, Not Just the Symptoms. Prostaglandins & Other Lipid Mediators, 96, 90-93.
4. Lands, B. (2014) Historical Perspectives on the Impact of n-3 and n-6 Nutrients on Health. Progress in Lipid Research, 55, 17-29. http://www.sciencedirect.com/science/article/pii/S0163782714000253
5. Lands, B. (2015) Omega-3 PUFAs Lower the Propensity for Arachidonic Acid Cascade Overreactions. Biomed Research International, 2015, Article ID 285135.http://www.hindawi.com/journals/bmri/2015/285135/
6. Lands, B. (2016) Fatty Acids: Essential Fatty Acids. In: Caballero, B., Finglas, P. and Toldrá, F., Eds., The Encyclopedia of Food and Health, Academic Press, Oxford, Vol. 2, 615-622.
7. Ameur, A., Enroth, S., Johansson, A., Zaboli, G., Igl, W., Johansson, A.C.V., Rivas, M.A., Daly, M.J., Schmitz, G., Hicks, A.A., Meitinger, T., Feuk, L., van Duijn, C., Oostra, B., Pramstaller, P.P., Rudan, I., Wright, A.F., Wilson, J.F., Campbell, H. and Gyllensten, A. (2012) Genetic Adaptation of Fatty-Acid Metabolism: A Human-Specific Haplotype Increasing the Biosynthesis of Long-Chain Omega-3 and Omega-6 Fatty Acids. The American Journal of Human Genetics, 90, 809-820.

8. Centers for Disease Control and Prevention (CDC) (2015) Minority Health. http://www.cdc.gov/minorityhealth/ populations/REMP/black.html

9. Clark, C. and Lands, B. (2016) What Financial Motivations Support Preventive Nutrition? Nutrition and Health, Unpublished. [Paper reference:6]

10. Centers for Disease Control and Prevention (2015) Chronic Disease Overview. http://www.cdc.gov/chronic disease/overview/

11. Gerteis, J., Izrael, D., Deitz, D., LeRoy, L., Ricciardi, R., Miller, T. and Basu, J., Agency for Healthcare Research and Quality (AHRQ) (2014) Multiple Chronic Conditions Chartbook. http://www.ahrq.gov/sites/default/files/wysiwyg/professiona ls/prevention-chronic-care/decision/mcc/mccchartbook.pdf

12. Health Spending Explorer (2015) Peterson-Kaiser Health System Tracker.http://www.healthsystemtracker. org/interactive/health-spending-explorer/?display=U.S.%2520%2524%2520Billions&service=H ospitals%252CPhysicians%2520%2526%2520Clinics%252CPr escription%2520Drug

13. Keehan, S.P., Cuckler, G.A., Sisko, A.M., Madison, A.J., Smith, S.D., Stone, D.A., Poisal, J.A., Wolfe, C.J. and Lizonitz, J.M. (2015) National Health Expenditure Projections, 2014-24: Spending Growth Faster than Recent Trends. Health Affairs, 8, 1707-1717. (Exhibit 3)

14. Kaiser Family Foundation (2012) Health Care Costs: A Primer. (Figure 1) http://kff.org/report-section/health-care-costs-a-primer-2012-report/

15. Fries, J.F., Koop, C.E., Sokolov, J., Beadle, C.E. and Wright, D. (1998) Beyond Health Promotion: Reducing Need and Demand for Medical Care. Health Affairs, 17, 70-84.

16. Centers for Disease Control and Prevention (CDC) (2009) The Power of Prevention Chronic Disease . . . the Public Health Challenge of the 21st Century. http://www.cdc.gov/chronicdisease/pdf/2009-Power-of-Prevention.pdf

17. Hibbeln, J.R. and Davis, J.M. (2009) Considerations Regarding Neuropsychiatric Nutritional Requirements for Intakes of Mmega-3 Highly Unsaturated Fatty Acids. Prostaglandins, Leukotrienes and Essential Fatty Acids, 81, 179-186.

18. Centers for Disease Control and Prevention (CDC) (2015) Chronic Obstructive Pulmonary Disease. http://www.cdc.gov/copd/index.html

19. Lands, B. (2016) Omega-3 Fatty Acids Counterbalance Actions of Omega-6 Fatty Acids. In: Raatz, S. and Bibus, D., Eds., Fish and Fish Oils in Health and Disease, Elsevier, Philadelphia

20. Murphy, R.C., Pickett, W.C., Culp, B.R and Lands, W.E.M. (1981) Tetraene and Pentaene Leukotrienes: Selective Production from Murine Mastocytoma Cells after Dietary Manipulation. Prostaglandins, 22, 613-622.

21. Soderstrom, M., Mannervik, B., Garkov, V. and Hammarstrom, S. (1992) On the Nature of Leukotriene C4 Synthase in Human Platelets. Archives of Biochemistry and Biophysics, 294, 70-74.

22. Lee, T.H., Sethi, T., Crea, A.E.G., Peters, W., Arm, J.P., Horton, C.E., Walport, M.J. and Spur, B.W. (1988) Characterization of Leukotriene B3: Comparison of its Biological Activities with Leukotriene B4 and Leukotriene B5 in Complement Receptor Enhancement, Lysozyme Release and Chemotaxis of Human Neutrophils. Clinical Science, 74, 467-475.

23. Mohanan, S., Horibata, S., McElwee, J.L., Dannenberg, A.J. and Coonrod, S.A. (2013) Identification of Macrophage Extracellular Trap-like Structures in Mammary Gland Adipose Tissue: a Preliminary Study. Frontiers in Immunology, 4, 1-8. http://www.ncbi.nlm.nih.gov/pmc/articles/PMC3600535/

24. Li, P., Oh, D.Y., Bandyopadhyay, G., Lagakos, W.S., Talukdar, S., Osborn, O., Johnson, A., Chung, H., Mayoral, R., Maris, M., Ofrecio, J.M., Taguchi, S., Lu, M. and Olefsky, J.M. (2015) LTB4 Promotes Insulin Resistance in Obese Mice by Acting on Macrophages, Hepatocytes and Myocytes. Nature Medicine, 21, 239-247.

25. Spite, M., Hellmann, J., Tang, Y., Mathis, S.P., Kosuri, M., Bhatnagar, A., Jala, V.R. and Haribabu, B. (2011) Deficiency of the Leukotriene B4 Receptor, BLT-1, Protects against Systemic Insulin Resistance in Diet-induced Obesity. The Journal of Immunology, 187, 1942-1949.

26. Alvheim, A.R., Malde, M.K., Osei-Hyiaman, D., Lin, Y.H., Pawlosky, R.L., Madsen, L., Kristiansen, K., Frøyland, L. and Hibbeln, J.R. (2012) Dietary Linoleic Acid Elevates Endocannabinoids 2-AG and Anandamide and Induces Obesity. Obesity, 10, 1984-1994.

27. Alvheim A.R., Torstensen B.E., Lin Y.H., Lillefosse H.H., Lock E.J., Madsen L., Frøyland L., Hibbeln J.R. and Malde M.K. (2014)

Dietary Linoleic Acid Elevates the Endocannabinoids 2-AG and Anandamide and Promotes Weight Gain in Mice Fed a Low Fat Diet. Lipids, 49, 59-69.

28. Alvheim, A.R., Torstensen, B.E., Lin, Y.H., Lillefosse, H.H., Lock, E.J., Madsen, L., Hibbeln, J.R. and Malde, M.K. (2013) Dietary Linoleic Acid Elevates Endogenous 2-Arachidonoylglycerol and Anandamide in Atlantic Salmon (Salmo salar L.) and Mice, and Induces Weight Gain and Inflammation in Mice. British Journal of Nutrition, 109, 1508-1517.

29. The Look AHEAD Research Group, Wing, R.R., Bolin, P., Brancati, F.L., Bray, G.A., Clark, J.M., Coday, M., Crow, R.S., Curtis, J.M., Egan, C.M., Espeland, M.A., Evans, M., Foreyt, J.P., Ghazarian, S., Gregg, E.W., Harrison, B., Hazuda, H.P., Hill, J.O., Horton, E.S., Hubbard, V.S., Jakicic, J.M., Jeffery, R.W., Johnson, K.C., Kahn, S.E., Kitabchi, A.E., Knowler, W.C., Lewis, C.E., Maschak-Carey, B.J., Montez, M.G., Murillo, A., Nathan, D.M., Patricio, J., Peters, A., Pi-Sunyer, X., Pownall, H., Reboussin, D., Regensteiner, J.G., Rickman, A.D., Ryan, D.H., Safford, M., Wadden, T.A., Wagenknecht, L.E., West, D.S., Williamson, D.F. and Yanovski, S.Z. (2013) Cardiovascular Effects of Intensive Lifestyle Intervention in Type 2 Diabetes. The New England Journal of Medicine, 369, 145-154.

30. Lands, W.E.M. (2003) Diets Could Prevent Many Diseases. Lipids, 38, 317-321.

31. Marugame, T. and Mizuno, S. (2005) Comparison of Prostate Cancer Mortality in Five Countries: France, Italy, Japan, UK and USA from the WHO Mortality Database (1960-2000). Japanese Journal of Clinical Oncology, 35, 690-691.

32. Howlader, N., Noone, A.M., Krapcho, M., Garshell, J., Miller, D., Altekruse, S.F., Kosary, C.L., Yu, M., Ruhl, J., Tatalovich, Z., Mariotto, A., Lewis, D.R., Chen, H.S., Feuer, E.J. and Cronin, K.A., Eds. (2015) Prostate Cancer: Cancer Statistics Review, 1975-2012, National Cancer Institute. http://seer.cancer.gov/statfacts/html/prost.html

33. Huang, R.Y., Li, S.S., Guo, H.Z., Huang, Y., Zhang, X., Li, M.Y., Chen, G.G. and Zeng, X. (2014) Thromboxane A2 Exerts Promoting Effects on Cell Proliferation Through Mediating Cyclooxygenase-2 Signal in Lung Adenocarcinoma Cells. Journal of Cancer Research and Clinical Oncology, 140, 375-386.

34. Ramsden, C.E., Faurot, K.R., Zamora, D., Suchindran, C.M., MacIntosh, B.A., Gaylord, S., Ringel, A., Hibbeln, J.R., Feldstein,

A.E., Mori, T.A., Barden, A., Lynch, C., Coble, R., Mas, E., Palsson, O., Barrow, D.A. and Mann, J.D. (2013) Targeted Alteration of Dietary n-3 and n-6 Fatty Acids for the Treatment of Chronic Headaches: A Randomized Trial. Pain, 154, 2441-2451.

35. EFAeducation.org (2015) Omega 3-6 Apps Use Balance Scores. http://efaeducation.org/omega-3-6-apps/

36. Bibus, D. and Lands, B. (2015) Balancing Proportions of Competing Omega-3 and Omega-6 Highly Unsaturated Fatty Acids (HUFA) in Tissue Lipids. Prostaglandins LeukotEssent Fatty Acids, 99, 19-23. Ramsden, C.E., Faurot, K.R., Zamora, D., Palsson, O.S., MacIntosh, B.A., Gaylord, S., Taha, A.Y., Rapoport, S.I., Hibbeln, J.R., Davis, J.M. and Mann, J,D. (2015) Targeted Alterations in Dietary n-3 and n-6 Fatty Acids Improve Life Functioning and Reduce Psychological Distress among Patients with Chronic Headache: A Secondary Analysis of a Randomized Trial. Pain, 156, 587-596.

37. MacIntosh, B.A., Ramsden, C.E., Faurot, K.R., Zamora, D., Mangan, M., Hibbeln, J.R. and Mann, J.D. (2013) Low-n-6 and Low-n-6 Plus High-n-3 Diets for Use in Clinical Research. British Journal of Nutrition, 110, 559-568.

38. Wood, K.E., Mantzioris, E., Gibson, R.A. and Muhlhausler, B.S. (2013) Incorporating Macadamia Oil and Butter to Reduce Dietary Omega-6 Polyunsaturated Fatty Acid Intake. Nutrition & Dietetics, 70, 94-100.

39. U.S. Department of Defense (2013) Defense Science Board Study on Technology Innovation Enablers for Superiority in 2030. 80-83. http://www.acq.osd.mil/dsb/reports/DSB2030.pdf

40. Marriott, B.P., Yu, K., Majchrzak-Hong, S., Johnson, J. and Hibbeln, J.R. (2014) Understanding Diet and Modeling Changes in the Omega-3 and Omega-6 Fatty Acid Composition of U.S. Garrison Foods for Active Duty Personnel. Military Medicine, 179, 168-175.

41. Lin, Y.H., Hanson, J.A., Strandjord, S.E., Salem, N.M., Dretsch, M.N., Haub, M.D. and Hibbeln, J.R. (2014) Fast Transmethylation of Total Lipids in Dried Blood by Microwave Irradiation and Its Application to a Population Study. Lipids, 49, 839-851.

42. DuPont Pioneer (2015) Plenish® High Oleic Soybeanshttps://www.pioneer.com/home/site/us/products/soybean/enhanced-oil-soybeans/

43. Branch, W.D. (2014) Registration of "Georgia-13M" Peanut. Journal of Plant Registrations, 8, 253-256.

44. Gorbet, D. (2003) SunOleic®/High Oleic Peanuts: A Step Forward. http://ufdcimages.uflib.ufl.edu/IR/00/00/15/85/00001/AG15900.pdf

45. Isleib, T.G., Pattee, H.E., Sanders, T.H., Hendrix, K.W. and Dean, L.O. (2006) Compositional and Sensory Comparisons between Normal- and High-Oleic Peanuts. Journal of Agricultural and Food Chemistry, 54, 1759-1763.

46. Derbyshire, E.J. (2014) A Review of the Nutritional Composition, Organoleptic Characteristics and Biological Effects of the High Oleic Peanut. International Journal of Food Sciences and Nutrition, 65, 781-790.

47. Haytowitz, D.B. (2012) List of Key Foods Based on NHANES 2007-08. http://www.ars.usda.gov/SP2UserFiles/Place/12354500/Data/KeyFoods/Keyfoods_0708.xlsx

3

THE ROLE OF FUNCTIONAL FOODS, NUTRACEUTICALS, AND FOOD SUPPLEMENTS IN INTESTINAL HEALTH

Avrelija Cencic [1,2,*] and Walter Chingwaru[1]

[1]Department of Microbiology, Biochemistry, Biotechnology and Biotechnology, University of Maribor, Faculty of Agriculture and Life Sciences, Pivola 10, 2311 Hoče, Slovenia; Email:

[2]University of Maribor, Faculty of Medicine, Slomškov trg 15, 2000 Maribor, Slovenia

ABSTRACT

New eating habits, actual trends in production and consumption have a health, environmental and social impact. The European Union is fighting diseases characteristic of a modern age, such as obesity, osteoporosis, cancer, diabetes, allergies and dental problems. Developed countries are also faced with problems relating to aging populations, high energy foods, and unbalanced diets. The potential of nutraceuticals/functional foods/food supplements in mitigating health problems, especially in the gastrointestinal (GI) tract, is discussed. Certain members of gut microflora (e.g., probiotic/protective strains) play a role in the host health due to its involvement in nutritional, immunologic and physiological functions. The potential mechanisms by which nutraceuticals/functional foods/food supplements may alter a host's health are also highlighted in this paper. The establishment of novel functional cell models of the GI and analytical tools that allow tests in controlled experiments are highly desired for gut research.

Keywords: nutraceutical; functional food; food supplement; intestinal health; probiotic; intestinal cell models; gut research

1. INTRODUCTION

Eating habits and trends in food production and consumption have health, environmental and social impacts. Diet has implications on gut health. Gut complications, such as ulcerative colitis, Crohn's disease, irritable bowel syndrome, and gluten therapy resistant celiac, result from overgrowth and imbalance of intestinal microbial flora, and are related to one's diet. Notably, the gastrointestinal tract is sterile at birth; intestinal microflora develops after birth, with the colonization rate varying according to factors such as the mode of birth, infant nutrition, antibiotic use, diet and age. Gut health determines an individual's overall health. The human gut has the following functions: (a) it breaks food down to nutrients, (b) it facilitates absorption of nutrients into the blood through intestinal walls, and (c) it prevents foreign and toxic molecules from entering the bloodstream. Gut malfunction, therefore, has a direct negative impact on human health. This review focuses on the role of functional foods, nutraceuticals, and food supplements in intestinal health.

Consumption patterns vary significantly across Europe, from more southern healthy diets (rich in fruits and vegetables), to the northern ones (rich in animal fat and animal food products). Another striking difference is the fact that in northern European countries, eating is an individual affair, whereas in continental and southern countries consumers attach importance to the social dimension of food and sharing a meal [1]. These nutritional/consumption differences across Europe contribute greatly to the apparent differences in the health of populations on the continent. In spite of the fact that today's consumers are increasingly attentive to food safety, quality and health-related issues, the population in the European Union (EU) is still fighting with the diseases of a modern age such as obesity, osteoporosis, cancer, diabetes, allergies, stress and dental problems.

Furthermore, food additives, toxins and emerging food pathogens potentially present in fresh products and processed food present another threat, with their real effects being confounded by their adverse and synergistic effects. On the other hand, the increasingly aging populations in Europe require different foods for healthy aging [2]. Increased energy uptake, unbalanced diets, and highly processed foods used in fast food products are huge problems, which the EU [3] and other developed countries such as the United States of America [4,5,6] have to overcome. Nevertheless, economic crises and high food prices tend to favor unbalanced "cheap" food intake. Attributes such as educational inequalities also contribute to obesity in Europe [7]. However, the USA diet, notably, has the highest amount of calories for the lowest cost worldwide [8]. The USA also has the highest availability of large-scale agricultural commodities, and refined and processed food products.

Based on the European Food Safety Authority (EFSA) Food-Based Dietary Guidelines, it is evident that in most EU member countries, the most frequent country-specific diet-related health problems are still cardiovascular diseases, overweight/obesity, dyslipidemia, hypertension, type 2 diabetes, osteoporosis and dental caries [9]. In 93% of EU countries, the EFSA reported that the average intake of total fat is above 30% of the energy intake, with the highest intake in Latvia, Lithuania and Slovenia [9]. Only in Italy the intake of saturated fat acids is below 10% [9]. However, overall, females tend to have lower dietary fat and higher carbohydrate intakes than males. Also notable is the fact that more females tend to consume fruits and vegetables within the recommended levels than males in Europe, based on data obtained in Central and Eastern Europe [10]. Moreover, it is a common observation in the EU that among the food groups (bread/cereals, rice/pasta/potatoes, vegetables, fruit, milk/dairy products, meat, fish, oils/fats, legumes and eggs), fruits and vegetables are not prioritized among consumers [11,12]. While consumers are aware of the link between eating and health, they expect visible implications of consumption of a particular product on health [13] and tend to acquire food based on convenience [14]. Recently, food manufacturers have embarked on a health criterion in the development of "functional foods", the latter being defined as food products that have an added positive health benefit [15]. While some functional ingredient benefits may be perceived to enhance short-term well-being or performance ability, many such benefits concern the long-term mitigation of certain diseases [15]. Long term health benefits are generally invisible to the average consumer. Traditional foods are increasingly considered healthy and wholesome, and as a result, public interest in their nutritional and health impact has increased, as has their demand [15].

2. FOOD AND HEALTH

Food habits develop in early infancy. In fact, it is known that initial phases of life (intra-uterine period and the first year of life) are sensitive to nutritional factors [16]. Exclusive breastfeeding up to six months, with breastfeeding lasting up to two years or longer in combination with the introduction of balanced complementary feeding (CF), are emphasized by the World Health Organization (WHO) as important measures of public health, with effective impact on the reduction in the risk of developing chronic diseases. It is now known that children after the age of two years should be fed a nutritionally balanced diet similar to that of adults, particularly a diet low in sugar, salt and fat, and rich in complex carbohydrates, fruits and vegetables. Development of food habits is a complex process that may be influenced by such factors as region, religion, family structure and habits, income, prices, stress levels and technological advancements. Several epidemiologic studies over the last 50 years have clearly shown that diets dominated by fruits, vegetables and dietary fibers (plant based foods) prevent and reduce the risk of chronic diseases (e.g. cardiovascular diseases, obesity, diabetes) and promote sound human health. The generation of scientific research linking foods of plant origin and health worldwide has resulted in acknowledgement that plant bioactive compounds have anti-oxidant and other healthy properties [17,18].

High dietary intake of fruits, vegetables and whole grains is strongly associated with reduced risk of developing chronic diseases, such as cancer and cardiovascular diseases (CVD), which are the highest causes of death in Europe, United States and in most industrialized countries [9,19]. It is estimated that one-third of all cancer deaths in industrialised countries could be avoided through appropriate dietary formulations. This suggests that dietary behavioral changes, such as increasing consumption of fruits, vegetables, and whole grains, and related changes in lifestyle, are practical strategies for significant reduction of the incidence of cancer [20]. There is a huge amount of scientific literature consistently, but not universally, linking consumption of diets rich in vegetables and fruits with reduced risk of cancer, particularly epithelial cancers of the alimentary and respiratory tracts [21]. Based on results from 206 human epidemiologic studies and 22 animal studies, similar effects of plant based diets are consistent for cancers of the stomach, esophagus, lung, oral cavity and pharynx, endometrium, pancreas, and colon [21]. The types of vegetables or fruit that most often appear to be protective against cancer are raw vegetables, followed by allium vegetables, carrots, green vegetables, cruciferous vegetables, and tomatoes [21].

In 1996 the American Dietetics Association produced a paper demonstrating protective effects of eating fruit and vegetables against several cancers.

Cardiovascular diseases (CVD, including heart disease and stroke), represent the primary cause of death, with high negative impact on both human health and community social costs in Western countries. Cardiovascular diseases and tumors, together, contribute to more than 60 % of deaths in economically-developed countries [22]. In economically-developed countries, CVDs acquire a character of epidemic proportions, and surpass infectious diseases in mortality. Recent studies implicate reactive oxygen species (ROS) in the pathogenesis of both acute and chronic heart diseases as a result of cumulative oxidative stress [23]. In particular, oxidation of low density lipoproteins (LDL), the latter emanating from saturated, trans fats and meat products, has a key role in the pathogenesis of atherosclerosis and cardiovascular heart diseases through the initiation of the plaque formation process [23].

Important risk factors for CVD include obesity, high blood cholesterol level, high blood pressure and type 2 diabetes. The risk of CVD is increased not only by the consumption of poor diets, but also by lifestyle habits such as smoking and alcohol intake [23]. It has been shown that people consuming healthy diets, living active lifestyles, not smoking and not indulging in excessive alcohol consumption tend to have a reduced risk of CVD [24]. It is also known that diets leading to elevated serum total cholesterol, LDL-cholesterol, and triacylglycerol concentrations, while leading to reduced HDL-cholesterol concentrations, lead to reduced risk of coronary artery disease. As a result, treatment of hypercholesterolemia has focused on increasing fecal excretion of cholesterol and bile acids, and reducing hepatic cholesterol synthesis through diet modification among the few optional strategies available [25,26].

Blood pressure control is important in the prevention of heart disease, kidney disease and stroke. Blood pressure is influenced by numerous factors including atherosclerosis, imbalances in the renin-angiotensin system, and hyperinsulinemia, the latter increasing sodium retention in the body and speeding up atherosclerosis [27]. Consequently, a general nutritional plan to minimize hypertensionrisk includes attaining and maintaining a healthy body weight; consuming a diet rich in calcium, phosphorus, and magnesium; and consuming alcoholic beverages and sodium in moderation [28].

Obesity is a medical condition characterized by accumulation of excess body fat. As a condition, obesity is associated with reduced life expectancy and/or increased health problems [29]. Obesity is therefore not just a cosmetic problem [29]. Numerous studies indicate that higher levels of body fat are associated with an increased risk of many adverse health conditions. Weight loss is increasingly recognized as bringing major health benefits to overweight people and is linked with increases in life expectancy of people having obesity-related complications [30]. Overweight and obesity have increased over the past 20 years in many regions of the world, particularly the prevalence of obesity in childhood. Obesity is not only restricted to the developed world; it is also becoming a growing burden for the developing countries [31]. Data from the International Obesity Task Force (IOTF) [32] indicate that, worldwide, over 20 million children under the age of six are obese or overweight. Obesity is a multi factorial problem and its development is due to multiple interactions between genes and environment. There is a need to identify aspects of behavior that curtail excessive energy intake while enhancing energy expenditure. These include making appropriate dietary choices, embarking on good eating behavior, and having an active lifestyle [32].

Cancer development, a dynamic and long-term process, involves many complex factors with stepwise progression, ultimately leading to an uncontrolled spreading and growth of cancerous cells throughout the body, called metastasis. Epidemiological studies have provided convincing evidence that dietary factors can modify carcinogenesis. Laboratory research has further demonstrated that a number of bioactive dietary components or natural products have the ability to prevent cancer [17,18]. In addition, many food constituents with yet undefined nutritional benefits have been found to possess anti-mutagenic and anti-carcinogenic properties. Such promising research provides a strong support for the acceptance in the future of bioactive components of food as chemopreventative agents [33].

3. FUNCTIONAL FOODS

Functional foods are similar in appearance to conventional foods; the former being consumed as part of the normal diet. In contrast to conventional foods, functional foods, however, have demonstrated physiological benefits and can reduce the risk of chronic disease beyond basic nutritional functions, including maintenance of gut health [34]. When food is being cooked or prepared using "scientific intelligence" with or without knowledge of how or why it is being used, the food is called "functional food". Thus, functional food provides the body with the required amount of vitamins, fats, proteins, carbohydrates,*etc.*, needed for its healthy survival [34].

4. PROBIOTICS, PREBIOTICS AND SYNBIOTICS

The human gut is populated by a wide array of bacterial species, the latter bearing important metabolic and immune functions, all leading to marked effects on the nutritional and health status of the host [35]. Probiotics, according to a consensus definition, are 'living micro-organisms, which upon ingestion in certain numbers, exert health benefits beyond inherent basic nutrition' [36,37], alternatively probiotics are loosely known as live microorganisms belonging to natural biota with low or no pathogenicity, but with functions of importance to the health and well being of the host [38,39]. Numerous probiotic microorganisms (e.g.,*Lactobacillus rhamnosus* GG, *Lactobacillus reuteri*, bifidobacteria and certain strains of *Lactobacillus casei*, the*Lactobacillus acidophilus*-group, *Escherichia coli* strain Nissle 1917, certain enterococci, especially *Enterococcus faecium* SF68, and the probiotic yeast *Saccharomyces boulardii*) are used in probiotic food, particularly fermented milk products, or have been investigated with regard to their medicinal use. New genera and strains of probiotics are emerging; some with high health benefits as in *Lactobacillus plantarum* isolates (PCS20, PCS22, PCS25 and PCS26) from Slovenian cheese with high antimicrobial [40] and immunomodulatory [38] capabilities. Probiotics were originally used to influence human health through intestinal microbiota alterations. At present, probiotics and their effects on human health have been demonstrated both within different food matrices and as single or mixed microbial culture preparations. Furthermore, the health-promoting properties of probiotics are now known to be strain-dependent [37,38,39]. An international expert group of the International Life Sciences Institute (ILSI) has evaluated the categorized and published evidence of functionality of different probiotics in four areas of (human) application, namely, (i) metabolism, (ii) chronic intestinal inflammatory and functionaldisorders, (iii) infections, and (iv) allergy [41]. The ILSI report gives concrete examples demonstrating benefits and gaps, and guidelines and recommendations on the design of next generation of probiotic studies, with the aim to substantiate the current body of information on probiotic benefits. The effects of probiotics on human health are positive and well defined in diarrhoea treatment, however there are no clinical results regarding the dose of probiotics or duration of such treatments [42]. The results from clinical studies have not been conclusive in that the effects of probiotics on the host are dependent on probiotic strains, type of infection (acute or chronic gastrointestinal infections, immunological or inflammatory disease), different doses used and duration of treatment [42]. Probiotics have been shown to have applications in alleviating symptoms of allergies [43,44], cancer [45], AIDS [46], respiratory and urinary tract infections [47]. Furthermore, various findings suggest that probiotics have beneficial effects in alleviating symptoms associated with aging, fatigue, autism, and in reducing the risks of osteoporosis, obesity and possibly type 2 diabetes [48]. Advantages of probiotics for health can only be realized if proper probiotic strain or product selection, and dose guidelines of commercial production, are followed in human food or medicine [44,48].

The concentration of probiotics needed to obtain a clinical effect is often quoted as $\geq 10^6$ colony forming units (cfu) per milliliter in the small bowel and $\geq 10^8$ cfu/g in the colon. The dose for treatment of an acute illness by a particular probiotic agent may be lower or higher, in the order of 10-fold or 100-fold or more in terms of cfu. In acute infectious diarrhoea, it seems that higher doses of probiotics given for short courses are more effective than lower doses. In chronic or immunological diseases (allergic, inflammatory and/or immune diseases), the effects of probiotics depend also on the interactions between the respective microorganisms and gut immune system, and duration of treatment. To evaluate the efficacy of probiotics it may be essential to identify specific target groups of individuals with more specific higher susceptibilities to the potential effects of probiotics.

A **prebiotic** is "a selectively fermented ingredient, or a fiber that allows specific changes, both in the composition and/or activity of the gastrointestinal microflora, resultantly conferring benefits on the well being and health of host " [37,48]. Other, more specific effects of prebiotics on health are indirect, namely prevention of diarrhoea or obstipation, modulation of the metabolism of the intestinal flora, cancer prevention, effects on lipid metabolism, stimulation of mineral adsorption and immunomodulatory properties. Prebiotics form a group of diverse carbohydrate ingredients that is poorly understood in regard to their origin, fermentation profiles, and dosages required for health effects, although providing nutraceutical and nutritional value [48]. Today, only bifidogenic, non-digestible oligosaccharides (particularly inulin, its hydrolysis product oligofructose, and (trans)galactooligosaccharides), fulfill all the criteria for prebiotic classification [37]. In the last few years, successful attempts have been reported to make infant formula more breast-milk-like by the addition of fructo- and (primarily) galactooligosaccharides.

Probiotics and prebiotics share unique roles in human nutrition, largely centered on manipulation of populations or activities of the microbiota that colonize the human GI tract [48]. Regular consumption of probiotics or prebiotics has health implications that include enhanced immune function, improved colonic integrity, decreased incidence and duration of intestinal infections, down-regulated allergic response, and improved digestion and elimination [48].

It is noteworthy that human subjects and their enteric microbiota have evolved together to reach a state of mutual tolerance. There is mounting evidence from both animal models and human studies to suggest that inflammatory bowel disease (IBD) is a result of a malfunction of this mutual relationship [49]. Probiotics and prebiotics, however, have been investigated in clinical trials as treatments for IBD, with conflicting results [49]. While there is general consensus about the value of probiotics and prebiotics, their influence on bowl health in terms of Crohn's disease is less convincing [49]. This may be attributed to variations in methodologies, differences in the range of probiotic, prebiotic and combination (synbiotic) treatments tested, and variability in test subjects used, such as different patient groups [49].

Synbiotics are synergistic combinations of pro- and prebiotics [37].

Mechanisms of probiotic actions

While probiotics are gaining significant interest as alternatives for antibiotics or anti-inflammatory drugs, their mode of action is poorly understood [50]. Probiotics may act by modulating the host's immune system, affecting other microorganisms directly or acting on microbial products, host products or food components [50]. The effectiveness of a probiotic depends on its metabolic properties, the set of molecules presented at its surface, the components it secretes, and the integral parts of the microorganism such as its DNA or peptidoglycan [50].

Imbalance of Intestinal Microbial Flora

Modern lifestyles tend to impose stress on systems genetically adapted over millions of years. The consumption of food containing microorganisms has dramatically reduced, and as a consequence, the developing mucosal immune systems are faced with different microflora, particularly fewer pathogens than paleolithic man. Increases in observed incidence and severity of allergies and conditions such as IBD in the Western world have been linked with increases in standards of hygiene and sanitation, which have occurred concomitantly with decreases in the number and range of infectious challenges encountered by the growing and developing host. This lack of immune education impairs the development of the immune system and allows the host to over-react to non-pathogenic antigen-containing commensal flora, resulting in inflammatory damage, allergy and/or autoimmunity [51]. To combat these trends directly, the World Health Organisation currently advocates the implementation of alternative disease control strategies, such as exploiting the prophylactic and therapeutic potential of probiotic bacteria [52]. Most of these probiotic microorganisms, isolated from such sources as faeces of healthy individuals, are safe for human consumption and are available over the counter. Because of continued scepticism of such products, European Union funded research groups including medical, scientific and industrial interests, have agreed on criteria for selection and assessment of probiotics.

5. NUTRACEUTICALS

The term "nutraceutical" was coined from "nutrition" and "pharmaceutical" in 1989 by Stephen DeFelice, MD, founder and chairman of the Foundation for Innovation in Medicine (FIM), Cranford, NJ [53]. DeFelice proceeded to define nutraceutical as, "a food (or part of a food) that provides medical or health benefits, including the prevention and/or treatment of a disease" [53]. When functional food aids in the prevention and/or treatment of disease(s) and/or disorder(s) other than anaemia, it is called a nutraceutical [54]. It should be noted that the term nutraceutical, as commonly used in marketing, has no regulatory definition [55]. Thus, nutraceuticals differ from dietary supplements in the following aspects: (1) nutraceuticals must not only supplement the diet but should also aid in the prevention and/or treatment of disease and/or disorder; and (2) nutraceuticals are used as conventional foods or as sole items of a meal or diet [56]. Dietary components play beneficial roles beyond basic nutrition, leading to the development of the functional food concept and nutraceuticals [35]. A functional food for one consumer can act as a nutraceutical for another consumer.

Examples of nutraceuticals include fortified dairy products (e.g., milk) and citrus fruits (e.g., orange juice) [56].

Several naturally derived food substances have been studied in cancer therapies. Vitamin E, selenium, vitamin D, green tea, soy, and lycopene are examples of nutraceuticals widely studied in human health [53]. While many of these 'natural' compounds have been found to have high therapeutic potential; future studies should include well-designed clinical trials assessing combinations of these compounds to realize possible synergies they bring into human health.

Polyunsaturated fatty acids (PUFAs) (which include the omega-3 and omega-6 fatty acids) and phytochemicals also play an important role as healthy dietary bioactive compounds [35]. A balanced PUFA composition of food influences diverse aspects of immunity and metabolism [35]. Moreover, interactions between PUFAs and components of the gut microbiota may also influence their biological roles. Phytochemicals (bioactive non-nutrient plant compounds), have raised interest in human nutrition because of their potential effects as antioxidants, antiestrogenics, anti-inflammatory, immunomodulatory, and anticarcinogenics [17,35]. Gut microbiota can, for example, transform and influence the bioavailability and effects of polyphenols [35]. Phytochemicals and their metabolic products may also inhibit pathogenic bacteria [17,35] while stimulate the growth of beneficial bacteria, exerting prebiotic-like effects [34]. Interactions between functional food components, such as prebiotics, probiotics, phytochemicals, and intestinal microbiota, have consequences on human health [35].

6. FOOD SUPPLEMENTS

According to the US Dietary Supplement Health and Education Act (DSHEA) of 1994, the term "dietary supplement" can be defined using several criteria; namely (a) a product (other than tobacco) that is intended to supplement the diet that bears or contains one or more of the following dietary ingredients: a vitamin, a mineral, an herb or other botanical, an amino acid, a dietary substance for use by man to supplement the diet by increasing the total daily intake, or a concentrate, metabolite, constituent, extract, or combinations of these ingredients [55], (b) a product intended for ingestion in pill, capsule, tablet, or liquid form, (c) a product not represented for use as a conventional food or as the sole item of a meal or diet, (d) anything labeled as a "dietary supplement", and (e) products such as a newly approved drug, certified antibiotic, or licensed biologic that was marketed as a dietary supplement or food before approval, certification, or license (unless if this provision is waived by an authority such as Secretary of Health and Human Services, as in USA) [56].

Under the DSHEA (1994), the manufacturer of a dietary supplement is responsible for ensuring that the dietary supplement is safe before it is marketed [57]. It is also binding to the manufacturers that they make sure that product label information is truthful and not misleading [57].

Many European countries have adopted the highly restrictive CODEX standards for dietary supplements, which eliminate the consumer's ability to purchase dietary supplements in therapeutic or meaningful preventive dosages. Codex Alimentarius (Latin for "Food Code") is the United Nation's proposed set of international guidelines for nutritional supplements, food handling, production, and trade which is gradually being ratified in countries around the world, starting in the EU [58]. In comparison to most other industrialized countries, there is virtually no restriction on the type or strength of nutritional supplements that can be purchased in the United States [58]. The only significant limitation on the sale of supplements is that disease and cure related claims cannot be made by supplement manufacturers without USA Food and Drug Agency (FDA) approval. And the FDA has approved only a few disease related claims for supplements [58].

Questions can arise whether a nutrient used as part of a treatment for a defined disease can be considered a drug, whereas the same nutrient is used to enhance health (reduce the risk of disease), can be considered a functional food or dietary supplement? This overlap shows interlinks that exist between functional foods and medicines.

Mounting evidence supports the observation that functional foods containing physiologically active components, either from plant or animal sources, may enhance health [59]. Clearly, all foods are functional, as they provide taste, aroma, or nutritive value [59]. There has been an explosion of consumer interest in the health enhancing role of specific foods or physiologically-active food components, so-called functional foods [59]. It should be stressed, however, that functional foods are not a magic bullet or universal panacea for poor health habits [59]. There are no "good" or "bad" foods, but there are good or bad diets [59].

7. THE INTESTINAL HEALTH

Proper functioning of the digestive tract, with both its chemical and muscular activity, is essential to health. Digestive disorders are on the increase. About 38 million Americans suffer from a variety of digestive problems such as gastroesophageal reflux disease (GERD), irritable bowel syndrome, celiac disease, food allergies, diverticulitis, ulcerative colitis, and Crohn's disease [60]. Approximately 25 million Americans have daily heartburn, and it is estimated that 20% of the adult population have irritable bowel syndrome. Celiac disease, once considered rare, is now thought to affect 1 in 133 people, and food allergies have increased alarmingly [60].

8. THE GASTROINTESTINAL (GI) TRACT AS AN ECOSYSTEM

Co-evolution led to a symbiotic relationship between eukaryotes and prokaryotes with the development of sophisticated by-directional signaling systems of mucosal epithelia and lymphocytes in the intestinal tract [51]. It is estimated that over 400 species of bacteria, separated into two broad categories, namely beneficial (e.g., *Bifidobacterium* and *Lactobacillus*) and those considered detrimental (e.g., Enterobacteriaceae and*Clostridium* spp.) inhabit the human gastrointestinal tract. Bacterial end products of fermentation are essential mucosal nutrients including amino acids (arginine, cysteine and glutamine) and short chain fatty acids (SCFA: acetate, propionate and butyrate) [51]. These SCFAs serve as an energy source for the host, providing 10–30% of basal metabolic requirements including energy for liver cells, colonocytes and peripheral tissues with only about 5% excreted in the feces [51]. Besides fermentation, the metabolic products of the microflora includes vitamins K and B complex, secondary bile acid production, neutralization of dietary carcinogens such as nitrosamines, and conversion to active metabolites of some prodrugs. The indigenous intestinal (autochthonous) microbiota act as a further barrier against any transient (allochthonous) potential pathogens by competing for nutrients and mucosal adherence and by production of antigens (bacteriocins), which are active against pathogens. Furthermore, it has been clearly established that the gastrointestinal flora are essential for mucosal protection and immune education as it has been described as the most adaptable and renewable metabolic organ of the body. The composition and activities of gastrointestinal flora affect both intestinal and systemic physiology. The complex gastrointestinal microbial load is required for normal development and homeostasis of the humoral and cellular immune system. It is the interaction between the mucosal immune system and the enteric microflora which maintains the physiologically normal state or activation of immune organ, the latter resulting in secretion of antibodies against harmful antigens (pathogenic microorganisms) [51].

9. APPLICATION OF INTESTINAL CELL MODELS

Functional cell/co-culture models involve growth of cell lines in co-culture, either in direct contact with each other on the membrane or indirectly where one cell line is cultured on the apical side of a membrane and the other cell line on either the underside of the membrane (basolateral) or on the surface of the plastic feeder or receiver trays in multi-well cell plates [61,62,63,64]. Use of cells in co-culture systems mimics the natural existence of such cells in an organism, so that direct effects on cells, tissues or organs of chemicals, microorganisms and their products and so forth, can be tested *in situ*. The direct mixing of different cell types in culture is otherwise normally avoided in co-culture systems, allowing scientists to model such interactions *in vivo*. Functional/co-culture cell models are increasingly gaining recognition in science, as they mimic normal organ, tissue and physiological organization in human organism.

In a co-culture system, two or more cell types brought together in the same culture environment very likely interact and communicate [65]. Co-culture has proved to be a powerful *in vitro* tool in unravelling the importance of cellular interactions during normal physiology, homeostasis, repair and regeneration [65].

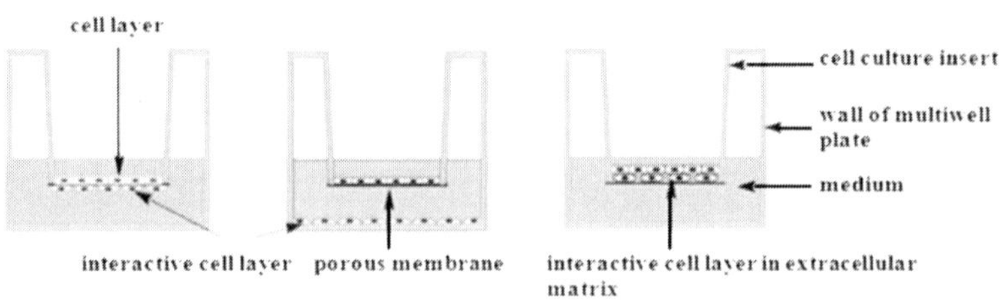

Figure 1. Co-culture set up system.

Co-culture cell systems have been used in a variety of applications such studies on disease pathogenesis, for example Crohn's disease [63] drug testing [64], study of xenobiotic kinetics [66], studies on cancer progression [67], to name a few examples. The advantages of studying effects of different substances *in vitro*on cell lines include: (i) the ability to manipulate cells in a defined environment and to retrieve and study specific cell types; (ii) ability to identify novel growth or inhibitory paracrine factors involved in regulation of growth; (iii) cell behavior is easier to reproduce in these *in situ* models than *in vivo*; (iv) they provide a physiological basis for future studies of molecular and genetic mechanisms of disease; and (v) they allow dissection of mechanisms of cell-cell and cell-matrix interactions involved in human disease, while avoiding extrapolation of data from studies using other species. Co-culture systems are therefore important developments with novel medical applications and resulting in reduced testing of substances on living animals.

Co-culture systems and studies of interactions between probiotic bacteria and intestinal epithelium

Recently Gradisnik *et al*., (2006) [68] reported establishment of a pig functional cell model involving two pig intestinal epithelial cell lines (PSI and CLAB) and macrophages from pig peripheral blood (PoMac), with possible applications in both human and animal studies. This model was developed in sight of the substantial lack of good intestinal cell culture models. It was noted that pig cell lines represented better animal models than rodents in human research. Recently Nissen *et al*., (2009) [39] have reported use of the pig functional cell model described by Gradisnik *et al*. [68] in studies of interactions between intestinal epithelium, macrophages and probiotic bacteria. Such a model has been found to give novel effects in such interactions. Current efforts are centred on development of human co-culture model systems, including use of three-dimensional co-culture systems for use in studying gut health, and development of nutraceuticals or functional ingredients of foods with useful protective effects on the GI tract.

10. CONCLUSION

Overall, this paper discusses nutraceuticals/functional foods/food supplements (broadly including probotics, prebiotics, synbioitcs, phytochemicals *etc*.), especially the need for consuming appropriate diets, health issues surrounding failure to adhere to the known healthy eating models, development of new nutraceuticals/functional foods/food supplements with novel health benefits, elucidation mechanisms of action of these products, development of study systems such as *in-vitro* co-culture cell models. Appropriate diet culminates in a healthy, properly functioning GI tract, resulting in attainment of proper human physiology, hence healthy living; otherwise the opposite becomes true. Modeling new eating habits using the existing knowledge is needed for the eventual ideal of 'health for all' vision.

REFERENCES

1. Bronzwaer, S. EFSA scientific forum "from safe food to healthy diets". EU risk assessment -Past, present and Future. Trends Food Sci. Technol. 2008, 19, S2–S8.
2. Roberts, S.B.; Rosenberg, I. Nutrition and aging: changes in the regulation of energy metabolism with aging. Physiol. Rev. 2006, 86, 651–667.
3. Perez-Cueto, F.J.; Verbeke, W.; de Barcellos, M.D.; Kehagia, O.; Chryssochoidis, G.; Scholderer, J.; Grunert, K.G. Food-related lifestyles and their association to obesity in five European countries.Appetite 2009, 54, 156–562.
4. The Analysis of Prehistoric Diets; Gilbert, R.L., Mielke, J.H., Eds.; Academic Press: Orlando, FL, USA, 1985.
5. Eaton, S.B.; Eaton, S.B., III; Konner, M.J.; Shostak, M. An evolutionary perspective enhances understanding of human nutritional requirements. J. Nutr. 1996, 126, 1732–1740.
6. Eaton, S.B.; Eaton, S.B., III; Konner, M.J. Paleolithic nutrition revisited: a twelve-year retrospective on its nature and implications. Eur. J. Clin. Nutr. 1997, 51, 207–216.
7. Roskam, A.J.; Kunst, A.E.; Van Oyen, H.; Demarest, S.; Klumbiene, J.; Regidor, E.; Helmert, U.; Jusot, F.; Dzurova, D.; Mackenbach, J.P. Comparative appraisal of educational inequalities in overweight and obesity among adults in 19 European countries. Int. J. Epidemiol. 2009. [Epub ahead of print].
8. Crawford, M.A.; Marsh, D. Nutrition and Evolution; Keats Publishing: New Canaan, CT, USA, 1995.
9. EFSA (European Food Safety Authority). Scientific Opinion of the Panel on Dietetic Products, Nutrition and Allergies on a

request from the EC on Food-Based Dietary Guidelines. The EFSA J. 2008, 1–44.

10. Boylan, S.; Welch, A.; Pikhart, H.; Malyutina, S.; Pajak, A.; Kubinova, R.; Bragina, O.; Simonova, G.; Stepaniak, U.; Gilis-Januszewska, A.; Milla, L.; Peasey, A.; Marmot, M.; Bobak, M. Dietary habits in three Central and Eastern European countries: the HAPIEE study. BMC Public Health. 2009, 9, 439.

11. Acheson, D. Independent Inquiry into Inequalities in Health, Foodaware Proposals for an EU Nutrition Policy, Comments on the Joint WHO/FAO Expert Consultation on Diet, Nutrition and the Prevention of Chronic Diseases. 2002. Available online: http://www.who.int/dietphysicalactivity/media/en/gsfao_cmo_035.pdf (accessed on 25 February 2010).

12. NHS. Exploration of Adult Food Portion Size Tools. NHS Health Scotland: Edinburgh, Scotland, 2008.

13. Brunso, K.; Fjord, T.A.; Grunert, K.G. Consumers' food choice and quality perception; Aarhus School of Business: Aarhus, Denmark, 2002; MAPP Working Paper No. 77.

14. Grunert, K.G.; Brunso, K.; Bredahl, L.; Bech, A.C. Food-Related Lifestyle: A Segmentation Approach to European Food Consumers. In Food, People and Society: A European Perspective of Consumers' Food Choices; Frewer, L.J., Risvik, E., Schifferstein, H.N.J., von Alvensleben, R., Eds.; Springer Verlag: Berlin, Germany, 2001; pp. 211–230.

15. Public Health Boon or 21st Century Quackery? International, Functional Foods, Center for Science in the Public. CSPI Reports, 1998. Available online: http://www.cspinet.org/reports/functional_foods/introduction.html/ (accessed on 25 February 2010).

16. Caetano, M.C.; Ortiz, T.T.; da Silva, S.G.; de Souza, F.I.; Sarni, R.O. Complementary feeding: inappropriate practices in infants. J. Pediatr. (Rio J). 2010, 86. [Epub ahead of print].

17. Cencic, A.; Chingwaru, W. Antimicrobial Agents Deriving from Indigenous Plants. RPFNA 2010, 2, 83–92.

18. Balsano, C.; Alisi, A. Antioxidant effects of natural bioactive compounds. Curr. Pharm. Des. 2009, 15, 3063–3073.

19. Liu, R.H. Potential synergy of phytochemicals in cancer prevention: mechanism of action. J. Nutr.2004, 134, 3479S–3485S.

20. Terry, P.; Giovannucci, E.; Michels, K.B.; Bergkvist, L.; Hansen, H.; Holmberg, L.; Wolk, A. Fruit, vegetables, dietary fiber, and risk of colorectal cancer. J. Natl. Cancer. Inst. 2001, 93, 525–533.

21. Denny, A.; Buttriss, J. Synthesis Report No 4: Plant Foods and Health: Focus on Plant Bioactives. British Nutrition Foundation, 2005. Available online: http://www.eurofir.net/temp/PLANTspFOODSspANDspHEALTHspFOCUSspONspPLANTspBIOACTIVEShs1hs.pdf (accessed on 11 October 2009).

22. Stramba-Badiale, M.; Fox, K.M.; Priori, S.G.; Collins, P.; Daly, C.; Graham, I.; Jonsson, B.; Schenck-Gustafsson, K.; Tendera, M. Cardiovascular diseases in women: a statement from the policy conference of the European Society of Cardiology. Eur. Heart. J. 2006, 27, 994–1005.

23. Wang, C.Z.; Mehendale, S.R.; Yuan, C.S. Commonly used antioxidant botanicals: active constituents and their potential role in cardiovascular illness. Am. J. Chin. Med. 2007, 35, 543–558.

24. Riccioni, G.; Mancini, B.; Di Ilio, E.; Bucciarelli, T.; D'Orazio, N. Protective effect of lycopene in cardiovascular disease. Eur. Rev. Med. Pharmacol. Sci. 2008, 12, 183–190.

25. The Expert Panel. Summary of the second report of the National Cholesterol Education Program (NCEP) Expert Panel on detection, evaluation, and treatment of high blood cholesterol in adults (Adult Treatment Panel II). JAMA 1993, 269, 3015–3023.

26. Austin, M.A. Plasma triglyceride and coronary heart disease. Arterioscler. Thromb. 1991, 11, 2–14.

27. Lampe, J.W. Health effects of vegetables and fruit: assessing mechanisms of action in human experimental studies. Am. J. Clin. Nutr. 1999, 70, 475S–490S.

28. Dwyer, J. Overview: dietary approaches for reducing cardiovascular disease risks. J. Nutr. 1995, 125, 656S–665S.

29. Haslam, D.W.; James, W.P. Obesity. Lancet 2005, 366, 1197–1209.

30. Rayalam, S.; Della-Fera, M.A.; Baile, C.A. Phytochemicals and regulation of the adipocyte life cycle. J. Nutr. Biochem. 2008, 19, 717–726.

31. Martorell, R.; Kettel Khan, L.; Hughes, M.L.; Grummer-Strawn, L.M. Overweight and obesity in preschool children from

developing countries. Int. J. Obes. Relat. Metab. Disord. 2000, 24, 959–967.

32. International Obesity TaskForce (IOTF). Obesity in Europe, EU Platform Briefing Paper, prepared by Lobstein, T.; Rigby, N.; in collaboration with European Association for the Study of Obesity. 2005. Available online: http://www.iaso.org/popout.asp?linkto=http%3A//www.iotf.org/media/euobesity3.pdf (accessed on 25 February 2010).

33. Pan, M.H.; Ghai, G.; Ho, C.T. Food bioactives, apoptosis, and cancer. Mol. Nutr. Food. Res. 2008, 52, 43–52.

34. Food and Agriculture Organization of the United Nations (FAO). Report on Functional Foods, Food Quality and Standards Service (AGNS). 2007. Available online: http://www.fao.org/ag/agn/agns/files/Functional_Foods_Report_Nov2007.pdf (accessed on 25 February 2010).

35. Laparra, J.M.; Sanz, Y. Interactions of gut microbiota with functional food components and nutraceuticals. Pharmacol. Res. 2010, 61, 219–225.

36. Guarner, F.; Schaafsma, G.J. Probiotics. Int. J. Food Microbiol. 1998, 39, 237–238.

37. de Vrese, M.; Schrezenmeir, J. Probiotics, prebiotics, and synbiotics. Adv. Biochem. Eng. Biotechnol.2008, 111, 1–66.

38. Bengmark, S. Ecological control of the gastrointestinal tract. The role of probiotic flora. Gut. 1998, 42, 2–7.

39. Nissen, L.; Chingwaru, W.; Sgorbati, B.; Biavati, B.; Cencic, A. Gut health promoting activity of new putative probiotic/protective Lactobacillus spp. strains: a functional study in the small intestinal cell model. Int. J. Food. Microbiol. 2009, 135, 288–294.

40. Maragkoudakis, P.A.; Chingwaru, W.; Gradisnik, L.; Tsakalidou, E.; Cencic, A. Lactic acid bacteria efficiently protect human and animal intestinal epithelial and immune cells from enteric virus infection. Int. J. Food. Microbiol. 2010. [Epub ahead of print]..

41. Rijkers, G.T.; Bengmark, S.; Enck, P.; Haller, D.; Herz, U.; Kalliomaki, M.; Kudo, S.; Lenoir-Wijnkoop, I.; Mercenier, A.; Myllyluoma, E.; Rabot, S.; Rafter, J.; Szajewska, H.; Watzl, B.; Wells, J.; Wolvers, D.; Antoine, J.M. Guidance for substantiating the evidence for beneficial effects of probiotics: current status and recommendations for future research. J. Nutr. 2010, 140, 671S–676S.

42. Minelli, E.B.; Benini, A. Relationship between number of bacteria and their probiotic effects. Microb. Ecol. Health Dis. 2008, 20, 1651–2235.

43. Yao, T.C.; Chang, C.J.; Hsu, Y.H.; Huang, J.L. Probiotics for allergic diseases: Realities and myths.Pediatr. Allergy Immunol. 2009. [Epub ahead of print].

44. Kalliomaki, M.; Antoine, J.M.; Herz, U.; Rijkers, G.T.; Wells, J.M.; Mercenier, A. Guidance for substantiating the evidence for beneficial effects of probiotics: prevention and management of allergic diseases by probiotics. J. Nutr. 2010, 140, 713S–721S.

45. Kumar, M.; Kumar, A.; Nagpal, R.; Mohania, D.; Behare, P.; Verma, V.; Kumar, P.; Poddar, D.; Aggarwal, P.K.; Henry, C.J.; Jain, S.; Yadav, H. Cancer-preventing attributes of probiotics: an update.Int. J. Food. Sci. Nutr. 2010. [Epub ahead of print].

46. Trois, L.; Cardoso, E.M.; Miura, E. Use of probiotics in HIV-infected children: a randomized double-blind controlled study. J. Trop. Pediatr. 2008, 54, 19–24.

47. Kaur, I.P.; Kuhad, A.; Garg, A.; Chopra, K. Probiotics: delineation of prophylactic and therapeutic benefits. J. Med. Food. 2009, 12, 219–235.

48. Douglas, L.C.; Sanders, M.E. Probiotics and prebiotics in dietetics practice. J. Am. Diet. Assoc. 2008,108, 510–521.

49. Hedin, C.; Whelan, K.; Lindsay, J.O. Evidence for the use of probiotics and prebiotics in inflammatory bowel disease: a review of clinical trials. Proc. Nutr. Soc. 2007, 66, 307–315.

50. Oelschlaeger, T.A. Mechanisms of probiotic actions -A review. Int. J. Med. Microbiol. 2010, 300, 57–62.

51. O'Sullivan, G.C.; Kelly, P.; O'Halloran, S.; Collins, C.; Collins, J.K.; Dunne, C.; Shanahan, F. Probiotics: An Emerging Therapy. Curr. Pharm. Design 2005, 11, 3–10.

52. Dunne, C.; O'Mahony, L.; Murphy, L.; Thornton, G.; Morrissey, D.; O'Halloran, S.; Feeney, M.; Flynn, S.; Fitzgerald, G.; Daly, C.; Kiely, B.; O'Sullivan, G.C.; Shanahan, F.; Collins, J.K. In vitro selection criteria for probiotic bacteria of human origin: correlation with in vivo findings. Am. J. Clin. Nutr. 2001,73, 386S–392S.

53. Brower, V. Nutraceuticals: poised for a healthy slice of the healthcare market? Nat. Biotechnol. 1998, 16, 728–731.

54. Trottier, G.; Bostrom, P.J.; Lawrentschuk, N.; Fleshner, N.E. Nutraceuticals and prostate cancer prevention: a current review. Nat. Rev. Urol. 2010, 7, 21–30.

55. Zeisel, S.H. Regulation of "Nutraceuticals". Science 1999, 285, 185–186.

56. Kalra, E.K. Nutraceutical -Definition and Introduction. AAPS PharmSci. 2003, 5, p. 25. Available online:http://www.aapsj.org/view.asp?art=ps050325 (accessed on 25 February 2010).

57. The Regulation of Dietary Supplements. United States Pharmacopeia (USP), 2006. Available online: http://www.usp.org/pdf/EN/USPVerified/dietarySupplementRegulation.pdf (accessed on 13 January 2010).

58. Hasler, C.M. Functional Foods: Their role in disease prevention and health promotion, Institute of Food Technologists' Expert Panel on Food Safety and Nutrition. Foodtechnology. 1998, 52, 63–70.

59. Gaffe, R. The Current and Future Regulation of Dietary Supplements. 2010. Available online: http://www.richardjaffeesq.com/jaffe/dietarysupplements.asp (accessed on 25 February 2010).

60. Biddle, J.; Dasgupta-O'Brien, S.; Walch, A. Gut Health, Asheville Integrative Medicine (undated). Available online: http://www.docbiddle.com/moreinfo/guthealth.pdf (accessed on 25 February 2010).

61. Mangum, J.B.; Everitt, J.I.; Bonner, J.C.; Moore, L.R.; Brody, A.R. Co-culture of primary pulmonary cells to model alveolar injury and translocation of proteins. In Vitro Cell. Dev. Biol. 1990, 26, 1135–1143.

62. Arnold, J.T.; Kaufman, D.G.; Seppala, M.; Lessey, B.A. Endometrial stromal cells regulate epithelial cell growth in vitro: a new co-culture model. Hum. Reprod. 2001, 16, 836–845.

63. Willemsen, L.E.; Schreurs, C.C.; Kroes, H.; Spillenaar Bilgen, E.J.; Van Deventer, S.J.; Van Tol, E.A. A co-culture model mimicking the intestinal mucosa reveals a regulatory role for myofibroblasts in immune-mediated barrier disruption. Dig. Dis. Sci. 2002, 47, 2316–2324.

64. Depasquale, I.; Wheatley, D.N. Action of Lovastatin (Mevinolin) on an in vitro model of angiogenesis and its co-culture with

malignant melanoma cell lines. Cancer Cell Int. 2006, 6, 1475–2867.

65. Hendriks, J.; Riesle, J.; van Blitterswijk, C.A. Co-culture in cartilage tissue engineering. J. Tissue Eng. Regen. Med. 2007, 1, 170–178.

66. Bhatia, S.N.; Balis, U.J.; Yarmush, M.L.; Toner, M. Effect of cell-cell interactions in preservation of cellular phenotype: cocultivation of hepatocytes and nonparenchymal cells. The FASEB J. 1999, 13, 1883–1900.

67. Brillet, B.; Petiot, S.; Iochmann, S.; Gaud, G.; Planque, C.; Blechet, C.; Heuze-Vourc'h, N.; Gruel, Y.; Courty, Y.; Reverdiau, P. 025 Tumor-stromal cell interactions modulate metalloproteinase and kalli Krein expression in direct and indirect co-culture cell models. Revue des Maladies Respiratoires 2008, 25, 1167, (translated).

68. Gradisnik, L.; Filipic, B.; de Vaureix, C.; Lefevre, F.; La Bonnardiere, C.; Cencic, A. Establishment of a functional cell culture model of the pig small intestine, LINZ, ALTEX 23. ALTEX Altern. Tierexp. 2006,23, 94.

4

SUPRAPHYSIOLOGICAL LEVELS OF QUERCETIN GLYCOSIDES ARE REQUIRED TO ALTER MINERALIZATION IN SAOS2 CELLS

Leslie A. Nash [1,2], Sandra J. Peters [2,3,†], Philip J. Sullivan [3,†] and Wendy E. Ward [1,2,3,]

[1]Department of Health Sciences, Faculty of Applied Health Sciences, Brock University, 1812 Sir Isaac Brock Way, St. Catharines, ON L2S 3A1, Canada

[2]Centre for Bone and Muscle Health, Brock University, 1812 Sir Isaac Brock Way, St. Catharines, ON L2S 3A1, Canada

[3]Department of Kinesiology, Faculty of Applied Health Sciences, Brock University, 1812 Sir Isaac Brock Way, St. Catharines, ON L2S 3A1, Canada

ABSTRACT

Flavonoid intake is positively correlated to bone mineral density (BMD) in women. Flavonoids such as quercetin exhibit strong anti-oxidant and anti-inflammatory activity that may be beneficial for bone health. Quercetin, previously shown to positively influence osteoblasts, is metabolized into glycosides including rutin and hyperoside. We compared the effects of these glycosides on mineralization in human osteoblast (Saos2) cells. Administration of rutin (≥25 μM) and hyperoside (≥5 μM) resulted in higher mineral content, determined using the alizarin red assay. This was accompanied by higher alkaline phosphatase activity with no cell toxicity. The expression of osteopontin, sclerostin, TNFα and IL6, known stimuli for decreasing osteoblast activity, were reduced with the addition of rutin or hyperoside. In summary, rutin and hyperoside require supraphysiological levels, when administered individually, to positively influence osteoblast activity. This information may be useful in developing nutraceuticals to support bone health.

Keywords: flavonoids; hyperoside; mineral; rutin; osteoblasts; tea

1. INTRODUCTION

Osteoporosis is defined by low BMD [1], a high risk of fragility fracture [2] and diminished quality of life [3]. Dietary strategies may help prevent osteoporosis by supporting peak bone mass as well as the maintenance of healthy bone after the growth period [4,5,6]. Flavonoids present in food and beverages such as tea [7], are emerging as potential bioactives for bone health [8]. Many studies show a positive association between flavonoid intake or habitual tea consumption and BMD in women [7,9,10,11,12,13,14]. One study showed an inverse association between flavonoid intake and a bone resorption marker [7] while most studies have not investigated whether bone formation, resorption or both are associated with habitual tea consumption and BMD.

Flavonoids have a wide-range of biological effects due to anti-oxidant [15] and anti-bacterial properties [16] and may thereby benefit bone health [17,18]. Rutin (quercetin-3-*O*-rutinoside) and hyperoside (quercetin-3-*O*-galactoside) are flavonoids found in green [19], black [19] and rooibos tea [20] and other foods [21,22,23]. They are also derivatives from quercetin, another flavonoid found in a variety of food and beverages [24]. Quercetin increases alkaline phosphatase activity (ALP) in mouse osteoblasts [25], and BMD at the lumbar spine and femur in ovariectomized mice [26]. Derivatives of quercetin (quercetin-6-C-β-D-glucopyranoside) have been shown to increase ALP and mineral formation *in vitro*, and BMD in female rats [27]. Hyperoside was recently shown to promote differentiation in U2O2 and MG63 cells without promoting cellular death [28].

A few studies have shown that rutin and hyperoside stimulate osteoblast activity [28,29] but no study has directly compared the effects of these main metabolites of quercetin within the same model. The objective of this research was to identify and compare, in the same model using a wide range of concentrations, if the addition of rutin or hyperoside, results in greater mineral content in Saos2 cells. Structure-function relationships between these two flavonoids were also assessed.

2. MATERIALS AND METHODS

Saos2 cells [30] were purchased from Cedarlane (Supplier ATCC, Burlington, ON, Canada). HAM-F12, 10× Trypsin, PBS, fetal bovine serum (FBS), antibiotic-antimycotic and flasks were purchased from Lonza (Mississauga, ON, Canada). Rutin trihydrate (≥97%) and 3-(4,5-dimethy-2-lthiazolyl)-2,5-diphenyl-2H-tetrazolium bromide were purchased from Alfa Aesar (Reston, VA, USA) and hyperoside (≥98%) from Aktin Chemicals (Sichuan, China). Human Milliplex bone magnetic bead panels for bone metabolism were purchased from EMD Millipore (Billerica, MA, USA) and read by xPONENT software on Magpix Luminex (Austin, TX, USA). Optical density (OD) measurements were analyzed using a BIO-TEK Synergy HT Multi-Detection Microplate Reader (Winooski, VT, USA). Other chemicals were purchased from Sigma-Aldrich (Oakville, ON, USA).

Cells were maintained and differentiated as previously described [31]. Following one week of differentiation in plates, differentiation cell media was supplemented with 0.01 M β-glycerophosphate (day 8) until day 21 (Media 3) in addition to either vehicle (0.1% DMSO) or flavonoid dissolved in DMSO to 0.1%.

For all experiments, a DMSO control was compared to flavonoid treated cells. All experiments were normalized to cell count using Trypan Blue staining.

2.1. Mineral Content

Mineral content was quantitatively assessed using the alizarin red assay [31]. Cells plated at 5 × 10^3cells/well in 24 well plates. On day 21 cells were fixed in 4% paraformaldehyde and kept at 4 °C for 24 h. Following, cells were washed with PBS and replaced with 0.04 M alizarin red S stain for 20 min on a plate shaker at room temperature. Cells were washed with PBS. Extraction required the addition of a 10% cetylpyridinium chloride solution for 1 h at room temperature. Mineral was quantified by measuring OD at 550 nm.

2.2. ALP Activity

Cells were grown in 12 well plates at 1 × 10^4 cells/well and lysed by mechanically homogenizing cells using ice cold 0.05% Triton X-100 solution dissolved in 0.05 M Tris-HCl. Cells were centrifuged at 10,000 rpm at 4 °C for 10 min. Cell lysates were introduced to p-nitrophenyl phosphate. P-nitrophenol production was monitored over 5 min and was stopped by the addition of 0.5 M NaOH. The OD was measured at 410 nm and normalized to protein concentration using the Bradford assay [32,33]. Cells were tested on days 3 (day 11), 7 (day 15) and 10 (day 18) after the addition of Media 3 and flavonoid.

2.3. Cell Activity

Mitochondrial reductase activity was measured by the reduction of 3-(4,5-dimethyl-2-thiazolyl)-2,5-diphenyl-2H-tetrazolium bromide (MTT). Cells were plated in 96 well plates at 1 × 10^4 cells/well, and allowed to adhere over 24 h. Media was replaced every 24 h. MTT reduction was measured at 24, 48, and 72 h following the addition of the flavonoid. Cells were washed three times with PBS and then supplemented with media sans flavonoid, with 5 mg/mL MTT for 4 h. Media was removed and crystals were dissolved in 0.04 M HCl-isopropanol. OD was taken at 570 nm with a reference measurement at 610 nm.

2.4. Cell Toxicity

Lactate dehydrogenase (LDH) was measured in cell media to quantify cell death. Cells were plated following the MTT protocol. LDH was measured by an *in vitro* toxicology assay kit from Sigma-Aldrich (Catalogue ID: Tox7). Media with flavonoid was replaced every 24 h and cells were harvested at 12, 24 and 48 h to be analyzed by Tox7 kits.

2.5. Osteoblast Regulatory Proteins

Levels were chosen based on their ability to promote significant mineralization without inducing toxicity. Cells were plated at 500,000 cells in 75 cm^2 flasks and allowed to adhere for 24 h. The addition of media 2 and media 3 followed differentiation guidelines indicated above. When the media was changed to media 3 (day 8), it was accompanied with the addition of vehicle (DMSO) or flavonoid. The cells, once exposed to media 3, were left for 3 days prior to media extraction (day 11). Media was examined early into mineralization to identify immediate changes in protein markers for osteoblast activity. Extraction of media at this time point, correlates with results obtained for ALP (day 3 into mineralization or day 11 total). All protein levels, OPG, OPN, SOST, IL6, TNFα were determined from a standard curve created with purified protein dissolved in media 3, using the ELISA reader. Cell media was analyzed using a commercial ELISA based assay for TNFα, IL6, SOST, OPG and OPN (Millipore, HBNMAG-51K, Billerica, MA, USA). Media was chosen to analyze as opposed to cell lysates to mimic the clinical scenario in which bone markers released into circulation are measured. Treated media was compared to cells exposed to vehicle (0.1% DMSO). In addition, media was added to each well within the ELISA to account for any background noise.

2.6. Statistics

Measurements of mineral content consisted of $n = 6$, with each sample corresponding to a separate experiment of three wells averaged together. Measurements for ALP, MTT and LDH consisted of $n = 6$ per time point, with each sample measured in triplicate. Protein measurements were completed using $n = 4$, with each sample measured in triplicate. Measurements are reported as an average ± SEM.

Statistical analyses were performed using IBM SPSS Statistics 21, utilizing 1 way-ANOVA with vehicle (rutin, hyperoside, or DMSO control) as the independent variable (IV). The dependent variable (DV) was expressed as per cent DMSO control and was a function of mineral, ALP activity, MTT reduced, LDH released or concentration of protein. If the 1 way-ANOVA was statistically significant ($p < 0.05$), *post-HOC*analysis was used to identify differences across groups ($p < 0.05$). Data was checked for homogeneity of variance. When homogeneity of variance was not statistically different ($p > 0.05$), *post-HOC* analysis utilized Bonferroni *t*-test. Where homogeneity of variance was statistically different across groups ($p < 0.05$), Games Howell *t*-test was utilized.

3. RESULTS

3.1. Mineral Content

Rutin (25 μM, 50 μM and 100 μM) resulted in higher mineral content ($p < 0.05$, $p < 0.001$, $p < 0.01$, respectively) compared to control (Figure 1). Hyperoside resulted in significantly higher mineral content at lower doses (5 μM through 100 μM, $p < 0.001$) compared to control.

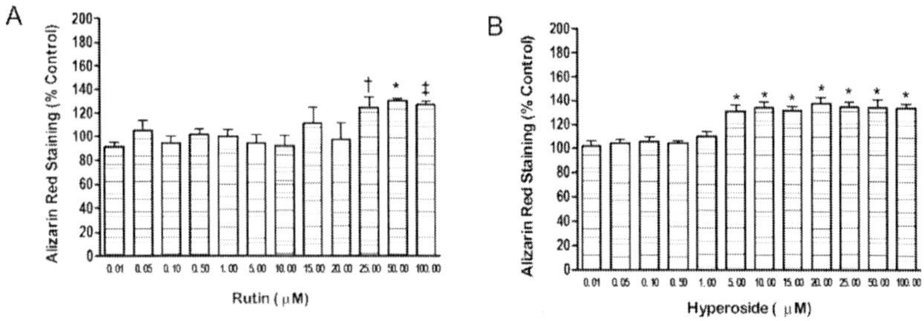

Figure 1. Mineral content produced by addition of (**A**) rutin or (**B**) hyperoside. Mineral content was measured by alizarin red staining. Significant differences are indicated by: † $p < 0.05$, ‡ $p < 0.01$, * $p < 0.001$ compared to control. Each bar represents $n = 6$.

3.2. ALP Activity

Two doses in which rutin or hyperoside resulted in higher mineral content were chosen along with one dose that did not (served as a negative control, Figure 2). Rutin (25 μM, 50 μM) resulted in higher ALP activity than control at day 3 ($p < 0.01$, $p < 0.01$, respectively), day 7 ($p < 0.01$, $p < 0.01$, respectively) and day 10 ($p < 0.01$, $p < 0.05$, respectively). Exposure to hyperoside (5 μM, 25 μM) resulted in higher ALP activity than control at day 3 ($p < 0.01$, $p < 0.05$, respectively), day 7 ($p < 0.05$, $p < 0.05$, respectively) and day 10 ($p < 0.05$, $p < 0.05$, respectively).

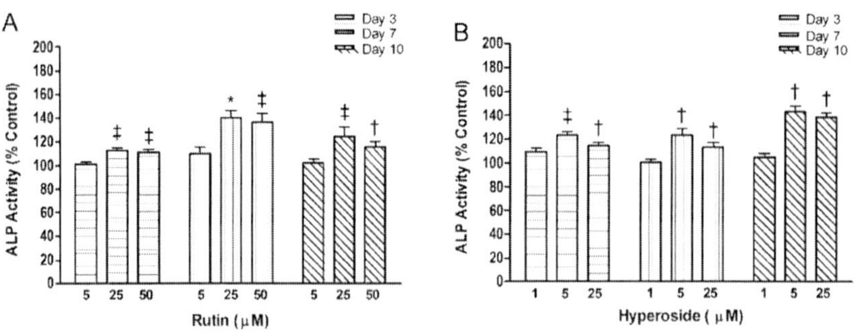

Figure 2. Alkaline phosphatase activity (ALP) activity with addition of (**A**) rutin or (**B**) hyperoside. Activity was measured by the rate of hydrolysis of p-nitrophenyl phosphate. Significant differences are indicated by: † $p < 0.05$, ‡ $p < 0.01$, * $p < 0.001$ compared to control within a day. Each bar represents $n = 6$.

3.3. Cell Mitochondrial Activity

Rutin (25 µM, 50 µM) increased mitochondrial activity after 48 h ($p < 0.05$, $p < 0.05$, respectively) and 72 h ($p < 0.01$, $p < 0.05$, respectively) compared to control (Figure 3). At 24 h, hyperoside (5.0 µM, 25.0 µM) increased mitochondrial activity ($p < 0.05$, $p < 0.05$, respectively) compared to control and was maintained for 48 h ($p < 0.01$, $p < 0.05$, respectively) and 72 h ($p < 0.01$, $p < 0.05$, respectively).

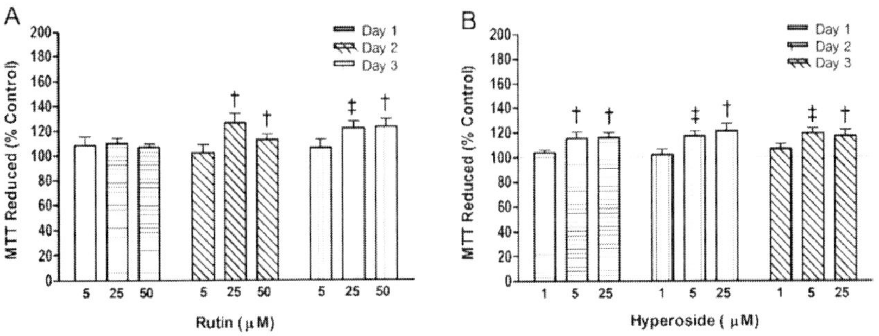

Figure 3. 3-(4,5-dimethyl-2-thiazolyl)-2,5-diphenyl-2H-tetrazolium bromide (MTT) levels reduced with addition of (**A**) rutin or (**B**) hyperoside. Activity was measured by the reduction of MTT. Significant differences are indicated by: † $p < 0.05$ and ‡ $p < 0.01$ compared to control within a day. Each bar represents $n = 6$.

3.4. Cell Toxicity

After 12 h of the initial flavonoid addition, rutin (25.0 µM or 50.0 µM) resulted in lower levels of LDH ($p < 0.05$, $p < 0.05$, respectively) compared to control (Figure 4), and was maintained at 24 h ($p < 0.05$, $p < 0.05$, respectively) and 48 h ($p < 0.001$, $p < 0.05$, respectively). Hyperoside did not alter LDH levels after 12 and 24 h of supplementation. After 48 h, hyperoside (5.0 µM, 25.0 µM) demonstrated lower LDH levels ($p < 0.05$, $p < 0.001$, respectively) than control.

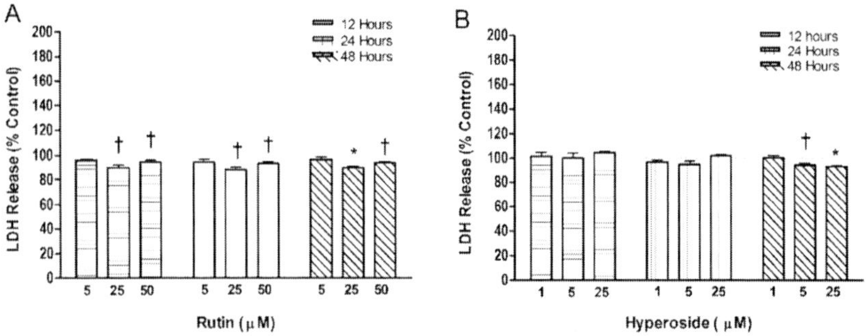

Figure 4. Lactate dehydrogenase (LDH) release by addition of (**A**) rutin or (**B**) hyperoside. LDH activity was measured by the reduction of NAD^+ to aid in the conversion of a tetrazolium dye to a formazan crystal. Significant differences are indicated by: † $p < 0.05$, and * $p < 0.001$ compared to control within a day. Each bar represents $n = 6$.

3.5. Quantification of Regulatory Proteins in Osteoblasts

Rutin and hyperoside resulted in lower levels of TNFα ($p < 0.001$, $p < 0.001$), IL6 ($p < 0.001$, $p < 0.001$), OPN ($p < 0.001$, $p < 0.001$), OPG ($p < 0.01$, $p < 0.01$), and SOST ($p < 0.001$, $p < 0.001$) than control. Direct comparison of rutin (50 μM) and hyperoside (25 μM) showed that rutin resulted in a greater reduction in TNFα ($p = 0.035$), IL6 ($p < 0.002$) and OPG ($p < 0.001$) compared to hyperoside. Normalizing the protein data to the amount of flavonoid added (per mol) using Equation (1) showed that hyperoside induced greater changes than rutin on a per mol basis (see Table 1).

$$|(\text{ProteinFlavonoid} - \text{ProteinControl})/(\text{molesFlavonoid})| \quad (1)$$

Table 1. Concentration of regulatory proteins involved in osteoblast activity.

Condition	TNFα	IL6	OPN	OPG	SOST
Control (pg/mL)	0.43 ± 0.01	3.24 ± 0.08	247.50 ± 10.71	1659.25 ± 107.78	810.00 ± 22.15
50 μM Rutin (pg/mL)	0.20 ± 0.02 ^{a,*}	1.36 ± 0.09 ^{a,*}	126.21 ± 10.78 *	431.25 ± 11.37 ^{a,‡}	572.00 ± 19.07 *
Rutin (pg/mL/mol) #	−46	−376	−24,258	−245,600	−47,600
25 μM Hyperoside(pg/mL)	0.25 ± 0.01 ^{b,*}	1.90 ± 0.06 ^{b,*}	145.75 ± 2.75 *	709.25 ± 25.28 ^{b,‡}	542.75 ± 10.01 *
Hyperoside pg/mL/mol #	−72	−536	−40,700	−380,000	−106,900

Data are expressed as mean ± SEM, $n = 4$; Significant differences in values, from control, are indicated by: ‡ $p < 0.01$ and * $p < 0.001$ within a column. Significant differences ($p < 0.05$) between rutin and hyperoside are indicated by [a] *vs.* [b] within a column. # The ability for a mol of flavonoid to change the expression of protein relative to DMSO control.

4. DISCUSSION

This study, the first to directly compare effects of two different glycosides of quercetin in a bone cell model, has shown that rutin (25–100 μM) and hyperoside (5–100 μM) stimulate a higher mineral content that is accompanied by higher alkaline phosphatase activity and cell mitochondrial activity with no cell toxicity. Moreover, expression of OPN, SOST, TNFα and IL6, known stimuli for decreasing osteoblast activity, were reduced with the addition of rutin or hyperoside. Of note is that basal levels of TNFα and IL6 were likely elevated because the Saos2 cell line is cancerous whereas unstimulated osteoblasts may have lower levels of these cytokines that may remain unchanged with the intervention. While rutin and hyperoside have not been previously studied in human Saos2 cells, in agreement with our findings, rutin has been shown to enhance mitochondrial activity in mouse bone marrow mesenchymal stem cells [29]. Similarly, hyperoside has been shown to increase ALP activity in a rat osteosarcoma cell line but mineral was not measured [34].

The down-regulation of TNFα and IL6 by rutin and hyperoside is important as high oxidative stress can inhibit differentiation and activity of osteoblasts and increase osteoclast activity [35,36] and such effects can be inhibited with pretreatment with antioxidants [37]. We also showed that OPG expression was altered by rutin and hyperoside. While OPG does not directly change osteoblast behavior and thus mineral formation, it is involved in bone turnover in the presence of osteoclasts. Specifically, it is the ratio of RANKL to OPG that determines osteoclastogenic potential, and since RANKL was not measured in this study, the effect of this ratio should be evaluated in a future study. Wnt3 inhibitors (DKK-1 and -2) reduce OPG expression in osteoblasts [38] and the production of the Wnt inhibitor SOST would lead to an increase in OPG levels. However, the addition of rutin and hyperoside resulted in lower levels of OPG. This may be an artifact of the Saos2 cell line as it is a cancerous cell line and high OPG levels are a marker for cancer. OPG acts as a decoy ligand for tumor necrosis factor related apoptosis ligand (TRAIL) [39] that is primarily in cancerous cells and stimulates apoptosis [39]. Also, it was previously shown that rutin (≥50 μM) increases OPG in mouse osteoblasts [29] Therefore, the difference seen between these two studies may be due to differences in OPG machinery found within the particular cell line. High OPG levels in a human osteosarcoma cell line are positively correlated with TNFα [40] and suggest that inflammatory cytokines may aid in tumor proliferation by stimulating the production of OPG. As the addition of rutin and hyperoside reduced both TNFα and IL6, and previous work has shown that levels of TNFα are related to levels of OPG in cancer [40], OPG may have decreased as a result of lower levels of TNFα and IL6.

OPN and SOST are markers of mineral inhibition. OPN is predominately recognized as an inhibitor for mineralization [41,42,43]. OPN knock-out mice have favorable bone outcomes: reduced osteoclast motility and bone resorption as well as higher trabecular bone area, and trabecular thickness with less trabecular spacing [44]. SOST inhibits the Wnt pathway and regulates bone formation [45]. Our study is the first to show that rutin and hyperoside down-regulate Wnt inhibitors in osteoblasts. Previous work in mouse osteoblasts has shown that the addition of rutin (≥25 μM) increased transcriptional levels of OPN [29] however protein levels were not measured. Another study demonstrated that carnosol from rosemary reduced OPN and IL6 in osteoblasts [46]. While our data demonstrates changes to osteoblast and inflammatory markers early into the mineralization phase, future work should examine changes in protein expression of these markers over differentiation, early mineralization and during the final end point. Establishment of these parameters at various time points would help determine whether greater or lower protein expression is transient, or whether changes occur with alterations in dose and/or time. The Saos2 cell line has been documented as an osteoblast line that mimics primary cells very closely [47,48]. However, comparison of data from this and other commonly used cancerous osteoblast cell lines (U2OS, UMR106, UMR, ROS, MG63) to primary cell lines is also necessary to determine key differences in bone metabolic markers after addition of bioactives.

A study using ovariectomized rats showed preservation of BMD in both total and distal femur with a diet of 0.25% rutin [49]. Higher femur peak load and a reduction in deoxypyridinoline, a marker of bone resorption was also observed [49]. However, ingestion of rutin leads to a variety of metabolites that may produce these biological effects, in which the authors identified quercetin and isorhamnetin in the low micromolar range [49]. Rutin has also been detected in human plasma after consuming tea [50] and pure rutin tablets [51] from low to high nM range. In contrast, hyperoside was not detectable in plasma after consumption of tea [50] but was detected in rat plasma in a dose-dependent manner after consumption of hyperoside tablets, but was quickly cleared by the hepatic system [52]. Hyperoside may therefore be a good candidate for encapsulation or chemical enhancement to improve its bioavailability. The bioavailability of rutin can be improved by conjugating it to 2-hydroxy-propyl-β-cyclodextrinin [53]. Bioavailability can also be improved by the presence of other bioactives that alters solubility and stability prior to absorption. Bioavailability of hypericin increases by 34% in the presence of hyperoside [54]. The mid to high micromolar ranges of these compounds, needed for biological effects, are not achieved through consumption of food and beverage. Thus, these results suggest studying the combination of flavonoids as opposed to individual flavonoids, as interactions of flavonoids with other flavonoids or food components may contribute to greater bioavailability.

As the addition of rutin or hyperoside led to an overall increase in mineral production, a dose-dependent effect was not observed. This may suggest that the individual flavonoids do not directly impact mineralization through binding to receptors, but instead act indirectly by providing osteoblasts with a more stable, enriched environment for mineralization to occur, by limiting pro-inflammatory cytokines that are known to be harmful to the mineralization process. Therefore, instead of a dose-response, a threshold of antioxidant activity must be reached to identify any benefit. This finding requires investigation in future studies.

Effective flavonoid concentrations may vary due to structure-function relationships. Rutin has greater hydrophobicity that modulates interactions at water-lipid interfaces and its ability to act as an antioxidant [55]. Quercetin [56,57] and rutin [57] have been shown to have high antioxidant potential. While we did not directly measure the antioxidant activity of rutin in our system, we indirectly showed this through down regulation of pro-inflammatory markers, TNFα and IL6. The C3 hydroxyl on the flavonoid backbone largely contributes to the antioxidant activity because of its close proximity to the 4C keto and the conjugated 2-3C leading to the aromatic B ring—this helps stabilize free radicals [58]. The loss of this C4 hydroxyl, due to the addition of sugars, results in significantly lower antioxidant capacity [56]. The addition of two sugars (*i.e.*, rutin) creates steric hindrance, further impacting the antioxidant capacity. The antioxidant capacity of quercetin is stronger than its glycosides [56,57]. The substitution of sugars at the C3 position (*i.e.*, rutin) in comparison to their aglycone (quercetin) with a hydroxyl group at that position, inhibited superoxide radical scavenging activity of flavonoids [59]. However, this free hydroxyl located on C3 can allow for quercetin to undergo auto-oxidation. Thus, quercetin can have pro-oxidant activity by increasing the levels of superoxide radicals and hydrogen peroxide within a local environment. Yet because of the disaccharide on C3 of rutin, it maintains potent antioxidant activity without acting as a pro-oxidant. This disaccharide also increases the hydrophobicity of rutin, allowing for easier uptake into membranes [59].

Isoquercetin is another glycoside of quercetin and has been shown to be toxic at levels as low as 10 μM in Saos2 cells [60]. Hyperoside and isoquercetin are epimers; the hydroxyl on the 4th carbon of the sugar ring is pointed in a different direction, thereby making them diastereomers. This difference results in a change in activity, and increases toxicity. The glucose ring of hyperoside may shield the C4 keto group on the flavonoid backbone, allowing a hydrogen bonding opportunity between the C4 hydroxyl on the galactoside and the keto group on the backbone. In contrast, the glucose of isoquercetin has its ring pointed away, leaving the C4 keto group open. This keto group is likely a key structure for pro-oxidant activity as it has the potential to create quinone, capable of generating reactive oxygen species [61]. This production of reactive oxygen species was identified with quercetin but failed to occur with rutin [62]. Flavonoids that are too strong of an antioxidant can have pro-oxidant activities. The position of a glycoside on the flavonoid can result in cellular death.

5. CONCLUSIONS

In closing, the levels of rutin and hyperoside required to enhance mineralization are greater than those present naturally in food, and the differing effects of these two metabolites highlight the need to consider whether it is provided in isolation or within a food source. Moreover, identification of key structural changes that lead to positive effects in osteoblast physiology may aid in the development of nutraceuticals that target bone. Future study in primary osteoblasts is warranted because Saos2 cells are derived from a primary osteosarcoma and may have genetic and epigenetic modifications that could alter their biology.

ACKNOWLEDGMENTS

We would like to acknowledge funding for the project provided to Wendy E. Ward through her NSERC Discovery Grant and to the funding provided to Leslie A. Nash through the Alexander Graham Bell Canadian Graduate Scholarship. Wendy E. Ward holds a Canada Research Chair in Bone and Muscle Development. The authors thank Leticia Rao for providing us with the Saos2 cell culture protocols.

AUTHOR CONTRIBUTIONS

Leslie A. Nash: designed and executed the study and wrote the manuscript. Sandra J. Peters: gave input into study design, reviewed and critiqued manuscript. Philip J. Sullivan: helped with the statistical analysis in the study design, reviewed and critiqued manuscript. Wendy E. Ward: conceived and funded the idea through her NSERC Discovery Grant, supervised the work and reviewed and edited the manuscript.

CONFLICTS OF INTEREST

The funding sponsors had no role in the design of the study, in the collection, analyses, or interpretation of data, in the writing of the manuscript, and in the decision to publish the results.

REFERENCES

1. National Osteoporosis Foundation (2014) Clinician's Guide to Prevention and Treatment of Osteoporosis; National Osteoporosis Foundation: Washington, DC, USA.
2. Bliuc, D.; Nguyen, N.D.; Nguyen, T.V.; Eisman, J.A.; Center, J.R. Compound risk of high mortality following osteoporotic fracture and refracture in elderly women and men. J. Bone Miner Res. 2013, 28, 2317–2324.
3. Dempster, D.W. Osteoporosis and burden of osteoporosis-related fractures. Am. J. Manag. Care 2011,17, S164–S169.
4. Lehtonen-Veromaa, M.; Mottonen, T.T.; Nuotio, I.; Irjala, K.M.; Leino, A.E.; Viikari, J.S. Vitamin D and attainment of peak bone mass among peripubertal Finnish girls: A 3-y prospective study. Am. J. Clin. Nutr. 2002, 76, 1446–1453.
5. Matkovic, V. Calcium and peak bone mass. J. Intern. Med. 1992, 231, 151–160.
6. Ward, W.E. Prevention of bone fragility: The role of diet. Int. J. Clin. Rheumatol. 2009, 4, 311–319.
7. Hardcastle, A.C.; Aucott, L.; Reid, D.M.; Macdonald, H.M. Associations between dietary flavonoid intakes and bone health in a Scottish population. J. Bone Miner. Res. 2011, 26, 941–947.

8. Nash, L.A.; Ward, W.E. Tea and bone health: Findings from human studies, potential mechanisms, and identification of knowledge gaps. Crit. Rev. Food Sci. 2015. in press.

9. Welch, A.; MacGregor, A.; Jennings, A.; Fairweather-Tait, S.; Spector, T.; Cassidy, A. Habitual flavonoid intakes are positively associated with bone mineral density in women. J. Bone Miner Res.2012, 27, 1872–1878.

10. Zhang, Z.Q.; He, L.P.; Liu, Y.H.; Liu, J.; Su, Y.X.; Chen, Y.M. Association between dietary intake of flavonoid and bone mineral density in middle aged and elderly Chinese women and men. Osteoporosis Int. 2014, 25, 2417–2425.

11. Devine, A.; Hodgson, J.A.; Dick, A.M.; Prince, R.L. Tea drinking is associated with benefits on bone density in older women. Am. J. Clin. Nutr. 2007, 86, 1243–1247.

12. Hoover, P.A.; Webber, C.E.; Beaumont, L.F.; Blake, J.M. Postmenopausal bone mineral density: Relationship to calcium intake, calcium absorption, residual estrogen, body composition and physical activity. Can. J. Physiol. Pharmacol. 1996, 74, 911–917.

13. Chen, Z.; Pettinger, M.B.; Ritenbaugh, C.; LaCroix, A.Z.; Robbins, J.; Caan, B.J.; Barad, D.H.; Hakim, I.A. Habitual tea consumption and risk of osteoporosis: A prospective study in the Women's Health Initiative observational cohort. Am. J. Epidemiol. 2003, 158, 772–781.

14. Myers, G.; Prince, R.L.; Kerr, D.A.; Devine, A.; Woodman, R.J.; Lewis, J.R.; Hodgson, J.M. Tea and flavonoid intake predict osteoporotic fracture risk in elderly Australian women: A prospective study.Am. J. Clin. Nutr. 2015, 102, 958–962.

15. Lee, K.W.; Lee, H.J.; Lee, C.Y. Antioxidant activity of black tea vs. green tea. J. Nutr. 2002, 132, 785.

16. Friedman, M. Overview of antibacterial, antitoxin, antiviral, and antifungal activities of tea flavonoids and teas. Mol. Nutr. Food Res. 2007, 51, 116–134.

17. Bertolini, D.R.; Nedwin, G.E.; Bringman, T.S.; Smith, D.D.; Mundy, G.R. Stimulation of bone resorption and inhibition of bone formation in vitro by human tumor necrosis factors. Nature 1986,319, 516–518.

18. Manolagas, S.C. Role of cytokines in bone resorption. Bone 1995, 17, S63–S67.

19. Stewart, A.J.; Mullen, W.; Crozier, A. On-line high-performance liquid chromatography analysis of the antioxidant activity of phenolic compounds in green and black tea. Mol. Nutr. Food Res. 2005, 49, 52–60.

20. Bramati, L.; Minoggio, M.; Gardana, C.; Simonetti, P.; Mauri, P.; Pietta, P. Quantitative characterization of flavonoid compounds in rooibos tea (Aspalathus linearis) by LC-UV/DAD. J. Agric. Food Chem. 2002, 50, 5513–5519.

21. Sun, J.; Feng, L.; Bin, Y.; Li, P.; Duan, C. Screening non-colored phenolics in red wines using liquid chromatography/ultraviolet and mass spectrometry/mass spectrometry libraries. Molecules 2007, 12, 679–693.

22. Makris, D.P.; Rossiter, J.T. Domestic processing of onion bulbs (Allium cepa) and asparagus spears (Asparagus officinalis): Effect on flavonol content and antioxidant status. J. Agric. Food Chem. 2001, 49, 3216–3222.

23. Zheng, W.; Wang, S.Y. Oxygen radical absorbing capacity of polyphenols in blueberries, cranberries, chokeberries and lingonberries. J. Agric. Food Chem. 2003, 51, 502–509.

24. Formica, J.V.; Regelson, W. Review of the biology of quercetin and related bioflavonoids. Food Chem. Toxicol. 1995, 33, 1061–1080.

25. Wong, R.W.K.; Rabie, A.B.M. Effect of quercetin on preosteoblasts and bone defects. Open Orthop. J.2008, 2, 27–32.

26. Tsuji, M.; Yamamoto, H.; Sato, T.; Mizuha, Y.; Kawai, Y.; Taketani, Y.; Kato, S.; Terao, J.; Inakuma, T.; Takeda, E. Dietary quercetin inhibits bone loss without effect on the uterus in ovariectomized mice. J. Bone Miner. Metab. 2009, 27, 673–681.

27. Siddiqui, J.A.; Swarnkar, G.; Sharan, K.; Chakravarti, B.; Gautam, A.K.; Rawat, P.; Kumar, M.; Gupta, V.; Manickavasagam, L.; Dwivedi, A.K.; et al. A naturally occurring rare analog of quercetin promotes peak bone mass achievement and exerts anabolic effect on osteoporotic bone. Osteoporosis Int. 2011, 22, 3013–3027.

28. Zhang, N.; Ying, M.D.; Wu, Y.P.; Zhou, Z.H.; Ye, Z.M.; Li, H.; Lin, D.S. Hyperoside, a flavonoid compound, inhibits proliferation and stimulates osteogenic differentiation of human osteosarcoma cells. PLoS ONE 2014, 9, e98973.

29. Srivastava, S.; Bankar, R.; Roy, P. Assessment of the role of flavonoids for inducing osteoblast differentiation in isolated bone marrow derived mesenchymal stem cells. Phytomedicine 2013, 20, 683–690.

30. Fogh, J.; Trempe, G. New human tumor cell lines. In Human Tumor Cells in Vitro; Plenum Press: New York, NY, USA; London, UK, 1975; pp. 115–159.

31. Nash, L.A.; Sullivan, P.J.; Peters, S.J.; Ward, W.E. Rooibos flavonoids, orientin and luteolin, stimulate mineralization in human osteoblasts through the Wnt pathway. Mol. Nutr. Food. Res. 2015, 59, 443–453.

32. Rao, L.G.; Kung-Sutherland, M.S.; Muzaffar, S.A.; Wylie, J.N.; McBroom, R.J.; Murray, T.M. Positive interaction between 17 beta-estradiol and parathyroid hormone in normal human osteoblasts cultured long term in the presence of dexamethasone. Osteoporosis Int. 1996, 6, 111–119.

33. Bradford, M.M. Rapid and sensitive method for the quantitation of microgram quantities of protein utilizing the principle of protein-dye binding. Anal. Biochem. 1976, 72, 248–254.

34. Yang, L.; Chen, Q.; Wang, F.; Zhang, G. Antiosteoporotic compounds from seeds of Cuscuta chinensis.J. Ethnopharmacol. 2011, 135, 553–560.

35. Bai, X.C.; Lu, D.; Bai, J.; Zheng, H.; Ke, Z.Y.; Li, X.M.; Luo, S.Q. Oxidative stress inhibits osteoblastic differentiation of bone cells by ERK and NF-kappa-b. Biochem. Biophys. Res. Commun. 2004, 314, 197–207.

36. Grassi, F.; Tell, G.; Robbie-Ryan, M.; Gao, Y.; Terauchi, M.; Yang, X.; Romanello, M.; Jones, D.P.; Weitzmann, M.N.; Pacifici, R. Oxidative stress causes bone loss in estrogen-deficient mice through enhanced bone marrow dendritic cell activation. Proc. Natl. Acad. Sci. USA 2007, 104, 15087–15092.

37. Wang, Y.; Zhao, L.; Wang, Y.; Xu, J.; Nie, Y.; Guo, Y.; Tong, Y.; Qin, L.; Zhang, Q. Curculigoside isolated from Curculigo orchioides prevents hydrogen peroxide-induced dysfunction and oxidative damage in calvarial osteoblasts. Acta Biochim. Biophys. Sin. 2012, 44, 431–441.

38. Fujita, K.; Janz, S. Attenuation of WNT signaling by DKK-1 and -2 regulates BMP2-induced osteoblast differentiation and expression of OPG, RANKL and M-CSF. Mol. Cancer. 2007, 6, 71.

39. Wang, S.; El-Deiry, W.S. TRAIL and apoptosis induction by TNF-family death receptors. Oncogene2003, 22, 8628–8633.

40. Brandstrom, H.; Jonsson, K.B.; Vidal, O.; Ljunghall, S.; Ohlsson, C.; Vidal, O.; Ljunghall, S.; Ljunggren, O. Regulation of osteoprotegerin mRNA levels by prostaglandin E2 in human bone marrow stroma cells. Biochem. Biophys. Res. Commun. 1998, 248, 454–457.

41. Hunter, G.K.; Kyle, C.L.; Goldberg, H.A. Modulation of crystal growth formation by bone phosphoproteins: Structural specificity of the osteopontin-mediated inhibition of hydroxyapatite formation. Biochem. J. 1994, 300, 723–728.

42. De Bruyn, J.R.; Goiko, M.; Mozaffari, M.; Bator, D.; Dauphinee, R.L.; Liao, Y.; Flemming, R.L.; Bramble, M.S.; Hunter, G.K.; Goldberg, H.A. Dynamic light scattering study of inhibition of nucleation and growth of hydroxyapatite crystals by osteopontin. PLoS ONE 2013, 8, e56764.

43. Hunter, G.K. Role of osteopontin in modulation of hydroxyapatite formation. Calcif. Tissue Int. 2013,93, 348–354.

44. Chellaiah, M.A.; Kizer, N.; Biswas, R.; Alvarez, U.; Strauss-Schoenberger, J.; Rifas, L.; Rittling, S.R.; Denhardt, D.T.; Hruska, K.A. Osteopontin deficiency produces osteoclasts dysfunction due to reduced CD44 surface expression. Mol. Biol. Cell 2003, 14, 173–189.

45. Manolagas, S.C.; Almeida, M. Gone with the Wnts: Beta-catenin, T-cell factor, forkhead box o, and oxidative stress in age-dependent disease of bone, lipid, and glucose metabolism. Mol. Endocrinol.2007, 21, 2605–2614.

46. Horcajada, M.N.; Sanchez, C.; Scalfo, F.; Ameye, L.; Henrotin, Y.; Offord, E. Effect of rosemary extract and related flavonoid carnosol on chondro-protection and on the bone-cartilage crosstalk. Osteoarthr. Cartil. 2010, 18, S38–S39.

47. Prideaux, M.; Wijenayaka, A.R.; Kumarasinghe, D.D.; Ormsby, R.T.; Evdokiou, A.; Findlay, D.M.; Atkins, G.J. Saos2 osteosarcoma cells as an in vitro model for studying the transition of human osteoblasts to osteocytes. Calif. Tissue Int. 2014, 95, 183–193.

48. Czekanska, E.M.; Stoddart, M.J.; Richards, R.G.; Hayes, J.S. In search of an osteoblast cell model for in vitro research. Eur. Cell. Mater. 2012, 24, 1–17.

49. Horcajada-Molteni, M.N.; Crespy, V.; Coxam, V.; Davicco, M.J.; Remesy, C.; Barlet, J.P. Rutin inhibits ovariectomy-induced osteopenia in rats. J. Bone Miner Res. 2000, 15, 2251–2258.

50. Breiter, T.; Laue, C.; Kressel, G.; Groll, S.; Engelhardt, U.H.; Hahn, A. Bioavailability and antioxidant potential of rooibos flavonoids in humans following the consumption of different rooibos formulations. Food Chem. 2011, 128, 338–347.

51. Ishii, K.; Furuta, T.; Kasuya, Y. Determination of rutin in human plasma by high performance liquid chromatography utilizing solid-phase extraction and ultraviolet detection. J. Chromatogr. B.-Biomed. Sci. Appl. 2001, 759, 161–168.

52. Ying, X.; Meng, X.; Wang, S.; Wang, D.; Li, H.; Wang, B.; Du, Y.; Liu, X.; Zhang, W.; Kang, T. Simultaneous determination of three polyphenols in rat plasma after orally administering hawthorn leaves extract by the HPLC method. Nat. Prod. Res. 2012, 26, 585–591.

53. Miyake, K.; Arima, H.; Hirayama, F.; Yamamoto, M.; Horikawa, T.; Sumiyoshi, H.; Noda, S.; Uekama, K. Improvement of solubility and oral bioavailability of rutin by complexation with 2-hydroxypropyl-beta-cyclodextrin. Pharm. Dev. Technol. 2000, 5, 399–407.

54. Butterweck, V.; Lieflander-Wulf, U.; Winterhoff, H.; Nahrsedt, A. Plasma levels of hypericin in presence of procyanidin b2 and hyperoside: A pharmacokinetic study in rats. Planta Medica 2003, 69, 189–192.

55. Ross, A.A.; Kasum, C.M. Dietary flavonoids: Bioavailability, metabolic effects and safety. Annu. Rev. Nutr. 2002, 22, 19–34.

56. Ioku, K.; Tsushida, T.; Takei, Y.; Nakatani, N.; Terao, J. Antioxidant activity of quercetin and quercetin monoglucosides in solution and phospholipid bilayers. Biochim. Biophys. Acta 1995, 1234, 99–104.

57. Jo, S.; Ka, E.; Lee, H.; Apostolidis, E.; Jang, H.; Kwon, Y. Comparison of antioxidant potential and rat intestinal a-glucosides inhibitory activities of quercetin, rutin and isoquercetin. Int. J. Appl. Res. Nat. Prod. 2010, 2, 52–60.

58. Silva, M.M.; Santos, M.R.; Caroco, G.; Rocha, R.; Justino, G.; Mira, L. Structure-antioxidant activity relationships of flavonoids: A re-examination. Free Radic. Res. 2002, 36, 1219–1227.

59. Kessler, M.; Ubeaud, G.; Jung, L. Anti- and pro-oxidant activity of rutin and quercetin derivatives. J. Pharm. Pharmacol. 2003, 55, 131–142.

60. Wang, X.; Schroder, H.C.; Feng, Q.; Diehl-Seifert, B.; Grebenjuk, V.A.; Muller, W.E. Isoquercetrin and polyphosphate co-enhance mineralization of human osteoblast-like SaOs-2 cells via separate activation of two RUNX2 cofactors AFT6 and Ets1. Biochem. Pharmacol. 2014, 89, 413–421.

61. Awad, H.M.; Boersma, M.G.; Boeren, S.; Bladeren, P.J.; Vervoort, J.; Rietjens, I.M.C.M. Structure-activity study of the quinone/quinone methide chemistry of flavonoids. Chem. Res. Toxicol. 2001, 14, 398–408.

62. Canada, A.T.; Giannella, E.; Nguyen, T.D.; Mason, R.P. The production of reactive oxygen species by dietary flavonols. Free Radic. Biol. Med. 1990, 9, 441–449.

5

POLYPHENOLS: BENEFITS TO THE CARDIOVASCULAR SYSTEM IN HEALTH AND IN AGING

Sandhya Khurana [1], Krishnan Venkataraman [2], Amanda Hollingsworth [1,3], Matthew Piche [1] and T. C. Tai[1,3,4,5]

[1]Medical Sciences Division, Northern Ontario School of Medicine, Sudbury, ON P3E 2C6, Canada

[2]Department of Gerontology, Huntington University, Sudbury, ON P3E 2C6, Canada

[3]Department of Biology, Laurentian University, Sudbury, ON P3E 2C6, Canada

[4]Department of Chemistry and Biochemistry, Laurentian University, Sudbury, ON P3E 2C6, Canada

[5]Biomolecular Sciences Program, Laurentian University, Sudbury, ON P3E 2C6, Canada

ABSTRACT

Numerous studies have demonstrated the importance of naturally occurring dietary polyphenols in promoting cardiovascular health and emphasized the significant role these compounds play in limiting the effects of cellular aging. Polyphenols such as resveratrol, epigallocatechin gallate (EGCG), and curcumin have been acknowledged for having beneficial effects on cardiovascular health, while some have also been shown to be protective in aging. This review highlights the literature surrounding this topic on the prominently studied and documented polyphenols as pertaining to cardiovascular health and aging.

Keywords: cardiovascular; ROS; polyphenols; aging, resveratrol; EGCG; curcumin; olive oil; quercetin; berries

1. INTRODUCTION

1.1. Consequences of Diet on Health

The consequences of nutrition on health and well-being are quite well established. In fact, a popular saying that "you are what you eat" emerged from nutritionist Henry Lindlahr's observations of a link between a healthy diet and better health, which was written in his book titled "You Are What You Eat: how to win and keep health with foods" (originally published in 1942) [1]. A quest to understand how increased consumption of certain foods leads to better health has generated an interest in polyphenols, natural compounds that are found in several edibles. Polyphenols are synthesized by plants as secondary metabolites and are usually synthesized as defense mechanisms against stressors such as pathogens [2]. Based on the number of phenolic rings as well as the structural moiety that holds these together, polyphenols are classified into four categories: phenolic acids, flavonoids, stilbenes and lignans, with the flavonoids further classified into six subclasses (flavonols, flavones, isoflavones, flavanones, anthocyanidins and flavonols) [3]. From two decades, these compounds have been extensively researched for their capacity to improve human health. These analyses include a wide variety of clinical and nutritional epidemiological studies that indicate that populations whose diets are rich in polyphenols are less susceptible to cardiovascular diseases along with their complications and related mortality [4,5]. The French diet with copious amounts of red wine, the culture of green tea consumption in far eastern diets, the centrality of turmeric in South Asian diet and the Mediterranean diet rich in olive oil allow for cuisines that are all dense in polyphenols [4,5,6,7].

1.2. Reactive Oxygen Species in Cardiovascular Diseases: Polyphenols as Potential Therapeutics

1.2.1. Role of Reactive Oxygen Species in Disease

Numerous studies have supported a role for oxidative stress in the development and pathogenesis of a wide variety of diseases such as diabetes, Alzheimer's disease, chronic lung disease and cardiovascular diseases; the principal contributor to oxidative stress in the body being the generation of excess reactive oxygen species (ROS) [8,9]. Typically, ROS production occurs during physiological processes like respiration and metabolism and is usually well regulated and monitored by the cellular defense mechanisms such as superoxide dismutase (SOD), catalase (CAT) and glutathione reductase (GSR) [10]. Under situations of stress, exposure to environmental pollution and in aging for example, ROS levels increase and the cell's antioxidant system may be overwhelmed with excessive ROS, thus becoming deleterious to cell health and integrity. ROS are free radicals and highly reactive oxidizers that can bind DNA, lipids and proteins to attain stability, thereby turning a physiological condition into a pathological state [11]. ROS have been implicated in the development of diabetes, cardiovascular disorders and a variety of age-associated disorders like Parkinson's and Alzheimer's disease [10,11,12,13].

1.2.2. Polyphenols as Potential Therapeutics for Cardiovascular Diseases

In the case of cardiovascular disorders, oxidative stress and ROS have been vastly implicated in endothelial damage, progression to atherosclerosis, and injury in sustained myocardial infarction, as well as in ischemia reperfusion [8,12,14]. A deterioration in nitric oxide (NO) dependent vasorelaxation is a well-established risk factor that can predispose individuals to cardiovascular disease, and has been accepted as a feature with tremendous value in the prognosis of cardiovascular health [15]. A decreased NO bioavailability can occur due to reduction in expression of endothelial NOS (eNOS), the enzyme that is responsible for NO biosynthesis in the endothelium, as well as reduction in the available NO due to degradation by ROS amongst other reasons [15]. The sources of ROS in the vasculature are many, with mitochondrial enzymes NADH/NADPH oxidase, xanthine oxidase and others being significant culprits [15,16].

The oxidation of LDL and thereafter its entry across the endothelial barrier is the initiating factor in the generation of atherosclerotic plaques. Further, the interplay between hypercholesterolemia, oxidative stress radicals and inflammatory molecules generates an environment prone to massive endothelial damage, a hallmark of atherosclerotic progression [17]. Vascular endothelial adhesion molecule-1 (VCAM-1), intercellular cell adhesion molecule-1 (ICAM-1) and *E*-selectin are membrane proteins that facilitate the adhesion of leukocytes to the vascular endothelium and atherosclerotic lesions thereby stimulating signal transduction cascades [17]. These pathways lead to infiltration of leukocytes and macrophages into atherosclerotic plaques and ultimately the release of proinflammatory cytokines like tumor necrosis factor α (TNFα), interferon γ (IFNγ) and migratory factors such as monocyte chemoattractant protein-1 (MCP-1). Eventually upon upregulation of the key transcription factor NFκB, interleukins (IL-6 and IL-8) and gelatinolytic enzymes like metalloproteinases (MMPs) and others are synthesized, all known to play a role in atherosclerosis development [18]. ROS-mediated early events in atherosclerosis also includes activation of platelets by the endothelial adhesion molecule P-selectin, followed by upregulation of thromboxane (TX) A2 and platelet derived factors such as CD40 [19]. Upon atherosclerotic plaque rupture, platelets can bind to the endothelium leading to tethering, aggregation, and thrombus formation, ultimately to embolism and vasoconstriction, both hallmarks of myocardial infarction [20]. Moreover, the migration and proliferation of vascular smooth muscle cells (VSMCs) at an exaggerated proliferative rate and migration into the intima are both critical factors in the pathogenesis of atherosclerosis [21].

Diseases such as hypertension, pressure overload and vascular stenosis can lead to structural changes in the heart such as hypertrophy which are exemplified by increases in ROS, potent vasoconstrictor molecules like endothelin-1 (ET-1) and angiotensin II (AngII), and activation of signaling pathways activated via MAP38 kinases and NFκB [22]. ET-1 has been implicated in the pathogenesis of ROS mediated vascular abnormalities including proliferation and hypertrophy in VSMCs by ROS mediated activation of protein kinase B (PKB), extracellular signal-regulated kinase 1/2 (ERK1/2) and protein tyrosine kinase (Pyk2) signaling [23]. ET-1 is found to be elevated in patients with hypertension [24]. Ang II, the fundamental determinant in the renin-angiotensin system is formed by the action of angiotensin converting enzyme (ACE) on angiotensin I, and is a crucial factor in the etiology of hypertension and resultant changes in cardiac morphology and remodeling [25].

Lastly, I/R injuries encountered in the heart, consequently leading to arrhythmias, cardiac stunning, microvascular damage and cardiac cell death by apoptosis, is more damaging since several ROS are increased in the heart following reperfusion [8,26]. Also, ischemic heart disease is accompanied by myocardial infarction leading to myocardial hypoxia, generation of ROS, and accumulation of waste metabolites which ultimately leads to cell death and atherosclerotic tissue [8]. Sirtuins, critical factors in cell division, aging and response to stress, especially SIRT1, is found to be dysregulated during hypertrophy and myocardial stress in the heart, is also a new target identified in the pathogenesis of CVD [27].

Antioxidant therapies have been gaining recognition as strategies to reduce ROS in the vasculature thereby diminishing their detrimental effects [9]. Inhibitors of ACE that reduce circulating AngII, have been shown to reduce oxidative stress in addition to their antihypertensive properties; statins have been employed for the same purpose in addition to their cholesterol reducing properties by virtue of modulating HMG CoA reductase and lastly, vitamin E and C have been used extensively as dietary aids in conjunction with other drugs to reduce oxidative stress [9]. Polyphenols on the other hand are beginning to gain recognition and acceptance as potential therapeutic agents that could be beneficial in combating oxidative stress and thereby protect individuals from cardiovascular diseases [28,29]. Historically, the beneficial effects of polyphenols have been attributed primarily to their antioxidant capacity and their ability to modulate cellular antioxidant defense mechanisms by inducing the synthesis of detoxification enzymes like SOD, CAT, glutathione *S*-transferase (GST), glutathione peroxidase (GPx), NAD(P)H quinone oxidoreductase1 (NQO1) amongst others [30,31,32]. However, recent research provides evidence of polyphenols as modulators of signaling pathways [33,34,35,36]. A variety of studies encompassing clinical trials, epidemiological data as well as *in vitro* and *in vivo* studies with animals have been performed to firstly establish a cause and effect link between a diet rich in polyphenols and improvement in health, and secondly to gain insight into the mechanisms of the mode of action and protection bestowed by these compounds [4,35,36,37]. A significant mechanism to prevent the development of atherosclerosis is to protect the endothelium, reduce the oxidation of LDL, reduce cholesterol levels and repress the synthesis of proinflammatory cytokines and adhesion molecules [2,6]. In this scenario, polyphenols have been shown to modulate a variety of targets which include eNOS and NO, inflammatory cytokines like TNFα, IL-6 and IL-8 in addition to VCAM-1 and ICAM-1, and modulating signaling pathways by altering SIRT1, MAP38 kinase, NFκB, AP-1 amongst many others [2,33,38,39,40,41].

1.3. An Aging Cardiovascular System—Role of ROS

As mammalian cardiovascular systems age, there are several changes in morphology, anatomy, physiology and biochemistry of the heart and associated vessels. Morphologically, the heart undergoes thickening of the left ventricle and hypertrophy of the left ventricle and interventricular septum. There is stiffening, scarring and calcification of aortic valve leaflets and aortic sclerosis. Mitral annular calcification (MAC) and apoptotic reduction of the SA and AV node's pacemaker cells along with deposition of collagen, adipose tissue and amyloid occurs, changes electrical activity over the myocardium [42,43].

From the perspective of cardiac tissues, cardiomyocyte dimensions increase with an actual decrease in cell numbers. The sympathetic nerve supply decreases, resulting in reduced responsiveness to the beta-adrenergic pathway. Aging arteries are thickened, with the changes primarily in the intima and media and the sub-endothelial space may contain exaggerated deposits of collagen, elastin and proteoglycans [42,43]. VSMCs in the tunica intima are rounded with larger amounts of organelles [44]. Often, smooth muscle cells, macrophages and leukocytes migrate to the sub-endothelial space and are associated with increased levels of proinflammatory cytokines [44,45,46]. The consequent low-grade inflammation and endothelial damage is correlated with coronary artery disease and stroke in the elderly. The primary culprit for the considerable amount of tissue remodeling in the cardiovascular system is recognized to be ROS which have been implicated in both apoptosis and senescence of various cell types of the cardiovascular system [47].

ROS are generated primarily due to increased NAD(P)H oxidase activity and dysfunctional mitochondria [47,48]. A recent review by Ungvari and colleagues summarizes age related changes in signaling to the mitochondria, wherein reduced levels of NO, growth hormone (GH), insulin-like growth factor (IGF) and adiponectin combined with an increase in angiotensin II result in reduced mitochondrial turnover and biogenesis and an increase in ROS [48]. Mitochondria show reduced biogenesis and increased ROS production in aging cells and this impacts cells in multiple ways ranging from altered Ca^{2+} signaling, signaling stress induced protein kinases and TOR associated pathways. The increased ROS production is attributed to a combination of inactivation of MnSOD, cellular reduction of GSH levels, lower levels of Nrf2/ARE along with a dysfunctional electron transport chain [48].

The cellular targets for ROS in the aging cardiovascular system are many-fold. Targets include mitochondrial proteins and mitochondrial DNA amongst several other factors associated with apoptosis and inflammation. The impact of ROS on numerous targets manifests as inflammation, vascular rarefaction, and an increased rate of apoptosis in endothelial and smooth muscle cells. Ungvari and colleagues suggest that dysregulated mitochondrial turnover in an aging vasculature can contribute to an altered redox state in cells, leading to additional oxidative damage [48]. Targets identified thus far for ROS are transcription factors AP2, NFκB, Nrf2 and p53. Additionally, studies involving quenching of ROS with resveratrol, results in deacetylation and activation of PGC1α by SIRT1 and Nrf2, both of which are associated with mitochondrial biogenesis and mitigation of oxidative stress and redox homeostasis [48]. Additionally, ROS has also been linked with damage to essential factors in various fundamental cellular pathways such as glycolysis, nuclear transport, translation, proteasome function and chaperones [49].

1.4. The Focus of This Review

This review will highlight key studies and describe how polyphenols can counteract ROS as well as modulate signaling pathways to enhance health outcomes in the realm of cardiovascular disorders and aging. For the purpose of this discussion, this review will focus on evidence from literature supporting rescue from cardiovascular disease and aging as a result of oxidative damage, by dietary polyphenols. All the phenolics will be discussed with the objective of identifying studies that delineate their role in antioxidant defenses, anti-inflammation, VSMC proliferation and migration, anti-thrombolytic activity and finally protection in prevention or rejuvenation of damaged cardiac morphology as seen in ischemia reperfusion and hypertrophy in cardiac heart failure. The studies identified here are representative of broader findings that indicate the same biological phenomena.

The focus of this review is on food as natural sources of cardioprotective phenolic compounds, identifying the predominant phenolic compounds amongst the most potent foods that are acknowledged to be "superfoods" for the heart. Most of the well-studied phenolic compounds are polyphenolic in structure. The foods that comprise our categorization of "superfoods" are green tea, red wine, turmeric, capers, olive oil and berries. With the exception of olive oil and berries, the other "superfoods" have at least one well-studied polyphenol that they are abundant in, which have been highlighted here—resveratrol, EGCG, curcumin and quercetin, and will be discussed under bioactive components of polyphenol rich foods. As for olive oil, berries and fruits, which have been discussed in literature primarily as foods containing multiple phenolics, not necessarily all polyphenols, this review will address these foods and their effects based on findings using the whole food or extracts thereof as a collective of mixed phenolics.

2. BIOACTIVE COMPONENTS OF POLYPHENOL RICH FOODS

2.1 Resveratrol

2.1.1 Dietary Sources of Resveratrol

Resveratrol is a stilbene compound, and a phytoalexin, synthesized by plants in response to stressful stimuli. In addition to its noteworthy and acclaimed presence in red wine, ports and sherries, resveratrol is found in red grapes, blueberries, peanuts, itadori tea, as well as hops, pistachios and in grape and cranberry juices [41,50]. The content of resveratrol varies depending on the source and processing of the fruit; for example, boiled peanuts have a much higher content (5.1 μg/g) than roasted ones (0.055 μg/g) while dried grapes skins have a much higher content (24.06 μg/g) than red grapes themselves (0.16–3.54 μg/g). Additionally, red grapes have much more resveratrol than white ones [50]. Also, resveratrol content in red wine is reported to be 0.1–14 mg/L while in white wines, it is <0.1–2.1 mg/L [41]. Furthermore the quantity of resveratrol in red wine varies depending on the type and the source of grapes used to produce the wine; the Pinot Noir has a higher quantity of resveratrol than a Merlot with an added difference in Pinot Noirs dependent on the origin of the grapes; Pinot Noir from Oregon being higher than the ones from Upstate New York [51]. According to Goncalves and Camara, employing a newer sophisticated method for quantification, the quantity of resveratrol can be up to 50 μg/mL in certain red wines which would translate to 15 mg in two glasses of red wine (300 mL) [52,53]. Tomato skin has also been found to have resveratrol, but the study also noted the differences in the content depending on the variety of the tomato, with the beefsteak having negligible resveratrol content compared to the MicroTom [54]. Recently, cocoa and dark chocolate were also identified as minor sources of resveratrol [55].

2.1.2. Epidemiological Data and Clinical Studies on Resveratrol

The World Health Organization's MONItoring trends and determinants in CArdiovascular diseases (MONICA) study collected data on food intake and parameters of cardiovascular health from individuals of 26 countries [56]. Some of the findings of the MONICA study suggested an inverse correlation of dietary fat intake and the risk of cardiovascular diseases attributed to the consumption of wine in French and Swiss populations; however in populations of the US, UK and Australia that consumed similar amounts of dietary fat but not an equivalent amount of wine, the rate of mortality from cardiovascular diseases was much higher [5]. The findings suggested that the detrimental effects of a fat rich diet were counteracted by the high consumption of wine, often referred to as the "French paradox". Since then, resveratrol, the primary polyphenol found in red wine has come into the limelight, particularly to study its effects on risk parameters that are considered hallmarks of cardiovascular and other diseases. Numerous clinical trials have been undertaken to assess the correlation between wine consumption/resveratrol intake and the risk parameters for cardiovascular diseases [57]. Recent clinical trials in patients with stable coronary artery disease (CAD) investigated the effect of a daily oral intake of 10 mg resveratrol capsule for 3 months. The results showed a drastic improvement in flow-mediated vasodilation (FMD), which is dependent on vasodilation and is an indicator of endothelial function. Further, Low Density Lipoprotein (LDL) as well as platelet aggregation was significantly reduced in these patients [58]. In another more recent study, the effect of grape extract intake was analyzed in CAD patients. Resveratrol containing grape extracts decreased Apolipoprotein B and oxidized LDL, increased circulating serum adiponectin, an anti-inflammatory molecule also involved in lipid and glucose metabolism. Also plasminogen activator-1 (PA-1) levels that can be modulated by adiponectin were decreased in these CAD patients. Further, the production of proinflammatory cytokines like IL-6 and TNF-α were also reduced in PBMCs [59,60,61]. In another clinical trial evaluating the effect of resveratrol, exposure of endothelial cells to plasma obtained from healthy subjects consuming 400 mg/day of resveratrol for a month, demonstrated a reduction in the mRNA of inflammatory and adhesion molecules. The study noted a significant decrease in the expression of VCAM-1 and ICAM-1. The secretion of IL-8 was also repressed. All these inflammatory markers are directly correlated with atherosclerosis progression and their reduction demonstrates that consumption of resveratrol can be a preventative measure that can modulate plasma content and the onset of atherosclerosis [62].

2.1.3. Mechanisms of Resveratrol Action—Cell and Animal Studies

Resveratrol has been extensively researched for its ability to modulate determinants that are linked with increased cardiovascular risk. Improvement in lipid profiles and cholesterol levels, reductions in blood pressure and platelet aggregation as well increase in lifespan have all been demonstrated with resveratrol intake [41,63]. Resveratrol can stimulate the activity of sirtuins, particularly SIRT1 a histone deacetylase which regulates expression of genes involved in the stress response and cellular aging as well as modulates the adenosine monophosphate kinase (AMPK) signaling pathway, that influences fatty acid and lipid metabolism [64,65]. Mitochondrial biogenesis and enhanced mitochondrial function has been demonstrated in endothelial cells treated with resveratrol, by inducing nuclear respiratory factor-1 (Nrf-1), mitochondrial transcription factor A (Tfam) and peroxisome proliferator activated receptor gamma co-activator 1α (PGC1α) [66]. In coronary arterial cells, resveratrol stimulated the activity of nuclear factor-2 (Nrf-2), a transcription factor which can bind to antioxidant response elements (ARE) and upregulate a variety of antioxidant enzymes such as NQO1, HO-1 and control γ-glutamylcysteine synthetase (GCLC), the enzyme that regulates glutathione synthesis [32].

In the endothelium, resveratrol can stimulate eNOS activity increasing the amount of NO, thereby increasing vasodilation in endothelial cells as well as in isolated rat aortas [67,68]. Resveratrol can also modulate the biosynthesis of thromboxanes TXA2 and TXB2, molecules involved in platelet aggregation, by inhibiting p38 MAP kinase and PKC activity thereby reducing platelet adhesion and aggregation, consequently being antithrombotic and atheroprotective [69,70,71]. It can also contribute to reduction in inflammatory markers by inhibition of NFκB, TNFα and IL-6 as well as ICAM-1 and VCAM-1 expression in coronary endothelial cells [72,73]. Also, it decreases STAT-1 activation thereby downregulating interferon-γ inducible genes in macrophages [74]. In C57BL/6J mice, a high fat diet renders these animals susceptible to dyslipidemia with increased cholesterol and oxidized LDL in the serum. Upon administration of 200 mg/kg diet/day resveratrol for 8 weeks, these parameters were reversed with a reduction in cholesterol and increased in HDL. This was mediated in part by the increase in cholesterol 7alpha hydroxylase (CYP7A1) in the liver, an enzyme that is important in bile synthesis and cholesterol homeostasis in the body [75].

A critical mechanism by which resveratrol can protect from cardiovascular diseases is by preventing structural changes in the heart precipitated by hypertension, pressure overload and vascular stenosis and preventing this hypertrophy and remodeling [41]. Numerous animal studies have also demonstrated that administration of resveratrol improves cardiac function and preserves cardiac anatomy. In the spontaneously hypertensive rat (SHR), resveratrol dose of 2.5 mg/kg/day for 10 weeks prevented cardiac concentric hypertrophy, improved systolic and diastolic function but without any change in blood pressure, as well as reduced arterial stiffening and increased compliance by inhibiting the ERK1/2 pathway thereby denoting that an intervention with resveratrol may prove beneficial in protecting from remodeling of heart tissue [76,77]. Further, this improvement in the SHR was demonstrated to be a consequence of increased serum NO due to an activation of the AMPK pathway in the heart tissue of these animals and an impediment in the norepinephrine induced hypertrophy in cardiomyocytes [78]. In another hypertensive model of heart failure, the Dahl salt sensitive (DSS) rats, a high salt diet induced high blood pressure, ventricular dysfunction and cardiac remodeling with loss in body mass and increased mortality. However, in the group that received 20 mg/kg/day of resveratrol, there was no reduction in the body weight with an improved survival rate of the animals fed a high salt diet [79]. The animals showed normal eNOS levels as compared to those high salt fed rats that didn't receive resveratrol, with improved vasodilation and endothelial function. Moreover, resveratrol stimulated an upregulation of the expression of PPARα and its co-activator PGC1α, both involved in lipid metabolism [79]. Although there was no prevention of ventricular wall thickening as reported in the SHR model, this could be because of the differing antecedents of cardiac dysfunction in the different models. In Sprague Dawley rats, treatment with 5 mg/kg/day of resveratrol for 1 week prior and then after induction of myocardial infraction by ligation of the coronary artery, resveratrol suppressed the ventricular tachycardia and fibrillation by inhibiting L-type calcium current. Moreover, by week 14 resveratrol reduced infarct size by 20% and the overall mortality by 33% likely by suppressing remodeling of the left ventricle [80]. Resveratrol has been shown to be beneficial in protecting from damage caused by I/R injuries [41]. In neonatal cardiomyocytes, resveratrol can protect cells from I/R mediated cell apoptosis by reducing Bax and caspase3 expression and improving cell survival [81].

A more advanced and rapidly growing area of scientific exploration in understanding the molecular mechanisms involved in cardiovascular disease, is to comprehend the alteration of microRNA in disease and healthy states. MicroRNA are regulatory RNA sequences that can influence gene expression. For example, the microRNA profile of patients who suffer from coronary artery disease is markedly different from healthy subjects [82]. Therefore, the modulation of microRNA by resveratrol is an area of increasing interest and scientific research [83,84]. Specifically, an interesting study on global miRNA expression in hearts of rats that got exposed to ischemia followed by reperfusion, demonstrated that pretreatment of these animals with resveratrol or longivinex, a multicomponent resveratrol containing formulation, reestablished miRNA signatures to the same as baseline vehicle controls as compared to the miRNA expression patterns seen in the group that received no pretreatment [85]. This study emphasizes that resveratrol can modulate miRNA pathways and signaling mechanisms that might be critical in the cardioprotection offered by this polyphenol.

2.1.4. Resveratrol in Cardiovascular Aging

Probably the most extensively studied polyphenol, proponents of resveratrol have ascribed longevity enhancing, anti-cancer as well as cardioprotective properties to it. All three properties may merely be a consequence of mitigation of oxidative stress [40,47]. The conundrum of low bioavailability of resveratrol and its rapid metabolism has prompted researchers to seek other stable analogs to understand the impact of this polyphenol. Regardless, it is widely accepted that resveratrol lowers lipid peroxidation and increases plasma antioxidant capacity directly or indirectly. Additionally, elevated plasma levels of resveratrol mimic effects of caloric restriction in older adults, the cardiovascular benefits of which are well documented. Resveratrol is a COX1 inhibitor. The selective inhibition of COX1 over COX2 results in reduced platelet aggregation and vasoconstriction. COX1 inhibition also translates to reduced endothelial inflammation [41]. Recent reports have additionally identified SIRT1 regulated genes as well as Nrf2 regulated genes to be modulated by resveratrol [47]. In a study on middle-aged mice fed a high calorie diet supplemented with resveratrol, the polyphenol was found to prevent the detrimental effects of the diet and alter the physiology of these animals to parallel those fed the standard diet. As the mice aged, resveratrol increased their lifespan, insulin sensitivity and modulated PGC1α and mitochondrial number [86]. Resveratrol is also a vasorelaxant as a consequence of being able to stimulate Ca^{2+} associated K^+ channels and increasing NO signaling in the endothelium. It is not apparent if the antioxidant pathways of resveratrol are a consequence of direct binding of ROS or if it is directly involved in stimulating cellular antioxidant pathways. Regardless, there is evidence of favorable serum lipid profiles being induced by resveratrol. In rat models, resveratrol has been additionally demonstrated to protect against I/R injury [41]. Resveratrol has also been demonstrated to be anti-proliferatory, impacting migration of VSMCs and the remodeling of arterial walls, implicated in atherosclerotic lesions [87,88,89]. The age associated increases in synthesis of proinflammatory cytokines from arterial VSMC isolated from aged rhesus monkeys as compared to that from the young ones was dramatically reduced with resveratrol treatment, likely by inhibiting NFκB [90]. Briefly, resveratrol has been demonstrated to impact all the hallmarks of cardiovascular aging and disease and unquestionably has been the most studied polyphenol.

2.2 Epigallocatechin Gallate—EGCG

2.2.1. Dietary Sources of EGCG

Epigallocatechin gallate (EGCG) is a polyphenol belonging to the catechin family, a group of polyphenolic compounds that are abundant within green tea [91]. Black and oolong teas also contain catechins including EGCG as well as epicatechin, epicatechin gallate and epigallocatechin. These three teas originate from the leaves of the *Camellia sinenis* plant but are distinct due to processing and fermentation. As a result of manufacturing, catechins encompass only 3%–10% of the solid content of black tea but 30%–42% of green tea [91]. Catechins are also found in a variety of food sources including fruits, vegetables, tea, wine, and chocolate among others; however, EGCG is almost exclusive to tea [92,93].

2.2.2. Epidemiological Data and Clinical Studies on EGCG

There is evidence for tea polyphenols to be the bioactive components contributing to the beneficial health effects observed in tea drinkers. Consumption of catechin-rich tea positively affected body weight, body-mass-index (BMI), waist circumference, body fat mass and subcutaneous fat of individuals following a 12 week intervention period [94]. Epidemiological observations highlight the association between heavy tea consumption and the apparent risk reduction in cardiovascular disease [95]. For example, tea consumption was found to be inversely associated with mortality due to all causes, including cardiovascular disease, in a study of 40,000 Japanese individuals. Lower risk of mortality was observed with consumption of greater than five cups of green tea per day in comparison to less than one cup per day [95]. Similarly, risk of developing hypertension in a Chinese population drinking 120–599 mL of tea per day was 46% lower than occasional tea drinkers and 65% lower when tea was consumed at a rate of 600 mL or more per day [96]. Tea consumption within elderly populations, as observed in participants of the Zutphen Elderly Study and the Rotterdam Study, is inversely related to mortality from coronary heart disease and incidence of a first myocardial infarction, with the risk of coronary heart disease and myocardial infarction being lower in heavy tea drinkers [97,98,99]. The inverse association of green tea intake in these studies and the incidence of cardiovascular disease might be associated with the decrease in triglycerides, total and LDL cholesterol as well as HDL cholesterol increase observed in tea drinkers [100]. A compilation of epidemiological studies examining green tea intake and cardiovascular risk revealed that of the 30 studies examined, 17 showed significant benefits of green tea consumption, 11 indicated no effects and the remaining studies documented negative effects [101,102]. Studies revealing negative or no effects of tea intake might be due to lack of consideration of other lifestyle factors and diet and the addition of milk to tea which may diminish its protective effect. Furthermore, the kind, preparation and strength of tea might also contribute to the lack of cardioprotective effects [101,103,104].

2.2.3. Mechanism of Action of EGCG—Cell and Animal Studies

The major tea polyphenol, EGCG, demonstrates beneficial cardiovascular effects, including: protection from endothelial dysfunction, hypertension, cardiac hypertrophy, cardiac cell damage and injury. Experimental studies demonstrate the anti-hypertensive effects of tea and its major catechin, EGCG. Blood pressure of SHRs was attenuated following black or green tea consumption likely through modulation of the production of eNOS and NO, increasing bioavailability of NO to improve endothelial dysfunction and mediate vasodilation [38,105]. EGCG treatment of human endothelial cell lines enhanced eNOS mRNA production and facilitated a 60% increase in NO levels [106]. Stimulation of NO production involves inhibition of p38 MAPK phosphorylation and a H_2O_2 mediated activation of fyn, a

Src family kinase that activates PI3 kinase/Akt and ultimately eNOS synthesis [33,107,108]. EGCG stimulation of NO via PI3 kinase induction was also shown in a study involving isolated mesenteric vascular beds (MVB) from SHRs wherein, the vasodilatory effect of EGCG was abolished after treatment with both a NO synthase inhibitor (L-NAME) and a PI3 kinase inhibitor (wortmannin) confirming the mechanism of action for EGCG [109]. The activation of PI3 kinase and p38 MAPK by EGCG also results in the upregulation of Nrf2 and activation of ERK 1/2, leading to an increase in the synthesis of HO-1 which in turn provides protection from H_2O_2 mediated oxidative stress and restricts expression of VCAM-1 [110,111,112]. Experimental models of atherosclerosis display upregulated inflammatory markers, including C-reactive protein (CRP), which is present in atherosclerotic lesions. Expression of CRP, a reliable marker of inflammation, was lower in animals subjected to an atherogenic diet supplemented with EGCG [113].

Rats fed a high-cholesterol diet exhibit poor lipid profiles, including high levels of serum and hepatic cholesterol, LDL and triglycerides along with low levels of HDL. Recovery of these lipid parameters were observed with green tea supplementation [114,115]. EGCG appears to affect cholesterol synthesis via the inhibition of hydroxyl-3-methyl-glutaryl-CoA (HMGR) activity, the rate-limiting enzyme in cholesterol synthesis [116]. Further, consumption of tea containing 58% EGCG reduced fatty plaque coverage within the aorta of ApoE-deficient mice [114]. EGCG treatment inhibited PKC and ERK 1/2 signaling pathways subsequently suppressing proliferation of VSMCs exposed to high glucose; EGCG also limits the migration of VSMCs, by inhibiting the activity of MMP-2 and MMP-9 [117,118,119]. Specifically, EGCG inhibits the activity of MMP-2 by blocking the activation of its catalytic subunit to reduce its gelatinolytic activity [119,120]. Platelet aggregation is repressed by EGCG by inhibiting p38 MAPK and ERK 1/2 while stimulating tyrosine phosphorylation of Syk and the adaptor protein SLP-76, which are requirements for intracellular Ca^{2+} elevation and platelet aggregation via the PKC pathway [121]. Synthesis of TXA_2, is also inhibited by EGCG [122]. Synthesis and secretion of ET-1 is regulated by the transcription factor, FOXO1, which binds to the promoter of ET-1 to facilitate activation. This process is impeded when FOXO1 is phosphorylated by AMP kinase and Akt rendering it incapable of activating ET-1. The inactivation of FOXO1 occurs through cytoplasmic targeting, upon treatment of endothelial cells with EGCG [123].

EGCG can attenuate cardiac hypertrophy, myocyte hypertrophy and fibrosis developing from aorta constriction. EGCG has been shown to further prevent increases in left ventricular dimensions as well as improve systolic dysfunction that is apparent in aortic-constricted animals [124]. Cardiac hypertrophy is accompanied by generation of ROS as is evident by increases in MDA and reductions of endogenous antioxidant enzymes including SOD and GPx; EGCG recovered these parameters indicating its potential role as an antioxidant to combat oxidative stress injuries related to cardiac hypertrophy [125]. In addition to cardiac hypertrophy, the progression of the pathophysiology of atherosclerosis via ROS production is significantly diminished with EGCG exposure. In response to oxidized LDL, EGCG exposure minimizes the activation of NFκB and p38 MAPK pathway via NADPH oxidase and Lox-1 expression [126]. Impairments of the coronary artery blood supply results in I/R injury, also accompanied by oxidative stress. Isolated rat hearts undergoing I/R injury exhibit increases in lipid peroxidation and decreases in mitochondrial and cytoplasmic SOD (Mn-SOD, Cu/Zn-SOD) and catalase levels [127]. Features characteristic of apoptosis were evident in perfused left ventricular tissue of male rats, including increases in cleaved caspase-3 and Bax, and decreases in Bcl-2 proteins. EGCG protected from subsequent apoptosis following I/R injury by regulating the Bcl-2/Bax ratio and blocking the cleavage of caspase-3 [127,128]. Moreover, in cardiac myocytes, EGCG impaired STAT-1 phosphorylation which is involved in I/R induced apoptosis thereby protecting from cell death and improving recovery [129]. EGCG perfusion increases coronary blood flow by means of decreasing LDH levels, reducing infarct size, and improving ventricular function [127,130]. Cardiac necrosis and stunning of the heart post-reperfusion were reduced when EGCG was administered at time of reperfusion [130]. An interesting recent study investigating the impact of EGCG on I/R injury revealed that higher doses did not equate to greater protection, indicating the importance of dosing to achieve optimal cardiovascular protection [128]. Injury to the myocardium following I/R is exemplified by neutrophil infiltration leading to an exaggerated oxidative stress response and an increase in infarct size, an indirect result of cardiac myocyte release of proinflammatory cytokines, such as TNFα and IL-6 [131]. EGCG reduced expression of IL-6 and TNFα in a model of I/R injury by inhibiting NFκB [132]. Additionally, EGCG has been shown to reduce the migration of neutrophils in a cell culture model [133,134]. Experimentally induced myocardial infarction leads to diminished endogenous antioxidants and antioxidant enzymes as well as increased plasma lipid peroxides and uric acid in animals; supplementation with EGCG reversed the effects thereby aiding in the protection against myocardial infarction injury [135].

The observations highlighted above illustrate the cardioprotective qualities of EGCG and suggests its potential use as a protective agent in the prevention and improvement of cardiovascular disease.

2.2.4. EGCG in Cardiovascular Aging

The most abundant catechin in green tea is EGCG. EGCG has been found to exert cardioprotective effects in several studies [95,136,137,138]. In a longitudinal study in 2006, Kuriyama *et al.*, discovered that cardiovascular disease associated mortality was greatly reduced in older adults consuming five or more cups of green tea every day [95]. EGCG was found to reduce cardiomyocyte apoptosis by inhibiting telomere attrition [139] and attenuated left ventricular remodeling, probably by decreasing oxidative stress [124,140,141]. EGCG was also found to improve endothelial function in patients with cardiovascular disease [136]. Similar findings amongst different cohorts have been summarized in a recent review [142]. EGCG reduces inflammation by indirectly regulating angiotensin II and consequently, NFκB. Other targets impacted by EGCG in smooth muscle cells (SMC) include IκB kinase, cJun, AP1, FAS receptor, STAT1, catalase, HO-I, and Nrf2 in endothelial and SMC. EGCG treatment also impacts migration and proliferation of SMC, thereby reducing progression of artherosclerosis. The mechanism for inhibition is believed to be EGCG incorporation into various cell compartments. EGCG has been shown to cause a G1 arrest by inhibiting cyclins D1 and E. Additionally, EGCG has also been shown to inhibit PCNA. Platelet function is also modulated by EGCG through regulation of PDGF. PDGF regulates several mitogenic genes such as ERK1/2, cFOS and EGR1. Factors down regulated in the inflammation pathway include TNFα, IL-12p40, p38 MAPK. All of this downregulation is accomplished through ERK1/2 activation, which breaks down IκBα and NFκB activation [33]. Endothelial function is improved by modulation of eNOS. Vasorelaxation is seen in both an NO dependent and an NO independent manner accompanied by an increase in cGMP levels [136]. The P13-Akt pathway is implicated along with estrogen receptor (ER) mediated pathways but no receptor for tea catechins or polyphenols have been identified in the cardiovascular system. Moreover, dietary intervention of aged Fischer 344 rats with EGCG was also found to lower the age-related oxidative damage in these animals by reducing oxidative stress, maintaining mitochondrial integrity while significantly declining the plasma level of 8-hydroxy-2′ deoxyguanosine, a critical biomarker of oxidative stress [143]. Most of the evidence of EGCG's antithrombotic activity comes from *in vitro* evidence. Multiple factors are attributed to the potential for EGCG as an anti-thrombolytic factor such as lower levels of platelet activation factor (PAF), the inhibition of related acetyl transferases, inhibition of thrombin induced phosphorylation of p38MAPK and ERK1/2, the inhibition of tyrosine phosphorylation of several platelet proteins, and reduction of intracellular Ca^{2+} level associated fibrinogen binding in platelets [33]. The impact of EGCG in mitigating cardiovascular disease development and in retardation of cardiovascular aging is unquestionable and its potential benefits as a component of daily diet cannot be overstated.

2.3 Curcumin

2.3.1. Dietary Sources of Curcumin

The polyphenol, curcumin, is the active component of turmeric, a common Indian spice, derived from the rhizome of the *Curcuma longa* plant [144,145]. Curcumin is the most abundant constituent of turmeric; comprising approximately 2%–5% of the compound [146].

2.3.2. Epidemiological Data and Clinical Studies on Curcumin

Clinical studies of volunteers on a week-long regimen of curcumin (500 mg) had decreased lipid peroxides and total serum cholesterol, and increased serum HDL levels [147]. Similarly, patients with acute coronary syndrome administered low doses of curcumin at 15 mg, three times daily for 2 months had greater reductions in LDL and greater elevations in HDL levels. However, triglyceride levels were higher compared to basal levels with the moderate dose of 30 mg, three times daily for 2 months, having a minimalist effect on increased levels [148].

2.3.3. Mechanism of Action of Curcumin—Cell and Animal Studies

Turmeric extract can influence the characteristic hypercholesterolemic effects of atherosclerosis reproduced in experimental models [149]. Rabbits administered a low dose (1.66 mg/kg body weight) of turmeric extract had a decreased susceptibility of LDL peroxidation, decreased total plasma cholesterol including lowered levels of LDL, triglycerides and phospholipids [149]. Further studies involving *Curcuma longa* extract supplementation in rabbits consuming an atherogenic diet revealed lessened plasma lipid peroxidation and fewer fatty streak lesions in the aorta. Additionally, α-tocopherol levels were greater with curcumin supplementation indicating the enhancement of endogenous antioxidant mechanisms [150]. This study also demonstrated the importance of dosing in the effectiveness of curcumin to attenuate cardiovascular complications since higher doses were not as effective as lower doses [149,150]. In addition, curcumin treatment of LDL-receptor knockout mice (LDL-KO) fed a high cholesterol diet increased plasma HDL and decreased LDL. Further, atherosclerosis biomarkers including atherogenic index, percent HDL:total cholesterol and ApoB:ApoA-1 ratio improved with curcumin treatment [151]. Atherosclerotic lesions subject to infiltration of lipids as well as the presence of ICAM-1 and VCAM-1 within aortic fatty plaques were detected in untreated LDL-KO mice consuming a high cholesterol diet but absent in mice administered curcumin [151]. In an alternate model, consumption of a high fat diet in hamsters demonstrated lower levels of free fatty acid, total cholesterol, triglyceride and leptins when supplemented with curcumin as well as elevations of plasma of HDL, apolipoprotein and paraoxonase activity [152].

Endothelial dysfunction modeled in porcine coronary arteries was attenuated with curcumin addition through impeding the homocysteine-induced impairment of endothelial-dependent vasorelaxation and eNOS levels as well as reducing superoxide anion production [153]. Curcumin relaxed pre-constricted porcine coronary arterial rings only in rings with intact endothelium and not when an inhibitor of NO synthesis, L-NNA (*N*-nitro-L-arginine) was introduced [154]. Furthermore, curcumin reduced transcript levels of TNFα receptors, diminished nuclear translocation of NFκB affecting gene regulation, and reduced TNFα-induced expression of adhesion molecules characteristic of atherosclerosis such as ICAM-1, MCP-1 and IL-8 mRNA and protein, as well as monocyte adhesion to HUVECs [145]. Curcumin also attenuates phosphorylation of PKB and ERK1/2 in VSMCs as well as inhibited c-Raf and insulin-like growth factor type 1 receptor (IGF-1R), all necessary for ET-1 activation thereby showing potential to modulate ET-1 effects in vascular physiology [155].

Curcumin possesses antioxidant properties that protect against oxidative effects on proteins and lipids [156]. Intracellular ROS levels within TNFα-stimulated HUVECs were attenuated with curcumin treatment [145]. Antioxidant abilities of curcumin were demonstrated in rats undergoing Adriamycin-induced myocardial toxicity [157]. Increased levels of lipid peroxidation products and catalase activity, in addition to, decreased myocardial glutathione and

GPx activity, accompanied myocardial toxicity in Adriamycin treated rats; the group receiving curcumin therapy did not present with ECG abnormalities seen with their Adriamycin-treated counterparts nor did they have increased serum lipid peroxides and lipid peroxidation products. Curcumin augmented the endogenous antioxidant systems as confirmed by increased glutathione levels, glutathione peroxidase activity and reduced catalase activity [157]. In addition, protection of aortic endothelial cells against H_2O_2 induced oxidative stress is mediated by a concentration- and time-dependent induction of HO-1 by curcumin, protection from cell injury and protein oxidation [158].

Remodeling of vasculature after injury can have pathogenic consequences leading to cardiovascular complications. Growth factors, including platelet-derived growth factor (PDGF), play an important role in vascular remodeling [159]. PDGF-stimulated VSMC migration, proliferation, cytoskeletal reorganization and collagen synthesis were inhibited with curcumin treatment. Mediation of remodeling events by curcumin is done through blockage of signaling events including: PDFGF receptor binding, increased phosphor-tyrosine levels on PDGF-receptor β, and phosphorylation of downstream effectors: Erk1/2 and Akt [159].

High cholesterol-induced VSMC proliferation was modeled via administration of Chol:MβCD, a water-soluble cholesterol, to primary rat VSMC. Chol:MβCD causes VSMC proliferation and downregulates caveolin-1, an important regulator of cell proliferation via MAPK signaling. Suppression of ERK signaling was observed following curcumin treatment and cell cycle arrest occurred at the G1/S phase to inhibit VSMC proliferation [160]. LOX-1, an oxidized LDL receptor, and angiotensin II type 1 receptor (AT1R) are involved in hypertrophy of cardiac myocytes [161]. AngII is thought to activate AT1R to upregulate LOX-1 and influence oxidative stress production via NADPH oxidase and NF-κB activation to ultimately influence cardiac myocyte hypertrophy. Curcumin treatment blocks AngII-stimulation of AT1R and LOX-1, ROS generation, upregulation of NADPH oxidase and expression of redox-sensitive, NFκB. Interestingly, curcumin treatment alone attenuated basal levels of ROS, NADPH oxidase and expression level of NF-κB [161].

Protective effects of curcumin have been demonstrated in a case of MI. Microarray analysis identified differential expression of genes in rats undergoing coronary artery ligation and those administered curcumin before surgery [162]. Specifically, differences were observed in expression of genes involved in cytokine-cytokine receptor interaction, focal adhesion, apoptosis and extracellular matrix (ECM) receptor interaction. Differential expression is important since cytokine-cytokine receptors affect heart failure, ECM components are elevated in atherosclerotic lesions and focal adhesions have a role in post-MI remodeling. Biomarkers for MI, creatine kinase and lactate dehydrogenase (LD), were also elevated in coronary artery ligated rats but reversed in rats administered curcumin prior to surgery [162].

In summary, curcumin, the polyphenol common to the Indian spice, turmeric, demonstrates beneficial health effects in the prevention of cardiovascular disorders as well as attenuating factors involved in the pathophysiology of cardiovascular disease. The protective effects of curcumin imply that supplementation within the diet can be beneficial for cardiovascular health.

2.3.4. Curcumin in Cardiovascular Aging

First identified as an anti-inflammatory agent in 1995, curcumin's ability to suppress inflammation by regulation of multiple cytokines such as beta-site APP-cleaving enzyme 1 (BACE-1), C-reactive protein (CRP), connective tissue growth factor (CTGF), endothelial leukocyte adhesion molecule-1 (ELAM-1), histone acetyl transferase (HAT), hypoxia inducible factor (HIF), ICAM-1, lipid peroxidation (LPO), MMPs, NFκB, ornithine decarboxylase (ODC), signal transducers and activator of transcription protein (STAT), TNFα, VCAM-1, vascular endothelial growth factor (VEGF), amongst others is evidence of the considerable potential for this polyphenol as a cardioprotective agent. In an extensive review published by Aggarwal and Harikumar in 2009 [163], the authors identified multiple sources of research that demonstrated physiological phenomena attributed to the role of curcumin in regulating the aforementioned factors. Some notable cardioprotective features of curcumin are inhibition of high glucose-induced foam cell formation by inhibition of NFκB, the inhibition of induced migration, proliferation and collagen synthesis in cultured VSMCs, the prevention of isoproterenol-induced myocardial infarction, decrease in the LPO of liver microsomes and mitochondria, inhibition of LDL oxidation, reduction of oxidative stress and reduction of aortic fatty streaks. Additionally, curcumin has been shown to decrease the levels of O^{2-}, XO, MPO and LPO in myocardium elevated the levels of GPx, SOD, CAT and GST, inhibits the development of atherosclerosis in ApoE/LDLR-DKO mice, attenuates global cardiac I/R injury; decreases myocardial MMP-9, IL-6, MCP-1, TNFα, decreases plasma IL-8, IL-10, and cardiac troponin 1 and decreased apoptosis in cardiomyocytes and myocardial

Myeloperoxidase (MPO). A detailed list of targets for curcumin as well as an extensive list of effect of curcumin on neurodegenerative, cardiovascular, neoplastic, pulmonary, metabolic, and autoimmune diseases is well documented [163]. A recent study supports the role for curcumin as a novel supplemental therapy for treatment of vascular aging by attenuating arterial stiffening and endothelial dysfunction preferentially in older mice [164]. In another study on postmenopausal women, curcumin ingestion for 8 weeks improved endothelial function as measured by flow mediated dilation [165]. Also, curcumin has been shown to mitigate cardiotoxicity due to adriamycin based anti-cancer treatments. An increase in cellular GST and reduced peroxidation of lipids due to curcumin's ability to scavenge ROS has been attributed to this phenomenon. In the case of older patients with a co-morbidity of diabetes and cardiomyopathy, curcumin down regulates NOS and NO production by chelating NO_2, an intermediate in production of NO. Abnormal accumulation of various connective tissue constituents in aging endothelia is a consequence of unstable lysosomal membranes. Curcumin reportedly stabilizes lysosomal membranes and decreases the activity of lysosomal acid hydrolases. It has additionally been suggested that curcumin may modulate hypertrophy in the aging heart by inhibiting the Adenoviral transcription co-activator, p300 [166].

The curcumin rich spice turmeric, prominently used in Indian cooking, is a promising candidate to aid in the healthy aging of the cardiovascular system.

2.4 Quercetin

2.4.1. Dietary Sources of Quercetin

Quercetin, a polyphenol belonging to the flavonoid group is found in a wide variety of fruits and vegetables. Apples and onions, having a concentration of 4.57 mg/100 g and 22 mg/100 g respectively, are the significant sources of this flavonoid in the Western diet [167]. In case of onions, it has been shown that the different colored onions, yellow, red, pink or white, have varied amounts of quercetin and that the storage temperature affects the amount of this phenolic [168]. The yellow Sweet Savannah onion had the highest amount of quercetin (286 mg/kg) while white onions had negligible amounts of quercetin [168]. Interestingly, the largest amount of quercetin is found in capers 233 mg/100 g, and it is also found in cocoa powder at 22 mg/100 g [167]. Broccoli and green and black tea are also sources of quercetin [167]. Plums also contain quercetin, it being the most prominent polyphenol accounting for about two-thirds of the polyphenolic content found in this fruit; the quantities vary based on the cultivar tested in the study by Mubarak *et al.* in 2012 [169]. The amount of quercetin in the 29 cultivars tested in Mubarak's study ranged from 9 mg/kg to 239.8 mg/kg. Plums also contain the glycoside of quercetin called Rutin ranging from 9.5 g/kg to 63.9 mg/kg [169]. Quercetin is also found in mulberry leaves, a medicinal plant used in China and Japan to aid in blood pressure reduction [170].

2.4.2. Epidemiological and Clinical studies with Quercetin

Intriguingly, a randomized, double-blind, placebo-controlled, crossover study involving human patients with stage 1 hypertension has shown that treatment with high dose quercetin led to a reduction in systolic, diastolic and mean arterial pressure, suggesting the potential for quercetin to be used therapeutically in the treatment of early stage hypertension. Subjects were given 730 mg/day of quercetin for 28 days with findings compared to placebo and those subjects who were stage 1 hypertensive displayed a significant reduction in their systolic and diastolic blood pressure by 7 ± 2 mmHg and 5 ± 2 mmHg respectively. This clearly suggests that quercetin may be a viable therapeutic option in early hypertension [171].

Moreover, quercetin was studied in an at-risk population of overweight or obese individuals aged 25–65 years of age with metabolic syndrome traits, for its effect on blood pressure, lipid metabolism, along with markers of oxidative stress, inflammation and body composition. This double-blind, placebo controlled cross-over trial randomized patients to 150 mg quercetin/day *versus* placebo for a 6-week treatment period followed by a 5 week wash-out period. This study revealed that quercetin significantly reduced systolic blood pressure in all subjects by 2–6 mmHg, by 2–9 mmHg in the hypertensive subgroup, and by 3–7 mmHg for those patients aged 25–50 years. Furthermore, quercetin treatment significantly reduced the concentration of oxidized LDL without any detrimental effect on serum electrolytes, hematology, or liver and kidney function [172]. Taken together, this clinical study suggests that quercetin supplementation at 150 mg/day may therapeutically alter systolic blood pressure and reduce the concentration of oxidized LDL in a patient profile that is significantly at risk for cardiovascular disease.

2.4.3. Mechanism of Action of Quercetin—Cell and Animal Studies

Quercetin can act as an indirect antioxidant, increasing the activities of phase 2 antioxidant enzymes GST, HO-1, NQO1 in cardiac ventricular myocytes isolated from WKY rats [173]. Using human umbilical vein endothelial cells, Balasuriya and Rupasinghe (2012) studied the effects of apple peel extracts rich in flavonoids and quercetin metabolites on ACE inhibition [174]. Interestingly, their work demonstrated that the flavonoid-rich apple peel extract as well as two quercetin metabolites inhibited ACE significantly with the flavonoids potentially acting as competitive inhibitors of ACE; notably, quercetin-3-*O*-glucoside and qyercetin-3-*O*-glucuronic acid significantly inhibited ACE [174].

Quercetin is a readily available flavonoid that has been suggested to be of benefit in ameliorating cardiovascular health via eNOS upregulation, and the reduction of oxidative stress [175]. Notably, studies involving rat aortic ring segments have demonstrated that quercetin treatment for 30 min enhanced relaxation of these aortic rings by virtue of NOS and endothelium derived hyperpolarizing factor. Moreover, this group demonstrated that bovine aortic endothelial cells, when treated with quercetin, exhibited an increase in intracellular calcium, eNOS phosphorylation and subsequent increase in NO. Taken together, these results suggest that quercetin induced phosphorylation of eNOS can increase availability of NO, thereby inducing protective vascular effects [176]. *In vivo* studies using SHRs have looked at the effects of quercetin administration on mean arterial pressure (MAP), heart rate and baroreflex sensitivity. SHR and their normotensive counterparts, the Wistar-kyoto rats (WKY), were treated with 2, 10 or 25 mg/kg/day oral quercetin or saline for 7 days. Notably, doses of 10 and 25 mg/kg/day were found to decrease MAP in SHR to 163 ± 4 and 156 ± 5 as compared to 173 ± 6 respectively with no change in WKY samples. Moreover, the dose of 25 mg/kg/day was found to decrease serum oxidative stress in SHR samples. This suggests that oral quercetin intake may play a protective role in decreasing blood pressure, perhaps via a mechanism linked to oxidative stress [177]. As Perez-Vizcaino *et al.* (2009) point out, quercetin has been studied in multiple rat models of hypertension and has been shown to induce a progressive and sustained reduction in blood pressure independently of the renin-angiotensin, oxidative stress or nitric oxide status without any effect in normotensive controls [178].

Lectin-like oxidized receptor 1 (LOX-1) is a receptor for oxidized LDL; activation of LOX-1 results in the subsequent increased expression of inflammatory cytokines as well as the decrease in the release of NO thereby disrupting the proper functioning of the endothelium [179]. LOX-1 is upregulated in physiologic circumstances highly linked to atherosclerotic disease such as hypertension, hyperlipidemia and diabetes [179]. Utilizing an *in vitro* model with Chinese hamster ovary cells expressing LOX-1, apple polyphenols inhibited uptake of oxidized LDL by 88%. Furthermore, SHR-SP rats were given oligomeric procyanidins purified from apples. At termination, the mesenteric artery of the rats displayed a significant reduction in the amount of lipid deposits in the arterial wall even in the context of a high fat diet [179]. Supplementation of diet in WKY rats with 0.5% quercetin, for 2 weeks resulted in altered serum lipid profile with an increase in LDL and decrease in HDL [180]. In ApoE deficient mice, a diet supplemented with Mulberry leaves (1%) reduced atherosclerotic lesions in the aorta by 40% as well as demonstrating a lag time in the onset of LDL oxidation [181]. Quercetin is also anti-atherosclerotic by inhibiting platelet aggregation [182]. In bovine aortic endothelial cells, treatment with mulberry leave extract inhibited the TNFα mediated activation of NFκB thereby repressing the inflammatory response, as well inhibiting the expression of LOX-1 [183]. Moreover, rabbits fed a high cholesterol diet (1% cholesterol supplement) displayed significant increases in CRP, total cholesterol, triglycerides and LDL, fibrinogen, nitrite, nitrate levels and a reduction in HDL levels [184]. Notably, administration of both high and low doses of apple juice, 10 mL and 5 mL respectively, lead to a decrease in total cholesterol, triglycerides, CRP, fibrinogen, and factor VII. On the other hand, 10 mL of apple juice supplementation lead to a significant decrease in LDL levels and an increase in the protective HDL levels. Taken together, these data suggest that apple juice supplementation may have a protective effect on the blood lipid profile *in vivo* [184]. Histologically, those groups supplemented with apple juice displayed a significant reduction in atherosclerotic lesions of the coronary arteries when compared to the high cholesterol diet group [184].

Quercetin treatment has been shown to prevent morphological and functional changes within organ systems such as blood vessels, kidney and heart secondary to hypertension. Quercetin also diminished the production of ROS associated with hypertension in the aforementioned rat models of the disease [185]. In Sprague Dawley rats undergoing myocardial I/R via coronary artery occlusion, infarct size was significantly reduced with quercetin treatment and inflammation was prevented by reduction of TNFα and IL-10 [186].

2.4.4. Quercetin in Cardiovascular Aging

Quercetin is found in several different foods and it is one of the polyphenols that is not limited considerably in terms of bioavailability, evidenced by lower levels of peroxidation of plasma lipids. Consumption of quercetin in animal models as well as in humans correlated inversely to hypertension [171]. Quercetin appears to improve endothelial function in a NOS independent pathway [187]. Quercetin has anti-clotting abilities due to its ability to competitively bind plasminogen and also modulates plasmin concentration via urokinase plasminogen activator (uPA) modulation [188]. Quercetin's anti-proliferative effect on vascular smooth muscle cells occurs primarily through inhibition of the JNK and AP-1 signaling pathways [185,189]. Quercetin has also been demonstrated to reduce ventricular hypertrophy, acting primarily to modulate Ang II [190,191]. Quercetin was also found to reduce cardiac myocyte apoptosis by preventing telomere shortening [139]. Thus, quercetin rich apples and onions can prove beneficial in protection of an aging cardiovascular system.

3. FUNCTIONAL FOODS RICH IN POLYPHENOLS

3.1 Berry and Fruit Polyphenols—Anthocyanins, Flavonoids, Tannins

3.1.1. Dietary Sources

The range of polyphenolic compounds that are found in berries is quite vast and encompass the flavonoids, namely, anthocyanins, flavanols and flavonols, condensed tannins (proanthocyanidins), hydrolysable tannins (ellagitannins and gallotannins), stilbenes and phenolic acids [192]. Berries are rich in anthocyanins and flavonoids, the most commonly found polyphenols in these fruits. The most widely consumed berries in the USA being blueberry, blackberry, raspberry, cranberry and strawberry while the less popular ones are acai and mulberry amongst others [39]. The anthocyanins are responsible for imparting the deep color to the berries and their concentration can range from 437.2 mg/100 g in raw chokeberries to 90.46 mg/100 g in blackberries [39]. The significant portion of the anthocyanin content is in the skin for most berries, but in a few like strawberries, they are contained in the flesh of the fruit. Grapes contain high amounts of polyphenols both in their skin and in their flesh. Also, polyphenols are found in grape seed extracts and in grape juice [193]. The polyphenols in grapes are phenolic acids, anthocyanins and flavonoids and their composition and content can vary depending on the location of grape cultivation [193]. The amount of resveratrol, which is one of the polyphenols in grapes, has been discussed in detail in the previous sections. Other dietary sources of anthocyanins include vegetables like red cabbage that contain 322 mg/100 g, whereas juices like pomegranate contain 15–252 mg/L and fruits like plum and grapefruit have lower content 2–25 mg/100 g and 5.9 mg/100 g respectively [194]. Other dietary sources of flavonols include apples (0.1–45 mg/100 g), plums (3.7–79 mg/100 g), and cherries (6.3–23 mg/100 g) to name a few [194]. Tannins are found in grape extracts and in red wine polyphenols (RWPs), in Indian blackberries (*Jamun*), plums, pomegranate *etc.* [192,195,196].

3.1.2. Epidemiological Data and Clinical Studies on Berries and Fruit Polyphenols

Numerous human intervention studies have been undertaken to assess the relationship between the consumption of fruits and vegetables in reducing CVD related risks. This has been reviewed extensively elsewhere [197]. In brief, purple grape juice was found to be most potent in reducing platelet aggregation; a diet rich in flavonoids, for example intake of 50 mL/day pomegranate juice or 150 g/day mixed berry juice (bilberry, ligonberry, black currant, strawberry, and raspberry) significantly reduced blood pressure in hypertensives. Purple grape juice and pomegranate juice improved vascular function as well as improved blood lipid profiles [197]. In the Zutphen elderly study, an inverse correlation was found between consumption of flavonoid rich fruits and vegetables and mortality from coronary heart disease in elderly male subjects [98,198]. Another study on an elderly cohort, a subset of the CPSII nutrition study in the USA, also came to the same conclusions about fruits and vegetable consumption and CVD related mortality [199].

The FINRISK study was undertaken initially in 1972 to understand the reasons for the highest coronary heart disease (CHD) related death in Finnish men in the 1960s. The study went on until 2007 to analyze trends and monitor risk factors via a survey every 5 years, and to assess the association of lifestyle and dietary trends with mortality in Finland. The study reported that the intervention after the initial survey (in 1972 and 1977) resulted in a gradual decline in CHD related mortality in this population underscored by a reduction in blood pressure and improvement in blood lipid profiles. The reduction in mortality index over the 30 years (from 1977 to 2007) was attributed to increased awareness and changes in health behavior attributable to major changes in dietary patterns with increase in intake of vegetables and fruit and a change in type of fat consumed [200].

In another study in Finland, the Kuopio Ischemic Heart Disease Study (KIHD) analyzed whether a diet rich in fruits and vegetables is associated with a decreased risk of cardiovascular disorders. In this study the dietary intake of a population of men from Eastern Finland was analyzed by a qualitative assessment of nutritional intake using a questionnaire to record dietary intake over 4 days. The intake of fruits, berries and vegetables was 41% lower in the population that had the highest mortality at the 5 year follow up. The key findings of the study points to the increased occurrence of CVD and non-CVD related mortality in the group with the lowest consumption of fruits, berries and vegetables at the follow up after 12.8 years [201]. Further, the measures of cardiovascular health like serum HDL and cholesterol levels were also significantly higher in the group that consumed the least amount of fruits, berries and vegetables, and parameters for metabolic disorders such as insulin levels were increased as well [201].

The INTERHEART study involved participants from 52 countries to assess the relationship between diet and risk for acute myocardial infarction (AMI) globally. The diet of the subjects was classified as Oriental, Western or prudent with the Oriental diet being high in tofu and soy, the Western diet being high in fried food, salty snacks and meat while the prudent diet was high in fruits and vegetables. The study observed an inverse correlation between the risk for AMI and the prudent diet [202]. Interestingly, participants of the INTERHEART study were also analyzed in another report that studied the effect of gene-environment interactions and the predisposition to CVD. Four SNPs from chromosome 9p21 that had been previously identified as being associated with increased risk in MI were assessed in the INTERHEART participants and it was found that diet modified the risk associated with these SNPs, reducing it in individuals who consumed the prudent diet [203]. The same study also expanded to analyzing individuals from the FINRISK study, with the same conclusion that with increased consumption of vegetable and fruits, the risk of CVD, associated with alleles at chromosome 9p21, was significantly reduced [203].

3.1.3. Mechanism of Action of Berry and Fruit Polyphenols—Cell and Animal Studies

The cardioprotective effects of berry and fruit polyphenols range from their anti-atherogenic and anti-inflammatory properties to their ability to modulate platelet aggregation and aid in recovery from ischemia reperfusion injury [39,197]. A few examples of cell and animal studies that aided evidence support of these cardioprotective properties are summarized here.

Apolipoprotein E deficient mice (Apo E) have an increased capacity for the intake of oxidized LDL into their macrophages, a hallmark of the early stages of atherosclerosis and foam cell formation [17]. Consumption of pomegranate byproduct by such mice resulted in 57% reduction in atherosclerotic lesion size. Further, in macrophages obtained from ApoE mice, the cellular lipid content was lowered by 53% and uptake of oxidized LDL was reduced by 19%, suggesting that pomegranate byproduct significantly attenuated the development of atherosclerosis [204]. ApoE deficient mice fed a diet rich in blueberries showed a recession in the symptoms of atherosclerosis by reducing the number of atherosclerotic lesions and importantly upregulating the synthesis of 4 key antioxidant enzymes in the liver and serum namely SOD 1 and 2, GSR, Thioredoxin (Tnxrd1) and serum Paraoxonase (PON1). Astonishingly, all these anti-atherosclerotic effects were observed without alterations in the lipid composition of serum; in fact both total and LDL cholesterol levels were higher in the blueberry diet group [205]. ApoE deficient mice fed a diet of added cholesterol and a low (4.75%) or high (9.5%) amount of dried plum powder showed no changes in serum cholesterol despite the added cholesterol in the diet, but demonstrated significant reduction in atherosclerotic lesions in the aortic arch and arterial tree [206]. Similarly, a diet supplemented with apple polyphenols and apple fiber as part of their diet also proved to be anti-atherosclerotic in ApoE mice by reducing size of atherosclerotic lesions, improving lipid profile and reducing oxidative stress parameters [207].

Polyphenolic grape extracts (PGE) are inhibitory toward platelet aggregation. These PGE, containing a high amount of gallic acid, inhibit thrombin receptor activating peptide (TRAP) induced platelet aggregation by reduced Ca^{2+} mobilization and an activation of platelet endothelial cell adhesion molecule-1 (PECAM-1), a molecule which is known to reduce thrombus formation [208,209]. Pomegranate juice is also inhibitory toward platelet activation by reduction in aggregation, H_2O_2 production and Ca^{2+} mobilization in addition to reduced TxA2 production in washed platelets stimulated with collagen or arachidonic acid [210]. Peroxisome Proliferator Activated Receptors (PPARs) are a family of nuclear receptors and transcription factors that are important in lipid metabolism, cell differentiation and have also been shown to play role in inflammation; agonists to PPARs have been useful in reducing cardiac pathologies due to hypertension and inflammation [211]. In the Dahl salt sensitive rat model, the animals that received dietary supplementation of grape seed powder showed an increase in cardiac PPAR activity and reduction in the PPAR agonist NFκB. The decreased NFκB activity also reduced the cardiac expression of the cytokine TNFα and the growth factor transforming growth factor β1 (TGFβ1) [212]. In a different study, the consumption of freeze dried tart cherries (1% w/w in the diet) by the Dahl-SS animals for 90 days, was also shown to enhance hepatic PPAR and improve the condition of hyperlipidemia and hyperinsulinemia in these animals [213].

In the SHRs fed an extract of ligonberry, cranberry and blackcurrant as part of their drinking fluid ad libitum for 8 weeks showed vastly improved vascular health and reduced inflammation. The mRNA expression of COX2, MCP-1, P-selectin, VCAM-1, and ACE were notably reduced in the cranberry and ligonberry extract fed animals [214]. The levels of circulating Ang II were significantly reduced, which otherwise leads to vasoconstriction. Flavanones can also modulate inflammatory process in atherosclerosis by reducing the binding of monocytes treated with Naringenin and Hesperitin, flavanones found primarily in citrus fruits, to TNFα activated endothelial cells [215].

Berry consumption may also be beneficial in reducing blood pressure. In a study utilizing the SHR model to analyze the effect of acetylcholine (Ach) induced vasorelaxation and phenylephrine induced vasoconstriction in animals fed a diet enriched with freeze dried blueberries (8% w/w with regular rat chow) for 7 weeks to assess the vasomotor tone in aortas of the animals. The study demonstrated that the Ach mediated vascular smooth relaxation was increased due to the blueberry diet, amplified when the NO pathway was blocked using L-NMMA and attenuated when the COX pathway was eliminated using Mefenamic acid a COX inhibitor, suggesting these berries affect the NO and COX pathway stimulated by Ach [216]. In the stroke prone SHRs, consumption of freeze dried blueberries (3% w/w) for 8 weeks reduced blood pressure by 19% by week 4 and 30% by week 6 relative to controls [217]. This reduction in blood pressure may in part be due to the inhibition of ACE activity and lowered Ang II levels in the plasma [218]. Reduction of blood pressure in SHR was also accomplished by intake of raspberry ethyl extracts; this was accompanied by increase in SOD and serum NO and lowered MDA and plasma ET-1 [219].

In a study of recovery from ischemia, Sprague Dawley rats were fed with an extract made from either grape skin or grape flesh (2.5 mg/kg/day) for 30 days. The hearts were isolated and ischemia induced for 30 min followed by a 2 h reperfusion. Post ischemic function was assessed by blood flow through the coronary artery, myocardial infarct size and estimation of ROS by measuring malonaldehyde (MDA) in the heart. The data showed that both grape skin and flesh were equally cardioprotective as evidenced by improved recovery from ischemia, smaller infarct size and reduced MDA content in the heart as compared to the control group [220]. Blueberry supplementation in rats that underwent coronary ligation induced myocardial infarction showed a 22% improvement in survival rates as well as reduction in the expansion of myocardial infarcts [221,222]. Mechanistically, this might be achieved by stimulating the synthesis of NOS via the Akt pathway, as was the case in chick embryonic cardiomyocytes stimulated with grape seed extract, thereby protecting from I/R induced cell death [223].

3.1.4. Berries and Fruits in Cardiovascular Aging

Berries contain a broad range of phenolics with strong antioxidant potential. Anthocyanins (billberries, blackberries, crowberries), hydroxycinnamic acid (currants, blueberries and sweet cherries), flavonol (blueberries), flavan-3-ol (red raspberries), caffeic acid, gallic acid, quercetin, rutin and naringenin (mulberry leaves) are some of the better studied phenolics with antioxidant function [224,225,226,227]. Pomegranates have also been demonstrated to have anti thrombolytic activity and a strong antioxidant ability [228]. Also, pomegranate juice improved antioxidant function in elderly subjects [229]. Antioxidant defenses stimulated by anthocyanins improved endothelial function by NO dependent relaxation of arteries. Anthocyanins are anti-thrombolytic by virtue of inhibiting thrombin receptor-activating peptide-induced platelet aggregation. They are anti-inflammatory and inhibit NFκB and CD40 signaling pathways. Anthocyanins reduce VEGF secretion and down regulate p38 MAPK and c-Jun *N*-terminal kinase pathways, thereby impacting proliferation and migration of VSMCs [194,230]. Hydroxycinnamic acid has been shown to be a strong free radical scavenging polyphenol [231]. Herperdin, the flavonone found in citrus fruits, improved the antioxidant enzymes in aged rat hearts by upregulation of SOD, CAT, and Gpx amongst others, reduced the levels of MDA and increased the level of Nrf-2 [232]. In summary, berries and fruits have several synergistically functioning polyphenols that offer significant cardioprotective functions. The Zutphen elderly study, and other studies on cohorts of elderly subjects have undoubtedly shown the importance of a diet rich in fruits and vegetables as an important parameter for healthy aging and reduced CVD risk [98,198,199].

3.2 Olive Oil Polyphenols—Hydroxytyrosol and Oleuropein

3.2.1. Dietary Sources

Previously; the beneficial health effects of olive oil were attributed primarily to its high monounsaturated fatty acid (MUFA) content; mainly in the form of oleic acid; MUFA content being 56%–84% of total fatty acid content [233]. When the antioxidant ability of olive oil was demonstrated in a variety of studies; it brought to limelight the most representative phenolics in extra virgin olive oil namely hydroxytyrosol and oleuropein [233,234]. There is a clear distinction among types of olive oil in terms of polyphenolic content; since extra virgin olive oil has a greater concentration of polyphenolic compounds than refined olive oil [233,235]. There are a variety of factors which affect the quality of the oil; primarily its oxidative stability which is in turn dependent on the MUFA/PUFA ratio; the higher the ratio; the better the oil; however, as the fruit ripens; this ratio falls [236]. Furthermore, the riper the olive; the lower the quantity of phenolics in the oil [237]. Also; some authors have argued that the oxidative stability of the oil is dependent on the phenolic content; therefore, a ripening index (RI) must be determined for each olive cultivar to extract oil with maximum stability in terms of high MUFA/PUFA ratio as well as higher phenolic content [238].

3.2.2. Epidemiological Data and Clinical Studies on Olive Oil

Large majority of studies attribute the beneficial health effects of the Mediterranean diet to olive oil because of its MUFA content. MUFAs are reported to improve heart disease risk factors by lowering total cholesterol levels as well as LDL cholesterol [239,240]. However, minor constituents of olive oil are also suggested to play a larger role in cardiovascular health, see review [241]. In fact, extra virgin olive oil has cholesterol lowering effects that are independent from the fatty acid content of the oil. For instance, diets enriched with virgin olive oil having a polyphenolic composition of 34.3 ± 1.5 mg/100 g resulted in a 7.3% reduction of LDL cholesterol in volunteers compared to baseline measurements [242]. Further, extra virgin olive oil had a greater antioxidant effect on the *in vitro* oxidation of LDL induced via peroxyl radicals and metals than refined olive oil [235]. Healthy male volunteers were administered a daily dose of olive oil containing any of the three varying levels of polyphenol content: low, medium or high. Volunteers with any intervention demonstrated increased HDL levels, decreased total cholesterol:HDL ratio and triglyceride levels, as well as an improved oxidized:reduced glutathione ratio. Interventions, excluding the low polyphenol olive oil, decreased LDL:HDL ratio and high polyphenol olive oil had reduced hydroxyl fatty acids and circulating oxLDL levels. Olive oil with increasing phenolic composition resulted in increasing HDL levels, decreasing total cholesterol:HDL ratio and oxidative biomarkers [243,244]. Similar studies indicate the beneficial effects of virgin olive oil compared to refined in terms of lipid profiles of healthy subjects [239,245,246]. Comparable doses of extra virgin olive oil to raw intake in some Spanish regions resulted in lower oxLDL and lipid peroxide levels and higher glutathione peroxidase activity in males with stable CHD. There is also evidence of anti-hypertensive effects of virgin olive oil since these males with CHD also had reduced systolic blood pressure [247]. In addition, extra virgin olive oil reduced inflammatory markers, TXB2 and LTB4, in 12 healthy participants consuming 150 g of mashed potatoes with 50mL of olive oil [248].

Antioxidant properties of the polyphenolic compounds found in olive oil were corroborated by Visioli, Bellomo, & Galli (1998) [234]. Radical scavenging activity, including that of superoxide anions, as well as protecting against hyperchlorite damage and inactivation of catalase were witnessed with hydroxtyrosol and oleuropein [234,249]. Importantly, there is evidence indicating that these major polyphenols, including tyrosol, have a high bioavailability in humans [240].

3.2.3. Mechanism of Action of Olive Oil—Cell and Animal Studies

The protective effects of the olive oil polyphenols, hydroxytyrosol and oleuropein, are reported in *in vitro*models of LDL oxidation. Hydroxytryosol inhibits the increase of lipid peroxidation markers, F2-isoprostanes and TBARS, as well as production of superoxide anion and H_2O_2, in addition to, preserving total glutathione content, GSR and GPx activity and transcript levels [250,251,252]. Oleuropein inhibited oxidation of lipoproteins, generation of superoxide anion and H_2O_2 as well, and reversed the decreased glutathione content, GSR and GPx activity observed with LDL oxidation [253].

Olive oil polyphenols have a potential role in improving the pathophysiology of atherosclerosis. For example, olive oil intervention improves endothelial function and reduces inflammation parameters, thereby, aiding in the treatment of atherosclerosis patients [254]. Experimental studies involving rabbits subjected to an atherogenic diet enriched with saturated fatty acids display hyperactivity of platelets, thrombogenicity and poor lipid profiles. Supplementation with olive oil improved the outcome of atherosclerosis via improving the lipid profile, reducing platelet hyperactivity and endothelial thrombogenicity and reducing the severity of endothelium and vascular wall lesions [255]. Similarly, rabbits fed a diet supplemented with hydroxytyrosol following an atherogenic diet had an improved lipid profile and a diminished total cross-sectional area and that of the intima layer of the aortic arch was observed [256]. Further, platelet aggregation is inhibited via the phenol component of olive oil [257]. Similar investigations have demonstrated the antioxidant and anti-atherogenic effects of olive oil polyphenols on the cardiovascular system [258]. However, it should be noted that hydroxytyrosol does not enhance eNOS or NO bioavailability in healthy circumstances. It is possible that hydroxytyrosol could preserve eNOS function indirectly under pro-inflammatory conditions only [259]. Inflammatory angiogenesis has a role in the progression of atherosclerosis, which is markedly reduced with *in vitro* treatment of olive oil polyphenols. The antioxidant effects of olive oil polyphenols are attributed to the inhibition of COX-2 and MMP-9 which are regulated by redox-sensitive signaling pathways and typically promote angiogenesis [260]. Extra virgin olive oil reduced cell surface expression of VCAM-1 and ICAM-1 in an *in vitro* model of inflammation [261,262]. Oleuropein and hydroxtyrosol reduced monocyte adhesion to the endothelial primarily due to the inhibition of VCAM-1 mRNA and protein expression. Further, transcriptional activation of the VCAM-1 gene via NF-κB and AP-1 was inhibited by the olive oil polyphenols screened [261,263]. Similar reductions were seen in the expression of adhesion molecules: *E*-selectin and ICAM [263]. Oleuropein demonstrates anti-proliferative properties on VSMCs by blocking cells in G1 to S phase via inhibition of ERK1/2 activation [264].

Oxidative stress is involved in myocardial damages associated with I/R, which suggests that the antioxidant capabilities of olive oil polyphenols might have a potential protective effect in the pathophysiology of I/R injury. For example, treatment with oleuropein prior to I/R induction in rat hearts resulted in a reduction in release of oxidize glutathione, a marker of the heart's exposure to oxidative stress. Additionally, oleuropein decreased creatine kinase activity, another measure of myocardial damage [265].

Polyphenols found in olive oil, particularly extra virgin olive oil, are recognized as having an important role in the protection of cardiovascular ailments including improvements in lipid profiles within clinical and experimental studies. It is important to note that these cardiovascular health benefits are not only attributed to the MUFA content of olive oil but to these polyphenols as well.

3.2.4. Olive Oil in Cardiovascular Aging

Olive oil is rich in MUFAs and over 30 different phenolic compounds, which together, make this potent super food likely to be a key player in lowered incidence of atherosclerosis and CVD in aging Mediterranean populations. A study on elderly people consuming the Mediterranean diet, reported that the proinflammatory markers NF-κB, MCP-1, TNF-α and IL-6 as well as atherogenic marker MMP-9 was reduced in PBMC from these subjects [266]. Additionally, the bioavailability of olive oil phenolics remains high after ingestion [267]. The predominant phenolic compounds are α-tocopherol, hydroxytyrosol, tyrosol, and oleuropein [268]. All four are potent antioxidants, with α-tocopherol and hydroxytyrosol being identified to have the greatest antioxidant scavenging potential [269]. Additionally, tyrosol has been implicated in stimulating antioxidant defenses by modulating the phosphorylation of Akt, eNOS and SIRT1 [270]. In a study on the senescence-accelerated mouse-prone 8 (SAMP8) mice, an animal model employed to understand the molecular mechanisms of age related changes, olive oil ingestion reduced cardiac oxidative stress by inducing Nrf2 and Nrf2 dependent genes as well as increased PON1 activity and SIRT1 mRNA [271]. The regulation of Akt and consequently the FOXO proteins as well as control of SIRT1 likely regulates cell viability of cardiomyocytes in the heart as well. In modulating the anti-inflammatory response, IL-1B levels are decreased by oleuropin [272] and COX1 and COX2 have been shown to be inhibited by another phenolic, oleocanthal in a dose dependent manner [273]. Extra virgin olive oil consumption (25 mL/day for 3 weeks) showed reduction in anti-inflammatory properties as a function of aging in healthy elderly subjects by modulating PON1 and decreasing age related atherogenic changes [274]. Proliferation of VSMCs in the aging arterial laminae are likely modulated by selective NO level based Akt inactivation by hydroxytyrosol [275]. Phenolics in olive oil have also been shown to modulate clotting, thereby adding to their cardioprotective value in an aging cardiovascular system [257,276]. A staple of Mediterranean communities, evidence suggests that olive oil clearly contributes considerably to a robust cardiovascular system.

4. THE POTENTIAL AND LIMITATIONS OF POLYPHENOLS IN TREATMENT OF HUMAN HEART DISEASE

Polyphenols can exert beneficial effects via their antioxidant capabilities yet interventions with antioxidants in clinical trials have been unsuccessful in the prevention and treatment of cardiovascular diseases. In particular, β-carotene, an antioxidant most commonly found in carrots, pumpkin, sweet potato, and others showed promise in experimental studies but failed in human trials. After 12 years of treatment, no significant benefit or harm of β-carotene treatment on myocardial infarction, stroke or cardiovascular death was determined [277,278]. Clinical trials of polyphenols as supplements for cardiovascular disease have also yielded inconsistent results, both positive and ineffectual. The following studies are a few examples of studies that demonstrated positive effects of polyphenol supplementation in heart disease patients. Consumption of resveratrol-rich grape supplement for 1 year improved inflammatory and fibrinolytic status of patients undergoing primary prevention of cardiovascular disease [59]. Additionally, blood pressure of 67 men at high cardiovascular risk was attenuated following a 4 week intervention of dealcoholized red wine [279]. Consumption of 7 mL/kg/day of purple grape juice inhibited platelet aggregation in 20 healthy subjects as well as increased NO production, α-tocopherol levels and decreased superoxide release [280]. Participants in a clinical study investigating the effects of freeze-dried blueberry beverage on cardiovascular risk factors showed positive results. These participants presenting with metabolic syndrome had a decrease in blood pressure with the 8 week blueberry intervention [281]. Positive effects on brachial artery vasomotor function were seen after consumption of black tea after 2 h and 4 weeks in 66 patients with coronary artery disease [282]. EGCG supplementation at 400mg reduced diastolic blood pressure in 46 overweight/obese males [283]. Additionally, throughout this review, various examples of other clinical as well as epidemiological studies have been highlighted that have emphasized the significance and correlation of diets rich in polyphenols and better cardiovascular health. However, some clinical trials have not had success with polyphenol and functional food intervention. For instance, capsules containing 800 mg polyphenols derived from either wine grape mix or grape seeds had no major impact on flow-mediated dilation in 35 healthy males [284]. Similarly, intervention with polyphenol-rich or polyphenol-poor apples did not affect flow-mediated dilation or other cardiovascular disease risk factors of 30 hypercholesterolemic volunteers [285]. Finally, biomarkers of cardiovascular disease risk were unchanged with a daily 3 week intervention of six capsules containing green tea extracts [286]. Similarly, green and black tea supplementation had no effect on cardiovascular disease risk parameters [287,288].

Further adverse effects of these compounds have also been indicated in a few studies. Though the studies reported are not necessarily all pertaining to cardiovascular conditions, it is important to note that polyphenols have been shown to be disadvantageous in certain circumstances related to interactions with other substances, pro-oxidant activity, toxicity and tumorigenesis [289]. Polyphenols can influence availability of a number of compounds, by binding to and forming complexes with proteins, and metal cations affecting their absorption [290]. For instance, the bioavailability of iron within humans was shown to be affected by tea, a major source of polyphenols [291,292]. However, two recent studies concluded that tea consumption does not influence iron status in populations where iron intake is adequate [293,294]. Polyphenols can have pro-oxidant effects, which normally aid in the plant's defense system. In the presence of oxygen and transition metals, such as copper and iron, redox cycling of polyphenols is initiated to generate ROS, leading to cellular injury including DNA damage [295]. Toxicity of polyphenols, particularly EGCG, was determined at a concentration of 2000 mg/kg/day in rats of which lethality was the measure of toxicity. In the same study, it was determined that doses up to 500 mg/kg/day for 13 weeks was not toxic in these animals [296]. Tumorigenesis has also been documented *in vitro* and *in vivo* models employing treatments with polyphenols. For example, carcinogen-exposed rats treated with 0.1% green tea catechins had an increase in average tumor size compared to controls. Interestingly, supplementation with 1% green tea catechins did not affect tumor size. Neither dose of green tea catechins contributed to incidence nor multiplicity of tumors in these animals [297]. Similarly to the animal study, cell proliferation in a cell culture model was stimulated with a lower concentration of quercetin yet a higher concentration decreased cell proliferation [298]. Thus, dosage of polyphenols is important to minimize harmful effects of their use.

Therefore, consideration for the bioavailability of these compounds, dosage parameters, and the interaction of polyphenols and other bioactive compounds in functional foods is important and may contribute to the effectiveness of interventions described in the clinic [299]. Bioavailability of these compounds as well as pharmacological properties and kinetics of absorption need to be further evaluated to improve our comprehension of their behavior within the body, and to aid in the investigation of intervention studies. More stable analogs with similar bioactivities but better bioavailability are being designed with the goal of developing functional nutraceuticals and to minimize harmful effects [300].

5. CONCLUSIONS

A number of epidemiological trends and clinical studies support the notion of a diet rich in fruits and vegetables being correlated with reduced cardiovascular complications and mortality. Polyphenol rich diets have been associated with reducing CVD risk thereby promoting optimal aging. The literature reviewed here validates that treatment of cells and animal models with polyphenols counteracts the burden of oxidative stress and influences signaling pathways to diminish the risk associated with cardiovascular diseases, and endorses their therapeutic efficacy in functioning as anti-aging molecules (Figure 1). These findings are sufficiently corroborated by longitudinal studies on human subjects, with some of the studies being reported in our review. It may not be single polyphenols but a combination found in a given food that may be responsible for the health benefit seen across populations. As Wersching (2011) points out, the direct interplay between nutrients in whole fruits and vegetables may be more important than the unique nutrients on their own in the reduction of risk in cardiovascular disease [301]. Further studies on bioavailability and kinetics of absorption need to be undertaken with the goal to find the combinatorial mix that acts synergistically upon the various targets, to then as a whole reduce the economic burden of cardiovascular disease and to promote healthy aging.

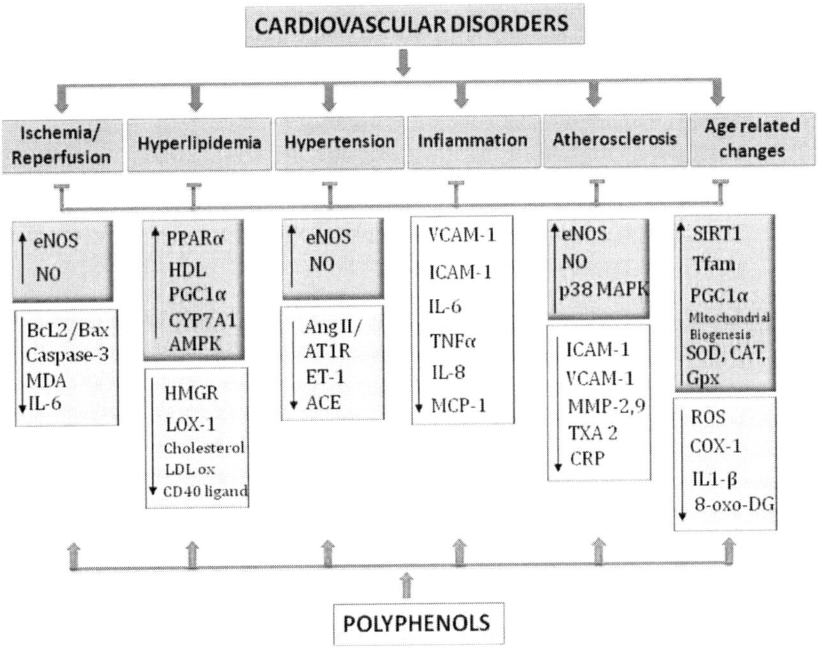

Figure 1. Mechanisms of protection by polyphenols in the cardiovascular system, in disease and in aging.

CONFLICTS OF INTEREST

The authors declare no conflict of interest.

REFERENCES

1. Lindlahr, V.H. How to Win and Keep Health with Foods; Kessinger Publishing: Whitefish, Montana, MT, USA, 2006; p. 132.
2. Pandey, K.B.; Rizvi, S.I. Plant polyphenols as dietary antioxidants in human health and disease. Oxid. Med. Cell. Longev. 2009, 2, 270–278.
3. Manach, C.; Scalbert, A.; Morand, C.; Rémésy, C.; Jiménez, L. Polyphenols: Food sources and bioavailability. Am. J. Clin. Nutr. 2004, 79, 727–747.
4. Arts, I.C.W.; Hollman, P.C.H. Polyphenols and disease risk in epidemiologic studies. Am. J. Clin. Nutr.2005, 81, 317S–325S.

5. Renaud, S.; de Lorgeril, M. Wine, alcohol, platelets, and the French paradox for coronary heart disease. Lancet 1992, 339, 1523–1526.

6. Opie, L.H.; Lecour, S. The red wine hypothesis: From concepts to protective signalling molecules. Eur. Heart J. 2007, 28, 1683–1693.

7. Huang, C.L.; Sumpio, B.E. Olive oil, the mediterranean diet, and cardiovascular health. J. Am. Coll. Surg. 2008, 207, 407–416.

8. Dhalla, N.S.; Temsah, R.M.; Netticadan, T. Role of oxidative stress in cardiovascular diseases. J. Hypertens. 2000, 18, 655–673.

9. Hamilton, C.A.; Miller, W.H.; Al-Benna, S.; Brosnan, M.J.; Drummond, R.D.; McBride, M.W.; Dominiczak, A.F. Strategies to reduce oxidative stress in cardiovascular disease. Clin. Sci. (Lond.) 2004,106, 219–234.

10. Brieger, K.; Schiavone, S.; Miller, F.J.; Krause, K.H. Reactive oxygen species: From health to disease.Swiss Med. Wkly. 2012, 142, w13659.

11. Selvaraju, V.; Joshi, M.; Suresh, S.; Sanchez, J.A.; Maulik, N.; Maulik, G. Diabetes, oxidative stress, molecular mechanism, and cardiovascular disease—An overview. Toxicol. Mech. Methods 2012, 22, 330–335.

12. Sugamura, K.; Keaney, J.F., Jr. Reactive oxygen species in cardiovascular disease. Free Radic. Biol. Med.2011, 51, 978–992.

13. Venkataraman, K.; Khurana, S.; Tai, T.C. Oxidative stress in aging-matters of the heart and mind. Int. J. Mol. Sci. 2013, 14, 17897–17925.

14. Raedschelders, K.; Ansley, D.M.; Chen, D.D.Y. The cellular and molecular origin of reactive oxygen species generation during myocardial ischemia and reperfusion. Pharmacol. Ther. 2012, 133, 230–255.

15. Cai, H.; Harrison, D.G. Endothelial dysfunction in cardiovascular diseases: The role of oxidant stress.Circ. Res. 2000, 87, 840–844.

16. Paravicini, T.M.; Touyz, R.M. NADPH oxidases, reactive oxygen species, and hypertension: Clinical implications and therapeutic possibilities. Diabetes Care 2008, 31, S170–S180.

17. Hansson, G.K.; Libby, P. The immune response in atherosclerosis: A double-edged sword. Nat. Rev. Immunol. 2006, 6, 508–519.

18. Libby, P. Inflammation and cardiovascular disease mechanisms. Am. J. Clin. Nutr. 2006, 83, 456S–460S.

19. Huo, Y.; Ley, K.F. Role of platelets in the development of atherosclerosis. Trends Cardiovasc. Med. 2004,14, 18–22.

20. Gawaz, M. Role of platelets in coronary thrombosis and reperfusion of ischemic myocardium.Cardiovasc. Res. 2004, 61, 498–511.

21. Iijima, K.; Yoshizumi, M.; Hashimoto, M.; Kim, S.; Eto, M.; Ako, J.; Liang, Y.Q.; Sudoh, N.; Hosoda, K.; Nakahara, K.; et al. Red wine polyphenols inhibit proliferation of vascular smooth muscle cells and downregulate expression of cyclin A gene. Circulation 2000, 101, 805–811.

22. Maulik, S.K.; Kumar, S. Oxidative stress and cardiac hypertrophy: A review. Toxicol. Mech. Methods2012, 22, 359–366.

23. Daou, G.B.; Srivastava, A.K. Reactive oxygen species mediate Endothelin-1-induced activation of ERK1/2, PKB, and Pyk2 signaling, as well as protein synthesis, in vascular smooth muscle cells. Free Radic. Biol. Med. 2004, 37, 208–215.

24. Schiffrin, E.L. Role of endothelin-1 in hypertension. 1999, 34, 876–881.

25. Williams, B. Angiotensin II and the pathophysiology of cardiovascular remodeling. Am. J. Cardiol.2001, 87, 10–17.

26. Dhalla, N.S.; Elmoselhi, A.B.; Hata, T.; Makino, N. Status of myocardial antioxidants in ischemia-reperfusion injury. Cardiovasc. Res. 2000, 47, 446–456.

27. Borradaile, N.M.; Pickering, J.G. NAD(+), sirtuins, and cardiovascular disease. Curr. Pharm. Des. 2009,15, 110–117.

28. Habauzit, V.; Morand, C. Evidence for a protective effect of polyphenols-containing foods on cardiovascular health: An update for clinicians. Ther. Adv. Chronic Dis. 2012, 3, 87–106.

29. Sies, H. Polyphenols and health: Update and perspectives. Arch. Biochem. Biophys. 2010, 501, 2–5.

30. Rodrigo, R.; Miranda, A.; Vergara, L. Modulation of endogenous antioxidant system by wine polyphenols in human disease. Clin. Chim. Acta 2011, 412, 410–424.

31. Cao, Z.; Li, Y. Potent induction of cellular antioxidants and phase 2 enzymes by resveratrol in cardiomyocytes: Protection against oxidative and electrophilic injury. Eur. J. Pharmacol. 2004, 489, 39–48.

32. Ungvari, Z.; Bagi, Z.; Feher, A.; Recchia, F.A.; Sonntag, W.E.; Pearson, K.; de Cabo, R.; Csiszar, A. Resveratrol confers endothelial protection via activation of the antioxidant transcription factor Nrf2.Am. J. Physiol. Heart Circ. Physiol. 2010, 299, H18–H24.

33. Stangl, V.; Dreger, H.; Stangl, K.; Lorenz, M. Molecular targets of tea polyphenols in the cardiovascular system. Cardiovasc. Res. 2012, 73, 348–358.

34. Vauzour, D.; Rodriguez-Mateos, A.; Corona, G.; Oruna-Concha, M.J.; Spencer, J.P.E. Polyphenols and human health: Prevention of disease and mechanisms of action. Nutrients 2010, 2, 1106–1131.

35. Rahman, I.; Biswas, S.K.; Kirkham, P.A. Regulation of inflammation and redox signaling by dietary polyphenols. Biochem. Pharmacol. 2006, 72, 1439–1452.

36. Middleton, E.; Kandaswami, C.; Theoharides, T.C. The effects of plant flavonoids on mammalian cells: Implications for inflammation, heart disease, and cancer. Pharmacol. Rev. 2000, 52, 673–751.

37. Scalbert, A.; Johnson, I.T.; Saltmarsh, M. Polyphenols: Antioxidants and beyond. Am. J. Clin. Nutr.2005, 81, 215–217.

38. Parks, D.A.; Booyse, F.M. Cardiovascular protection by alcohol and polyphenols—Role of nitric oxide.2002, 957, 115–121.

39. Basu, A. Berries: Emerging impact on cardiovascular health. Nutr. Rev. 2011, 68, 168–177.

40. Vita, J.A. Polyphenols and cardiovascular disease: Effects on endothelial and platelet function. Am. J. Clin. Nutr. 2005, 81, 292–297.

41. Baur, J.A.; Sinclair, D.A. Therapeutic potential of resveratrol: The in vivo evidence. Nat. Rev. Drug Dis.2006, 5, 493–506.

42. Karavidas, A.; Lazaros, G.; Tsiachris, D.; Pyrgakis, V. Aging and the cardiovascular system. Hell. J. Cardiol. 2010, 51, 421–427.

43. Maruyama, Y. Aging and arterial-cardiac interactions in the elderly. Int. J. Cardiol. 2012, 155, 14–19.

44. Orlandi, A.; Bochaton-Piallat, M.L.; Gabbiani, G.; Spagnoli, L.G. Aging, smooth muscle cells and vascular pathobiology: Implications for atherosclerosis. Atherosclerosis 2006, 188, 221–230.

45. Ferrari, A.U.; Radaelli, A.; Centola, M. Invited review: Aging and the cardiovascular system. J. Appl. Physiol. 2003, 95, 2591–2597.

46. Coleman, R.; Hayek, T.; Keidar, S.; Aviram, M. A mouse model for human atherosclerosis: Long-term histopathological study of lesion development in the aortic arch of apolipoprotein E-deficient (E0) mice. Acta Histochem. 2006, 108, 415–424.

47. Csiszar, A. Anti-inflammatory effects of resveratrol: Possible role in prevention of age-related cardiovascular disease. Ann. N. Y. Acad. Sci. 2011, 1215, 117–122.

48. Ungvari, Z.; Sonntag, W.E.; Csiszar, A. Mitochondria and aging in the vascular system. J. Mol. Med. (Berl.) 2010, 88, 1021–1027.

49. Avery, S.V. Molecular targets of oxidative stress. Biochem. J. 2011, 434, 201–210.

50. Burns, J.; Yokota, T.; Ashihara, H.; Lean, M.E.J.; Crozier, A. Plant foods and herbal sources of resveratrol. J. Agric. Food Chem. 2002, 50, 3337–3340.

51. Gu, X.; Creasy, L.; Kester, A.; Zeece, M. Capillary electrophoretic determination of resveratrol in wines. J. Agric. Food Chem. 1999, 47, 3223–3227.

52. Gonçalves, J.; Câmara, J.S. New method for determination of (E)-resveratrol in wine based on microextraction using packed sorbent and ultra-performance liquid chromatography. J. Sep. Sci. 2011,34, 2376–2384.

53. Netticadan, T. Why research on resveratrol-mediated cardioprotection should not decelerate. Can. J. Physiol. Pharmacol. 2012, 90.

54. Ragab, A.S.; van Fleet, J.; Jankowski, B.; Park, J.H.; Bobzin, S.C. Detection and quantitation of resveratrol in tomato fruit

(Lycopersicon esculentum Mill.). J. Agric. Food Chem. 2006, 54, 7175–7179.

55. Hurst, W.J.; Glinski, J.A.; Miller, K.B.; Apgar, J.; Davey, M.H.; Stuart, D.A. Survey of the trans-resveratrol and trans-piceid content of cocoa-containing and chocolate products. J. Agric. Food Chem.2008, 56, 8374–8378.

56. Bothig, S. WHO MONICA project: Objectives and design. Int. J. Epidemiol. 1989, 18, S29–S37.

57. Smoliga, J.M.; Baur, J.A.; Hausenblas, H.A. Resveratrol and health—A comprehensive review of human clinical trials. Mol. Nutr. Food Res. 2011, 55, 1129–1141.

58. Magyar, K.; Halmosi, R.; Palfi, A.; Feher, G.; Czopf, L.; Fulop, A.; Battyany, I.; Sumegi, B.; Toth, K.; Szabados, E. Cardioprotection by resveratrol: A human clinical trial in patients with stable coronary artery disease. Clin. Hemorheol. Microcirc. 2012, 50, 179–187.

59. Tomé-Carneiro, J.; Gonzálvez, M.; Larrosa, M.; Yáñez-Gascón, M.J.; García-Almagro, F.J.; Ruiz-Ros, J.A.; García-Conesa, M.T.; Tomás-Barberán, F.A.; Espín, J.C. One-year consumption of a grape nutraceutical containing resveratrol improves the inflammatory and fibrinolytic status of patients in primary prevention of cardiovascular disease. Am. J. Cardiol. 2012, 110, 356–363.

60. Tomé-Carneiro, J.; Gonzálvez, M.; Larrosa, M.; García-Almagro, F.J.; Avilés-Plaza, F.; Parra, S.; Yáñez-Gascón, M.J.; Ruiz-Ros, J.A.; García-Conesa, M.T.; Tomás-Barberán, F.A.; et al. Consumption of a grape extract supplement containing resveratrol decreases oxidized LDL and ApoB in patients undergoing primary prevention of cardiovascular disease: A triple-blind, 6-month follow-up, placebo-controlled, randomized trial. Mol. Nutr. Food Res. 2012, 56, 810–821.

61. Tomé-Carneiro, J.; Gonzálvez, M.; Larrosa, M.; Yáñez-Gascón, M.J.; García-Almagro, F.J.; Ruiz-Ros, J.A.; Tomás-Barberán, F.A.; García-Conesa, M.T.; Espín, J.C. Grape resveratrol increases serum adiponectin and downregulates inflammatory genes in peripheral blood mononuclear cells: A triple-blind, placebo-controlled, one-year clinical trial in patients with stable coronary artery disease.Cardiovasc. Drugs Ther. 2013, 27, 37–48.

62. Agarwal, B.; Campen, M.J.; Channell, M.M.; Wherry, S.J.; Varamini, B.; Davis, J.G.; Baur, J.A.; Smoliga, J.M. Resveratrol for primary prevention of atherosclerosis: Clinical trial evidence for improved gene expression in vascular endothelium. Int. J. Cardiol. 2012, 8, 9–11.

63. Borriello, A.; Cucciolla, V.; Della Ragione, F.; Galletti, P. Dietary polyphenols: Focus on resveratrol, a promising agent in the prevention of cardiovascular diseases and control of glucose homeostasis.Nutr. Metab. Cardiovasc. Dis. 2010, 20, 618–625.

64. Chung, S.; Yao, H.; Caito, S.; Hwang, J.W.; Arunachalam, G.; Rahman, I. Regulation of SIRT1 in cellular functions: Role of polyphenols. Arch. Biochem. Biophys. 2010, 501, 79–90.

65. Zang, M.; Xu, S.; Maitland-Toolan, K.A.; Zuccollo, A.; Hou, X.; Jiang, B.; Wierzbicki, M.; Verbeuren, T.J.; Cohen, R.A. Polyphenols stimulate AMP-activated protein kinase, lower lipids, and inhibit accelerated atherosclerosis in diabetic LDL receptor-deficient mice. Diabetes 2006, 55, 2180–2191.

66. Csiszar, A.; Labinskyy, N.; Pinto, J.T.; Ballabh, P.; Zhang, H.; Losonczy, G.; Pearson, K.; de Cabo, R.; Pacher, P.; Zhang, C.; et al. Resveratrol induces mitochondrial biogenesis in endothelial cells. Am. J. Physiol. Heart Circ. Physiol. 2009, 297, H13–H20.

67. Wallerath, T. Resveratrol, a polyphenolic phytoalexin present in red wine, enhances expression and activity of endothelial nitric oxide synthase. Circulation 2002, 106, 1652–1658.

68. Chen, C.K.; Pace-Asciak, C.R. Vasorelaxing activity of resveratrol and quercetin in isolated rat aorta.Gen. Pharmacol. 1996, 27, 363–366.

69. Pace-Asciak, C.R.; Hahn, S.; Diamandis, E.P.; Soleas, G.; Goldberg, D.M. The red wine phenolics trans-resveratrol and quercetin block human platelet aggregation and eicosanoid synthesis: Implications for protection against coronary heart disease. Clin. Chim. Acta 1995, 235, 207–219.

70. Olas, B.; Wachowicz, B. Resveratrol, a phenolic antioxidant with effects on blood platelet functions.Platelets 2005, 16, 251–260.

71. Shen, M.Y.; Hsiao, G.; Liu, C.L.; Fong, T.H.; Lin, K.H.; Chou, D.S.; Sheu, J.R. Inhibitory mechanisms of resveratrol in platelet activation: Pivotal roles of p38 MAPK and NO/cyclic GMP. Br. J. Haematol. 2007,139, 475–485.

72. Wung, B.S.; Hsu, M.C.; Wu, C.C.; Hsieh, C.W. Resveratrol suppresses IL-6-induced ICAM-1 gene expression in endothelial cells: Effects on the inhibition of STAT3 phosphorylation. Life Sci. 2005, 78, 389–397.

73. Csiszar, A.; Smith, K.; Labinskyy, N.; Orosz, Z.; Rivera, A.; Ungvari, Z.; Resveratrol, Z.U. Resveratrol attenuates TNF-α-induced activation of coronary arterial endothelial cells: Role of NF-κB inhibition.Am. J. Physiol. Heart Circ. Physiol. 2006, 291, H1694–H1699.

74. Chung, E.Y.; Kim, B.H.; Hong, J.T.; Lee, C.K.; Ahn, B.; Nam, S.Y.; Han, S.B.; Kim, Y. Resveratrol down-regulates interferon-γ-inducible inflammatory genes in macrophages: Molecular mechanism via decreased STAT-1 activation. J. Nutr. Biochem. 2011, 22, 902–909.

75. Chen, Q.; Wang, E.; Ma, L.; Zhai, P. Dietary resveratrol increases the expression of hepatic 7α-hydroxylase and ameliorates hypercholesterolemia in high-fat fed C57BL/6J mice. Lipids Health Dis.2012, 11, 56.

76. Thandapilly, S.J.; Wojciechowski, P.; Behbahani, J.; Louis, X.L.; Yu, L.; Juric, D.; Kopilas, M.A.; Anderson, H.D.; Netticadan, T. Resveratrol prevents the development of pathological cardiac hypertrophy and contractile dysfunction in the SHR without lowering blood pressure. Am. J. Hypertens. 2010, 23, 192–196.

77. Behbahani, J.; Thandapilly, S.J.; Louis, X.L.; Huang, Y.; Shao, Z.; Kopilas, M.A.; Wojciechowski, P.; Netticadan, T.; Anderson, H.D. Resveratrol and small artery compliance and remodeling in the spontaneously hypertensive rat. Am. J. Hypertens. 2010, 23, 1273–1278.

78. Thandapilly, S.J.; Louis, X.L.; Yang, T.; Stringer, D.M.; Yu, L.; Zhang, S.; Wigle, J.; Kardami, E.; Zahradka, P.; Taylor, C.; et al. Resveratrol prevents norepinephrine induced hypertrophy in adult rat cardiomyocytes, by activating NO-AMPK pathway. Eur. J. Pharmacol. 2011, 668, 217–224.

79. Rimbaud, S.; Ruiz, M.; Piquereau, J.; Mateo, P.; Fortin, D.; Veksler, V.; Garnier, A.; Ventura-Clapier, R. Resveratrol improves survival, hemodynamics and energetics in a rat model of hypertension leading to heart failure. PLoS One 2011, 6, e26391.

80. Chen, Y.R.; Yi, F.F.; Li, X.Y.; Wang, C.Y.; Chen, L.; Yang, X.C.; Su, P.X.; Cai, J. Resveratrol attenuates ventricular arrhythmias and

improves the long-term survival in rats with myocardial infarction.Cardiovasc. Drugs Ther. 2008, 22, 479–485.

81. Shen, M.; Wu, R.X.; Zhao, L.; Li, J.; Guo, H.T.; Fan, R.; Cui, Y.; Wang, Y.M.; Yue, S.Q.; Pei, J.M. Resveratrol attenuates ischemia/reperfusion injury in neonatal cardiomyocytes and its underlying mechanism. PLoS One 2012, 7, e51223.

82. Fichtlscherer, S.; de Rosa, S.; Fox, H.; Schwietz, T.; Fischer, A.; Liebetrau, C.; Weber, M.; Hamm, C.W.; Röxe, T.; Müller-Ardogan, M.; et al. Circulating microRNAs in patients with coronary artery disease.Circ. Res. 2010, 107, 677–684.

83. Mukhopadhyay, P.; Pacher, P.; Das, D.K. MicroRNA signatures of resveratrol in the ischemic heart.Ann. N. Y. Acad. Sci. 2011, 1215, 109–116.

84. Lançon, A.; Kaminski, J.; Tili, E.; Michaille, J.J.; Latruffe, N. Control of microRNA expression as a new way for resveratrol to deliver its beneficial effects. J. Agric. Food Chem. 2012, 60, 8783–8789.

85. Mukhopadhyay, P.; Mukherjee, S.; Ahsan, K.; Bagchi, A.; Pacher, P.; Das, D.K. Restoration of altered microRNA expression in the ischemic heart with resveratrol. PLoS One 2010, 5, e15705.

86. Baur, J.A.; Pearson, K.J.; Price, N.L.; Jamieson, H.A.; Lerin, C.; Kalra, A.; Prabhu, V.V; Allard, J.S.; Lopez-Lluch, G.; Lewis, K.; et al. Resveratrol improves health and survival of mice on a high-calorie diet. Nature 2006, 444, 337–342.

87. Kumerz, M.; Heiss, E.H.; Schachner, D.; Atanasov, A.G.; Dirsch, V.M. Resveratrol inhibits migration and Rac1 activation in EGF-but not PDGF-activated vascular smooth muscle cells. Mol. Nutr. Food Res.2011, 55, 1230–1236.

88. Ong, E.T.; Hwang, T.L.; Huang, Y.L.; Lin, C.F.; Wu, W.B. Vitisin B, a resveratrol tetramer, inhibits migration through inhibition of PDGF signaling and enhancement of cell adhesiveness in cultured vascular smooth muscle cells. Toxicol. Appl. Pharmacol. 2011, 256, 198–208.

89. Dubey, R.K.; Jackson, E.K.; Gillespie, D.G.; Zacharia, L.C.; Imthurn, B.; Rosselli, M. Resveratrol, a red wine constituent, blocks the antimitogenic effects of estradiol on human female coronary artery smooth muscle cells. J. Clin. Endocrinol. Metab. 2010, 95, E9–E17.

90. Csiszar, A.; Sosnowska, D.; Wang, M.; Lakatta, E.G.; Sonntag, W.E.; Ungvari, Z. Age-associated proinflammatory secretory

phenotype in vascular smooth muscle cells from the non-human primate Macaca mulatta: Reversal by resveratrol treatment. J. Gerontol. A Biol. Sci. Med. Sci. 2012, 67, 811–820.

91. Balentine, D.A.; Wiseman, S.A.; Bouwens, L.C. The chemistry of tea flavonoids. Crit. Rev. Food Sci. Nutr. 1997, 37, 693–704.

92. Arts, I.C.; van de Putte, B.; Hollman, P.C. Catechin contents of foods commonly consumed in The Netherlands. 2. Tea, wine, fruit juices, and chocolate milk. J. Agric. Food Chem. 2000, 48, 1752–1757.

93. Arts, I.C.; van de Putte, B.; Hollman, P.C. Catechin contents of foods commonly consumed in The Netherlands. 1. Fruits, vegetables, staple foods, and processed foods. J. Agric. Food Chem. 2000, 48, 1746–1751.

94. Nagao, T.; Komine, Y.; Soga, S.; Meguro, S.; Hase, T.; Tanaka, Y.; Tokimitsu, I. Ingestion of a tea rich in catechins leads to a reduction in body fat and malondialdehyde-modified LDL in men. Am. J. Clin. Nutr. 2005, 81, 122–129.

95. Kuriyama, S.; Shimazu, T.; Ohmori, K.; Kikuchi, N.; Nakaya, N.; Nishino, Y.; Tsubono, Y.; Tsuji, I. Green tea consumption and mortality due to cardiovascular disease. JAMA 2006, 296, 1255–1265.

96. Yang, Y.C.; Lu, F.H.; Wu, J.S.; Wu, C.H.; Chang, C.J. The protective effect of habitual tea consumption on hypertension. Arch. Intern. Med. 2004, 164, 1534–1540.

97. Geleijnse, J.M.; Launer, L.J.; van der Kuip, D.A.M.; Hofman, A.; Witteman, J.C.M. Inverse association of tea and flavonoid intakes with incident myocardial infarction: The Rotterdam Study. Am. J. Clin. Nutr. 2002, 75, 880–886.

98. Hertog, M.G.; Feskens, E.J.; Hollman, P.C.; Katan, M.B.; Kromhout, D. Dietary antioxidant flavonoids and risk of coronary heart disease: The Zutphen Elderly Study. Lancet 1993, 342, 1007–1011.

99. Hertog, M.G.; Feskens, E.J.; Kromhout, D. Antioxidant flavonols and coronary heart disease risk.Lancet 1997, 349, 699.

100. Imai, K.; Nakachi, K. Cross sectional study of effects of drinking green tea on cardiovascular and liver diseases. BMJ 1995, 310, 693–696.

101. Peters, U.; Poole, C.; Arab, L. Does tea affect cardiovascular disease? A meta-analysis. Am. J. Epidemiol.2001, 154, 495–503.

102. Kuriyama, S. The relation between green tea consumption and cardiovascular disease as evidenced by epidemiological studies. J. Nutr. 2008, 138, 1548–1553.

103. Mukamal, K.J.; MacDermott, K.; Vinson, J.A.; Oyama, N.; Manning, W.J.; Mittleman, M.A. A 6-month randomized pilot study of black tea and cardiovascular risk factors. Am. Heart J. 2007, 154, 724.

104. Woodward, M.; Tunstall-Pedoe, H. Coffee and tea consumption in the Scottish Heart Health Study follow up: Conflicting relations with coronary risk factors, coronary disease, and all cause mortality. J. Epidemiol. Community Health 1999, 53, 481–487.

105. Negishi, H.; Xu, J.W.; Ikeda, K. Black and green tea polyphenols attenuate blood pressure increases in stroke-prone spontaneously hypertensive rats. J. Nutr. 2004, 134, 38–42.

106. Appeldoorn, M.M.; Venema, D.P.; Peters, T.H.F.; Koenen, M.E.; Arts, I.C.W.; Vincken, J.P.; Gruppen, H.; Keijer, J.; Hollman, P.C.H. Some phenolic compounds increase the nitric oxide level in endothelial cells in vitro. J. Agric. Food Chem. 2009, 57, 7693–7699.

107. Kim, J.A.; Formoso, G.; Li, Y.; Potenza, M.A.; Marasciulo, F.L.; Montagnani, M.; Quon, M.J. Epigallocatechin gallate, a green tea polyphenol, mediates NO-dependent vasodilation using signaling pathways in vascular endothelium requiring reactive oxygen species and Fyn. J. Biol. Chem.2007, 282, 13736–13745.

108. Lorenz, M.; Wessler, S.; Follmann, E.; Michaelis, W.; Düsterhöft, T.; Baumann, G.; Stangl, K.; Stangl, V. A constituent of green tea, epigallocatechin-3-gallate, activates endothelial nitric oxide synthase by a phosphatidylinositol-3-OH-kinase-, cAMP-dependent protein kinase-, and -dependent pathway and leads to endothelial-dependent vasorelaxation. J. Biol. Chem. 2004, 279, 6190–6195.

109. Potenza, M.A.; Marasciulo, F.L.; Tarquinio, M.; Tiravanti, E.; Colantuono, G.; Federici, A.; Kim, J.A.; Quon, M.J.; Montagnani, M. EGCG, a green tea polyphenol, improves endothelial function and insulin sensitivity, reduces blood pressure, and protects against myocardial I/R injury in SHR. Am. J. Physiol. Endocrinol. Metab. 2007, 292, E1378–E1387.

110. Ludwig, A.; Lorenz, M.; Grimbo, N.; Steinle, F.; Meiners, S.; Bartsch, C.; Stangl, K.; Baumann, G.; Stangl, V. The tea flavonoid epigallocatechin-3-gallate reduces cytokine-induced VCAM-1

expression and monocyte adhesion to endothelial cells. Biochem. Biophys. Res. Commun. 2004, 316, 659–665.

111. Pullikotil, P.; Chen, H.; Muniyappa, R.; Greenberg, C.C.; Yang, S.; Reiter, C.E.N.; Lee, J.W.; Chung, J.H.; Quon, M.J. Epigallocatechin gallate induces expression of heme oxygenase-1 in endothelial cells via p38 MAPK and Nrf-2 that suppresses proinflammatory actions of TNF-α. J. Nutr. Biochem. 2012,23, 1134–1145.

112. Wu, C.C.; Hsu, M.C.; Hsieh, C.W.; Lin, J.B.; Lai, P.H.; Wung, B.S. Upregulation of heme oxygenase-1 by Epigallocatechin-3-gallate via the phosphatidylinositol 3-kinase/Akt and ERK pathways. Life Sci.2006, 78, 2889–2897.

113. Ramesh, E.; Geraldine, P.; Thomas, P.A. Regulatory effect of epigallocatechin gallate on the expression of C-reactive protein and other inflammatory markers in an experimental model of atherosclerosis.Chem. Biol. Interact. 2010, 183, 125–132.

114. Miura, Y.; Chiba, T.; Tomita, I. Tea catechins prevent the development of atherosclerosis in apoprotein E-deficient mice. J. Nutr. 2001, 131, 27–32.

115. Senthil Kumaran, V.; Arulmathi, K.; Sundarapandiyan, R.; Kalaiselvi, P. Attenuation of the inflammatory changes and lipid anomalies by epigallocatechin-3-gallate in hypercholesterolemic diet fed aged rats. Exp. Gerontol. 2009, 44, 745–751.

116. Cuccioloni, M.; Mozzicafreddo, M.; Spina, M.; Tran, C.N.; Falconi, M.; Eleuteri, A.M.; Angeletti, M. Epigallocatechin-3-gallate potently inhibits the in vitro activity of hydroxy-3-methyl-glutaryl-CoA reductase. J. Lipid Res. 2011, 52, 897–907.

117. Yang, J.; Han, Y.; Sun, H.; Chen, C.; He, D.; Guo, J.; Yu, C.; Jiang, B.; Zhou, L.; Zeng, C. (−)-Epigallocatechin gallate suppresses proliferation of vascular smooth muscle cells induced by high glucose by inhibition of PKC and ERK1/2 signalings. J. Agric. Food Chem. 2011, 59, 11483–11490.

118. Sartor, L.; Pezzato, E.; Dell'Aica, I.; Caniato, R.; Biggin, S.; Garbisa, S. Inhibition of matrix-proteases by polyphenols: Chemical insights for anti-inflammatory and anti-invasion drug design. Biochem. Pharmacol. 2002, 64, 229–237.

119. Maeda, K.; Kuzuya, M.; Cheng, X.W.; Asai, T.; Kanda, S.; Tamaya-Mori, N.; Sasaki, T.; Shibata, T.; Iguchi, A. Green tea catechins inhibit the cultured smooth muscle cell invasion through the basement barrier. Atherosclerosis 2003, 166, 23–30.

120. Cheng, X.W.; Kuzuya, M.; Nakamura, K.; Liu, Z.; Di, Q.; Hasegawa, J.; Iwata, M.; Murohara, T.; Yokota, M.; Iguchi, A. Mechanisms of the inhibitory effect of epigallocatechin-3-gallate on cultured human vascular smooth muscle cell invasion. Arterioscler. Thromb. Vasc. Biol. 2005, 25, 1864–1870.

121. Lill, G.; Voit, S.; Schrör, K.; Weber, A.A. Complex effects of different green tea catechins on human platelets. FEBS Lett. 2003, 546, 265–270.

122. Jin, Y.R.; Im, J.H.; Park, E.S.; Cho, M.R.; Han, X.H.; Lee, J.J.; Lim, Y.; Kim, T.J.; Yun, Y.P. Antiplatelet activity of epigallocatechin gallate is mediated by the inhibition of PLCgamma2 phosphorylation, elevation of PGD2 production, and maintaining calcium-ATPase activity. J. Cardiovasc. Pharmacol.2008, 51, 45–54.

123. Reiter, C.E.N.; Kim, J.; Quon, M.J. Green tea polyphenol epigallocatechin gallate reduces endothelin-1 expression and secretion in vascular endothelial cells: Roles for AMP-activated protein kinase, Akt, and FOXO1. Endocrinology 2010, 151, 103–114.

124. Hao, J.; Kim, C.H.; Ha, T.S.; Ahn, H.Y. Epigallocatechin-3 gallate prevents cardiac hypertrophy induced by pressure overload in rats. J. Vet. Sci. 2007, 8, 121–129.

125. Sheng, R.; Gu, Z.; Xie, M.; Zhou, W.; Guo, C. EGCG inhibits cardiomyocyte apoptosis in pressure overload-induced cardiac hypertrophy and protects cardiomyocytes from oxidative stress in rats. Acta Pharmacol. Sin. 2007, 28, 191–201.

126. Ou, H.C.; Song, T.Y.; Yeh, Y.C.; Huang, C.Y.; Yang, S.F.; Chiu, T.H.; Tsai, K.L.; Chen, K.L.; Wu, Y.J.; Tsai, C.S.; et al. EGCG protects against oxidized LDL-induced endothelial dysfunction by inhibiting LOX-1-mediated signaling. J. Appl. Physiol. 2010, 108, 1745–1756.

127. Piao, C.S.; Kim, D.S.; Ha, K.C.; Kim, H.R.; Chae, H.J.; Chae, S.W. The protective effect of epigallocatechin-3 gallate on ischemia/reperfusion injury in isolated rat hearts: An ex vivo approach.Korean J. Physiol. Pharmacol. 2011, 15, 259–266.

128. Yanagi, S.; Matsumura, K.; Marui, A.; Morishima, M.; Hyon, S.H.; Ikeda, T.; Sakata, R. Oral pretreatment with a green tea polyphenol for cardioprotection against ischemia-reperfusion injury in an isolated rat heart model. J. Thorac. Cardiovasc. Surg. 2011, 141, 511–517.

129. Townsend, P.A.; Scarabelli, T.M.; Pasini, E.; Gitti, G.; Menegazzi, M.; Suzuki, H.; Knight, R.A.; Latchman, D.S.; Stephanou, A. Epigallocatechin-3-gallate inhibits STAT-1 activation and protects cardiac myocytes from ischemia/reperfusion-induced apoptosis. FASEB J. 2004, 18, 1621–1623.

130. Kim, C.J.; Kim, J.M.; Lee, S.R.; Jang, Y.H.; Chun, K.J. Polyphenol (−)-epigallocatechin gallate targeting myocardial reperfusion limits infarct size and improves cardiac function. Korean J. Anesthsiol. 2010, 58, 169–175.

131. Duilio, C.; Ambrosio, G.; Kuppusamy, P.; DiPaula, A.; Becker, L.C.; Zweier, J.L. Neutrophils are primary source of O2 radicals during reperfusion after prolonged myocardial ischemia. Am. J. Physiol. Heart Circ. Physiol. 2001, 280, H2649–H2657.

132. Aneja, R.; Hake, P.W.; Burroughs, T.J.; Denenberg, A.G.; Wong, H.R.; Zingarelli, B. Epigallocatechin, a green tea polyphenol, attenuates myocardial ischemia reperfusion injury in rats. Mol. Med. 2004, 10, 55–62.

133. Takano, K.; Nakaima, K.; Nitta, M.; Shibata, F.; Nakagawa, H. Inhibitory effect of (−)-epigallocatechin 3-gallate, a polyphenol of green tea, on neutrophil chemotaxis in vitro and in vivo. J. Agric. Food Chem.2004, 52, 4571–4576.

134. Hofbauer, R.; Frass, M.; Gmeiner, B.; Handler, S.; Speiser, W.; Kapiotis, S. The green tea extract epigallocatechin gallate is able to reduce neutrophil transmigration through monolayers of endothelial cells. Wien. Klin. Wochenschr. 1999, 111, 278–282.

135. Devika, P.T.; Stanely Mainzen Prince, P. Protective effect of (−)-epigallocatechin-gallate (EGCG) on lipid peroxide metabolism in isoproterenol induced myocardial infarction in male Wistar rats: A histopathological study. Biomed. Pharmacother. 2008, 62, 701–708.

136. Widlansky, M.E.; Hamburg, N.M.; Anter, E.; Holbrook, M.; Kahn, D.F.; Elliott, J.G.; Keaney, J.F.; Vita, J.A. Acute EGCG supplementation reverses endothelial dysfunction in patients with coronary artery disease. J. Am. Coll. Nutr. 2007, 26, 95–102.

137. Deka, A.; Vita, J.A. Tea and cardiovascular disease. Pharmacol. Res. 2011, 64, 136–145.

138. Yamada, H.; Watanabe, H. Tea polyphenols in preventing cardiovascular diseases. Cardiovasc. Res.2007, 73, 439–440.

139. Sheng, R.; Gu, Z.L.; Xie, M.L. Epigallocatechin gallate, the major component of polyphenols in green tea, inhibits telomere attrition mediated cardiomyocyte apoptosis in cardiac hypertrophy. Int. J. Cardiol. 2011, 162, 199–209.

140. Li, H.L.; Huang, Y.; Zhang, C.N.; Liu, G.; Wei, Y.S.; Wang, A.B.; Liu, Y.Q.; Hui, R.T.; Wei, C.; Williams, G.M.; et al. Epigallocathechin-3 gallate inhibits cardiac hypertrophy through blocking reactive oxidative species-dependent and -independent signal pathways. Free Radic. Biol. Med. 2006, 40, 1756–1775.

141. Rickman, C.; Iyer, A.; Chan, V.; Brown, L. Green tea attenuates cardiovascular remodelling and metabolic symptoms in high carbohydrate-fed rats. Curr. Pharm. Biotechnol. 2010, 11, 881–886.

142. Wolfram, S. Effects of green tea and EGCG on cardiovascular and metabolic health. J. Am. Coll. Nutr.2007, 26, 373S–388S.

143. Meng, Q.; Velalar, C.N.; Ruan, R. Regulating the age-related oxidative damage, mitochondrial integrity, and antioxidative enzyme activity in Fischer 344 rats by supplementation of the antioxidant epigallocatechin-3-gallate. Rejuvenation Res. 2008, 11, 649–660.

144. Goel, A.; Kunnumakkara, A.B.; Aggarwal, B.B. Curcumin as "Curecumin": From kitchen to clinic.Biochem. Pharmacol. 2008, 75, 787–809.

145. Kim, Y.S.; Ahn, Y.; Hong, M.H.; Joo, S.Y.; Kim, K.H.; Sohn, I.S.; Park, H.W.; Hong, Y.J.; Kim, J.H.; Kim, W.; et al. Curcumin attenuates inflammatory responses of TNF-α-stimulated human endothelial cells.J. Cardiovasc. Pharmacol. 2007, 50, 41–49.

146. Kapakos, G.; Youreva, V.; Srivastava, A.K. Cardiovascular protection by curcumin: Molecular aspects.Indian J. Biochem. Biophys. 2012, 49, 306–315.

147. Soni, K.B.; Kuttan, R. Effect of oral curcumin administration on serum peroxides and cholesterol levels in human volunteers. Indian J. Physiol. Pharmacol. 1992, 36, 273–275.

148. Alwi, I.; Santoso, T.; Suyono, S.; Sutrisna, B.; Suyatna, F.D.; Kresno, S.B.; Ernie, S. The effect of curcumin on lipid level in patients with acute coronary syndrome. Acta Med. Indones. 2008, 40, 201–210.

149. Ramirez-Tortosa, M.C.; Mesa, M.D.; Aguilera, M.C.; Quiles, J.L.; Baro, L.; Ramirez-Tortosa, C.L.; Martinez-Victoria, E.; Gil, A. Oral

administration of a turmeric extract inhibits LDL oxidation and has hypocholesterolemic effects in rabbits with experimental atherosclerosis. Atherosclerosis 1999, 147, 371–378.

150. Quiles, J.L.; Mesa, M.D.; Ramirez-Tortosa, C.L.; Aguilera, C.M.; Battino, M.; Gil, A.; Ramirez-Tortosa, M.C. Curcuma longa extract supplementation reduces oxidative stress and attenuates aortic fatty streak development in rabbits. Arterioscler. Thromb. Vasc. Biol. 2002, 22, 1225–1231.

151. Shin, S.K.; Ha, T.Y.; McGregor, R.A.; Choi, M.S. Long-term curcumin administration protects against atherosclerosis via hepatic regulation of lipoprotein cholesterol metabolism. Mol. Nutr. Food Res. 2011,55, 1829–1840.

152. Jang, E.M.; Choi, M.S.; Jung, U.J.; Kim, M.J.; Kim, H.J.; Jeon, S.M.; Shin, S.K.; Seong, C.N.; Lee, M.K. Beneficial effects of curcumin on hyperlipidemia and insulin resistance in high-fat-fed hamsters.Metab. Clin. Exp. 2008, 57, 1576–1583.

153. Ramaswami, G.; Chai, H.; Yao, Q.; Lin, P.H.; Lumsden, A.B.; Chen, C. Curcumin blocks homocysteine-induced endothelial dysfunction in porcine coronary arteries. J. Vasc. Surg. 2004, 40, 1216–1222.

154. Xu, P.H.; Long, Y.; Dai, F.; Liu, Z.L. The relaxant effect of curcumin on porcine coronary arterial ring segments. Vasc. Pharmacol. 2007, 47, 25–30.

155. Kapakos, G. Attenuation of endothelin-1-induced PKB and ERK1/2 signaling, as well as Egr-1 expression, by curcumin in A-10 vascular smooth muscle cells. Can. J. Physiol. Pharmacol. 2012, 1285, 1277–1285.

156. Kolodziejczyk, J.; Olas, B.; Saluk-Juszczak, J.; Wachowicz, B. Antioxidative properties of curcumin in the protection of blood platelets against oxidative stress in vitro. Platelets 2011, 22, 270–276.

157. Venkatesan, N. Curcumin attenuation of acute adriamycin myocardial toxicity in rats. Br. J. Pharmacol.1998, 425–427.

158. Motterlini, R.; Foresti, R.; Bassi, R.; Green, C.J. Curcumin, an antioxidant and anti-inflammatory agent, induces heme oxygenase-1 and protects endothelial cells against oxidative stres. Free Radic. Biol. Med.2000, 28, 1303–1312.

159. Yang, X.; Thomas, D.P.; Zhang, X.; Culver, B.W.; Alexander, B.M.; Murdoch, W.J.; Rao, M.N.; Tulis, D.A.; Ren, J.; Sreejayan, N.

Curcumin inhibits platelet-derived growth factor-stimulated vascular smooth muscle cell function and injury-induced neointima formation. Arterioscler. Thromb. Vasc. Biol.2006, 26, 85–90.

160. Qin, L.; Yang, Y.B.; Tuo, Q.H.; Zhu, B.Y.; Chen, L.X.; Zhang, L.; Liao, D.F. Effects and underlying mechanisms of curcumin on the proliferation of vascular smooth muscle cells induced by Chol:MbetaCD. Biochem. Biophys. Res. Commun. 2009, 379, 277–282.

161. Kang, B.Y.; Khan, J.A.; Ryu, S.; Shekhar, R.; Seung, K.B.; Mehta, J.L. Curcumin reduces angiotensin II-mediated cardiomyocyte growth via LOX-1 inhibition. J. Cardiovasc. Pharmacol. 2010, 55, 417–424.

162. Hong, D.; Zeng, X.; Xu, W.; Ma, J.; Tong, Y.; Chen, Y. Altered profiles of gene expression in curcumin-treated rats with experimentally induced myocardial infarction. Pharmacol. Res. 2010, 61, 142–148.

163. Aggarwal, B.B.; Harikumar, K.B. Potential therapeutic effects of curcumin, the anti-inflammatory agent, against neurodegenerative, cardiovascular, pulmonary, metabolic, autoimmune and neoplastic diseases. Int. J. Biochem. Cell Biol. 2009, 41, 40–59.

164. Fleenor, B.S.; Sindler, A.L.; Marvi, N.K.; Howell, K.L.; Zigler, M.L.; Yoshizawa, M.; Seals, D.R. Curcumin ameliorates arterial dysfunction and oxidative stress with aging. Exp. Gerontol. 2013, 48, 269–276.

165. Akazawa, N.; Choi, Y.; Miyaki, A.; Tanabe, Y.; Sugawara, J.; Ajisaka, R.; Maeda, S. Curcumin ingestion and exercise training improve vascular endothelial function in postmenopausal women. Nutr. Res.2012, 32, 795–799.

166. Wongcharoen, W.; Phrommintikul, A. The protective role of curcumin in cardiovascular diseases. Int. J. Cardiol. 2009, 133, 145–151.

167. Larson, A.J.; Symons, J.D.; Jalili, T. Quercetin: A treatment for hypertension?—A review of efficacy and mechanisms. Pharmaceuticals 2010, 3, 237–250.

168. Patil, B.; Pike, L.; Yoo, K. Variation in the quercetin content in different colored onions (Allium cepa L.).J. Am. Soc. Hortic. Sci. 1995, 120, 909–913.

169. Mubarak, A.; Swinny, E.E.; Ching, S.Y.L.; Jacob, S.R.; Lacey, K.; Hodgson, J.M.; Croft, K.D.; Considine, M.J. Polyphenol composition of plum selections in relation to total antioxidant capacity. J. Agric. Food Chem. 2012, 60, 10256–10262.

170. Doi, K.; Kojima, T.; Makino, M. Studies on the constituents of the leaves of Morus alba L. Chem. Pharm. Bull. (Tokyo) 2011, 49, 151–153.

171. Edwards, R.L.; Lyon, T.; Litwin, S.E.; Rabovsky, A.; Symons, J.D.; Jalili, T. Quercetin reduces blood pressure in hypertensive subjects. J. Nutr. 2007, 137, 2405–2411.

172. Egert, S.; Bosy-Westphal, A.; Seiberl, J.; Kurbitz, C.; Settler, U.; Plachta-Danielzik, S.; Wagner, A.E.; Frank, J.; Schrezenmeir, J.; Rimbach, G.; et al. Quercetin reduces systolic blood pressure and plasma oxidised low-density lipoprotein concentrations in overweight subjects with a high-cardiovascular disease risk phenotype: A double-blinded, placebo-controlled cross-over study. Br. J. Nutr. 2009, 102, 1065–1074.

173. Angeloni, C.; Leoncini, E.; Malaguti, M.; Angelini, S.; Hrelia, P.; Hrelia, S. Role of quercetin in modulating rat cardiomyocyte gene expression profile. Am. J. Physiol. Heart Circ. Physiol. 2008, 294, H1233–H1243.

174. Balasuriya, N.; Rupasinghe, H.P. Antihypertensive properties of flavonoid-rich apple peel extract.Food Chem. 2012, 135, 2320–2325.

175. Chirumbolo, S. Role of quercetin in vascular physiology. Can. J. Physiol. Pharmacol. 2012, 90, 1652–1657.

176. Khoo, N.K.; White, C.R.; Pozzo-Miller, L.; Zhou, F.; Constance, C.; Inoue, T.; Patel, R.P.; Parks, D.A. Dietary flavonoid quercetin stimulates vasorelaxation in aortic vessels. Free Radic. Biol. Med. 2010, 49, 339–347.

177. Monteiro, M.M.; Franca-Silva, M.S.; Alves, N.F.; Porpino, S.K.; Braga, V.A. Quercetin improves baroreflex sensitivity in spontaneously hypertensive rats. Molecules 2012, 17, 12997–13008.

178. Perez-Vizcaino, F.; Duarte, J.; Jimenez, R.; Santos-Buelga, C.; Osuna, A. Antihypertensive effects of the flavonoid quercetin. Pharmacol. Rep. 2009, 61, 67–75.

179. Nishizuka, T.; Fujita, Y.; Sato, Y.; Nakano, A.; Kakino, A.; Ohshima, S.; Kanda, T.; Yoshimoto, R.; Sawamura, T. Procyanidins are

potent inhibitors of LOX-1: A new player in the French Paradox. Proc. Jpn. Acad. Ser. B Phys. Biol. Sci. 2011, 87, 104–113.

180. Zhao, L.; Wu, J.; Wang, Y.; Yang, J.; Wei, J.; Gao, W.; Guo, C. Cholesterol metabolism is modulated by quercetin in rats. J. Agric. Food Chem. 2011, 59, 1104–1108.

181. Harauma, A.; Murayama, T.; Ikeyama, K.; Sano, H.; Arai, H.; Takano, R.; Kita, T.; Hara, S.; Kamei, K.; Yokode, M. Mulberry leaf powder prevents atherosclerosis in apolipoprotein E-deficient mice.Biochem. Biophys. Res. Commun. 2007, 358, 751–756.

182. Mosawy, S.; Jackson, D.E.; Woodman, O.L.; Linden, M.D. Treatment with quercetin and 3′,4′-dihydroxyflavonol inhibits platelet function and reduces thrombus formation in vivo. J. Thromb. Thrombolysis 2012, 36, 50–57.

183. Shibata, Y.; Kume, N.; Arai, H.; Hayashida, K.; Inui-Hayashida, A.; Minami, M.; Mukai, E.; Toyohara, M.; Harauma, A.; Murayama, T.; et al. Mulberry leaf aqueous fractions inhibit TNF-alpha-induced nuclear factor kappaB (NF-kappaB) activation and lectin-like oxidized LDL receptor-1 (LOX-1) expression in vascular endothelial cells. Atherosclerosis 2007, 193, 20–27.

184. Setorki, M.; Asgary, S.; Eidi, A.; Rohani, A.H.; Esmaeil, N. Effects of apple juice on risk factors of lipid profile, inflammation and coagulation, endothelial markers and atherosclerotic lesions in high cholesterolemic rabbits. Lipids Health Dis. 2009, 8, 39.

185. Perez-Vizcaino, F.; Bishop-Bailley, D.; Lodi, F.; Duarte, J.; Cogolludo, A.; Moreno, L.; Bosca, L.; Mitchell, J.A.; Warner, T.D. The flavonoid quercetin induces apoptosis and inhibits JNK activation in intimal vascular smooth muscle cells. Biochem. Biophys. Res. Commun. 2006, 346, 919–925.

186. Jin, H.B.; Yang, Y.B.; Song, Y.L.; Zhang, Y.; Li, Y.R. Protective roles of quercetin in acute myocardial ischemia and reperfusion injury in rats. Mol. Biol. Rep. 2012, 39, 11005–11009.

187. Larson, A.J.; Symons, J.D.; Jalili, T. Therapeutic potential of quercetin to decrease blood pressure: Review of efficacy. Adv. Nutr. 2012, 3, 39–46.

188. Mozzicafreddo, M.; Cuccioloni, M.; Bonfili, L.; Eleuteri, A.M.; Fioretti, E.; Angeletti, M. Antiplasmin activity of natural occurring polyphenols. Biochim. Biophys. Acta 2008, 1784, 995–1001.

189. Yoshizumi, M.; Tsuchiya, K.; Suzaki, Y.; Kirima, K.; Kyaw, M.; Moon, J.H.; Terao, J.; Tamaki, T. Quercetin glucuronide prevents VSMC hypertrophy by angiotensin II via the inhibition of JNK and AP-1 signaling pathway. Biochem. Biophys. Res. Commun. 2002, 293, 1458–1465.

190. Qin, T.C.; Chen, L.; Yu, L.X.; Gu, Z.L. Inhibitory effect of quercetin on cultured neonatal rat cardiomyocytes hypertrophy induced by angiotensin. Acta Pharmacol. Sin. 2001, 22, 1103–1106.

191. Jalili, T.; Carlstrom, J.; Kim, S.; Freeman, D.; Jin, H.; Wu, T.C.; Litwin, S.E.; David Symons, J. Quercetin-supplemented diets lower blood pressure and attenuate cardiac hypertrophy in rats with aortic constriction. J. Cardiovasc. Pharmacol. 2006, 47, 531–541.

192. Seeram, N. Berry fruits: Compositional elements, biochemical activities, and the impact of their intake on human health, performance, and disease. J. Agric. Food Chem. 2008, 56, 627–629.

193. Leifert, W.R.; Abeywardena, M.Y. Cardioprotective actions of grape polyphenols. Nutr. Res. 2008, 28, 729–737.

194. De Pascual-Teresa, S.; Moreno, D.A.; García-Viguera, C. Flavanols and anthocyanins in cardiovascular health: A review of current evidence. Int. J. Mol. Sci. 2010, 11, 1679–1703.

195. Gil, M.I.; Tomás-Barberán, F.A.; Hess-Pierce, B.; Holcroft, D.M.; Kader, A.A. Antioxidant activity of pomegranate juice and its relationship with phenolic composition and processing. J. Agric. Food Chem.2000, 48, 4581–4589.

196. Aqil, F.; Gupta, A.; Munagala, R.; Jeyabalan, J.; Kausar, H.; Sharma, R.J.; Singh, I.P.; Gupta, R.C. Antioxidant and antiproliferative activities of anthocyanin/ellagitannin-enriched extracts fromSyzygium cumini L. (Jamun, the Indian Blackberry). Nutr. Cancer 2012, 64, 428–438.

197. Chong, M.F.F.; Macdonald, R.; Lovegrove, J.A. Fruit polyphenols and CVD risk: A review of human intervention studies. Br. J. Nutr. 2010, 104, S28–S39.

198. Huijbregts, P.P.; Feskens, E.J.; Kromhout, D. Dietary patterns and cardiovascular risk factors in elderly men: The Zutphen Elderly Study. Int. J. Epidemiol. 1995, 24, 313–320.

199. McCullough, M.; Peterson, J. Flavonoid intake and cardiovascular disease mortality in a prospective cohort of US adults. Am. J. Clin. Nutr. 2012, 95, 454–464.

200. Vartiainen, E.; Laatikainen, T.; Peltonen, M.; Juolevi, A.; Männistö, S.; Sundvall, J.; Jousilahti, P.; Salomaa, V.; Valsta, L.; Puska, P. Thirty-five-year trends in cardiovascular risk factors in Finland. Int. J. Epidemiol. 2010, 39, 504–518.

201. Rissanen, T.H.; Voutilainen, S.; Virtanen, J.K.; Venho, B.; Vanharanta, M.; Mursu, J.; Salonen, J.T. Low intake of fruits , berries and vegetables is associated with excess mortality in men: The Kuopio Ischaemic Heart Disease Risk Factor (KIHD). Nutr. Epidemiol. 2003, 133, 199–204.

202. Iqbal, R.; Anand, S.; Ounpuu, S.; Islam, S.; Zhang, X.; Rangarajan, S.; Chifamba, J.; Al-Hinai, A.; Keltai, M.; Yusuf, S. Dietary patterns and the risk of acute myocardial infarction in 52 countries: Results of the INTERHEART study. Circulation 2008, 118, 1929–1937.

203. Do, R.; Xie, C.; Zhang, X.; Männistö, S.; Harald, K.; Islam, S.; Bailey, S.D.; Rangarajan, S.; McQueen, M.J.; Diaz, R.; et al. The effect of chromosome 9p21 variants on cardiovascular disease may be modified by dietary intake: Evidence from a case/control and a prospective study. PLoS Med. 2011, 8, e1001106.

204. Rosenblat, M.; Volkova, N.; Coleman, R.; Aviram, M. Pomegranate byproduct administration to apolipoprotein E-deficient mice attenuates atherosclerosis development as a result of decreased macrophage oxidative stress and reduced cellular uptake of oxidized low-density lipoprotein. J. Agric. Food Chem. 2006, 54, 1928–1935.

205. Wu, X.; Kang, J.; Xie, C.; Burris, R.; Ferguson, M.E.; Badger, T.M.; Nagarajan, S. Dietary blueberries attenuate atherosclerosis in apolipoprotein E-deficient mice by upregulating antioxidant enzyme expression. J. Nutr. 2010, 140, 1628–1632.

206. Gallaher, C.M.; Gallaher, D.D. Dried plums (prunes) reduce atherosclerosis lesion area in apolipoprotein E-deficient mice. Br. J. Nutr. 2009, 101, 233–239.

207. Auclair, S.; Silberberg, M.; Gueux, E.; Morand, C.; Mazur, A.; Milenkovic, D.; Scalbert, A. Apple polyphenols and fibers attenuate atherosclerosis in apolipoprotein E-deficient mice. J. Agric. Food Chem. 2008, 56, 5558–5563.

208. De Lange, D.W.; Verhoef, S.; Gorter, G.; Kraaijenhagen, R.J.; van de Wiel, A.; Akkerman, J.W. Polyphenolic grape extract inhibits platelet activation through PECAM-1: An explanation for the French paradox. Alcohol. Clin. Exp. Res. 2007, 31, 1308–1314.

209. Falati, S.; Patil, S.; Gross, P.L.; Stapleton, M.; Merrill-Skoloff, G.; Barrett, N.E.; Pixton, K.L.; Weiler, H.; Cooley, B.; Newman, D.K.; et al. Platelet PECAM-1 inhibits thrombus formation in vivo. Blood 2006,107, 535–541.

210. Mattiello, T.; Trifirò, E.; Jotti, G.S.; Pulcinelli, F.M. Effects of pomegranate juice and extract polyphenols on platelet function. J. Med. Food 2009, 12, 334–339.

211. Berger, J.; Moller, D.E. The mechanisms of action of PPARs. Annu. Rev. Med. 2002, 53, 409–435.

212. Seymour, E.M.; Bennink, M.R.; Watts, S.W.; Bolling, S.F. Whole grape intake impacts cardiac peroxisome proliferator-activated receptor and nuclear factor kappaB activity and cytokine expression in rats with diastolic dysfunction. Hypertension 2010, 55, 1179–1185.

213. Seymour, E.M.; Singer, A.A.; Kirakosyan, A.; Urcuyo-Llanes, D.E.; Kaufman, P.B.; Bolling, S.F. Altered hyperlipidemia, hepatic steatosis, and hepatic peroxisome proliferator-activated receptors in rats with intake of tart cherry. J. Med. Food 2008, 11, 252–259.

214. Kivimäki, A.S.; Ehlers, P.I.; Siltari, A.; Turpeinen, A.M.; Vapaatalo, H.; Korpela, R. Lingonberry, cranberry and blackcurrant juices affect mRNA expressions of inflammatory and atherothrombotic markers of SHR in a long-term treatment. J. Funct. Foods 2012, 4, 496–503.

215. Chanet, A.; Milenkovic, D.; Claude, S.; Maier, J.A.; Kamran Khan, M.; Rakotomanomana, N.; Shinkaruk, S.; Bérard, A.M.; Bennetau-Pelissero, C.; Mazur, A.; Morand, C. Flavanone metabolites decrease monocyte adhesion to TNF-α-activated endothelial cells by modulating expression of atherosclerosis-related genes. Br. J. Nutr. 2013, 110, 587–598.

216. Kalea, A.Z.; Clark, K.; Schuschke, D.A.; Kristo, A.S.; Klimis-Zacas, D.J. Dietary enrichment with wild blueberries (Vaccinium angustifolium) affects the vascular reactivity in the aorta of young spontaneously hypertensive rats. J. Nutr. Biochem. 2010, 21, 14–22.

217. Shaughnessy, K.S.; Boswall, I.A.; Scanlan, A.P.; Gottschall-Pass, K.T.; Sweeney, M.I. Diets containing blueberry extract lower blood pressure in spontaneously hypertensive stroke-prone rats. Nutr. Res.2009, 29, 130–138.

218. Wiseman, W.; Egan, J.M.; Slemmer, J.E.; Shaughnessy, K.S.; Ballem, K.; Gottschall-pass, K.T.; Sweeney, M.I. Feeding blueberry diets inhibits angiotensin II-converting enzyme (ACE) activity in spontaneously hypertensive stroke-prone rats. Can. J. Physiol. Pharmacol. 2011, 89, 67–71.

219. Jia, H.; Liu, J.W.; Ufur, H.; He, G.S.; Liqian, H.; Chen, P. The antihypertensive effect of ethyl acetate extract from red raspberry fruit in hypertensive rats. Pharmacogn. Mag. 2011, 7, 19–24.

220. Falchi, M.; Bertelli, A.; Lo Scalzo, R.; Morassut, M.; Morelli, R.; Das, S.; Cui, J.; Das, D.K. Comparison of cardioprotective abilities between the flesh and skin of grapes. J. Agric. Food Chem. 2006, 54, 6613–6622.

221. Ahmet, I.; Spangler, E.; Shukitt-Hale, B.; Joseph, J.A.; Ingram, D.K.; Talan, M. Survival and cardioprotective benefits of long-term blueberry enriched diet in dilated cardiomyopathy following myocardial infarction in rats. PLoS One 2009, 4, e7975.

222. Ahmet, I.; Spangler, E.; Shukitt-Hale, B.; Juhaszova, M.; Sollott, S.J.; Joseph, J.A.; Ingram, D.K.; Talan, M. Blueberry-enriched diet protects rat heart from ischemic damage. PLoS One 2009, 4, e5954.

223. Shao, Z.H.; Wojcik, K.R.; Dossumbekova, A.; Hsu, C.; Mehendale, S.R.; Li, C.Q.; Qin, Y.; Sharp, W.W.; Chang, W.T.; Hamann, K.J.; et al. Grape seed proanthocyanidins protect cardiomyocytes from ischemia and reperfusion injury via Akt-NOS signaling. J. Cell. Biochem. 2009, 107, 697–705.

224. Kähkönen, M.P.; Hopia, A.I.; Heinonen, M. Berry phenolics and their antioxidant activity. J. Agric. Food Chem. 2001, 49, 4076–4082.

225. Heinonen, I.M.; Meyer, A.S.; Frankel, E.N. Antioxidant activity of berry phenolics on human low-density lipoprotein and liposome oxidation. J. Agric. Food Chem. 1998, 46, 4107–4112.

226. Heinonen, I.; Lehtonen, P.; Hopia, A. Antioxidant activity of berry and fruit wines and liquors. J. Agric. Food Chem. 1998, 46, 25–31.

227. Chan, K.C.; Ho, H.H.; Peng, C.H.; Lan, K.P.; Lin, M.C.; Chen, H.M.; Wang, C.J. Polyphenol-rich extract from mulberry leaf inhibits vascular smooth muscle cell proliferation involving upregulation of p53 and inhibition of cyclin-dependent kinase. J. Agric. Food Chem. 2010, 58, 2536–2542.

228. Cuccioloni, M.; Mozzicafreddo, M.; Sparapani, L.; Spina, M.; Eleuteri, A.M.; Fioretti, E.; Angeletti, M. Pomegranate fruit components modulate human thrombin. Fitoterapia 2009, 80, 301–305.

229. Guo, C.; Wei, J.; Yang, J.; Xu, J.; Pang, W.; Jiang, Y. Pomegranate juice is potentially better than apple juice in improving antioxidant function in elderly subjects. Nutr. Res. 2008, 28, 72–77.

230. Wallace, T.C. Anthocyanins in cardiovascular disease. Adv. Nutr. Int. Rev. J. 2011, 2, 1–7.

231. Chen, J.H.; Ho, C.T. Antioxidant activities of caffeic acid and its related hydroxycinnamic acid compounds. J. Agric. Food Chem. 1997, 45, 2374–2378.

232. Elavarasan, J.; Velusamy, P.; Ganesan, T.; Ramakrishnan, S.K.; Rajasekaran, D.; Periandavan, K. Hesperidin-mediated expression of Nrf2 and upregulation of antioxidant status in senescent rat heart.J. Pharm. Pharmacol. 2012, 64, 1472–1482.

233. Visioli, F.; Galli, C. Biological properties of olive oil phytochemicals. Crit. Rev. Food Sci. Nutr. 2002, 42, 209–221.

234. Visioli, F.; Bellomo, G.; Galli, C. Free radical-scavenging properties of olive oil polyphenols. Biochem. Biophys. Res. Commun. 1998, 247, 60–64.

235. Fitó, M.; Covas, M.I.; Lamuela-Raventós, R.M.; Vila, J.; Torrents, L.; de la Torre, C.; Marrugat, J. Protective effect of olive oil and its phenolic compounds against low density lipoprotein oxidation.Lipids 2000, 35, 633–638.

236. Beltrán, G.; Del Rio, C.; Sánchez, S.; Martínez, L. Influence of harvest date and crop yield on the fatty acid composition of virgin olive oils from cv. Picual. J. Agric. Food Chem. 2004, 52, 3434–3440.

237. Bonoli, M.; Bendini, A.; Cerretani, L.; Lercker, G.; Toschi, T.G. Qualitative and semiquantitative analysis of phenolic compounds in extra virgin olive oils as a function of the ripening

degree of olive fruits by different analytical techniques. J. Agric. Food Chem. 2004, 52, 7026–7032.

238. Rotondi, A.; Bendini, A.; Cerretani, L.; Mari, M.; Lercker, G.; Toschi, T.G. Effect of olive ripening degree on the oxidative stability and organoleptic properties of cv. Nostrana di Brisighella extra virgin olive oil. J. Agric. Food Chem. 2004, 52, 3649–3654.

239. Gimeno, E.; Fitó, M.; Lamuela-Raventós, R.M.; Castellote, A.I.; Covas, M.; Farré, M.; de la Torre-Boronat, M.C.; López-Sabater, M.C. Effect of ingestion of virgin olive oil on human low-density lipoprotein composition. Eur. J. Clin. Nutr. 2002, 56, 114–120.

240. Kafatos, A.G.; Zampelas, A. Olive oil intake in relation to cardiovascular diseases. Grasas Y Aceites2004, 55, 24–32.

241. Pérez-Jiménez, F.; Ruano, J.; Perez-Martinez, P.; Lopez-Segura, F.; Lopez-Miranda, J. The influence of olive oil on human health: Not a question of fat alone. Mol. Nutr. Food Res. 2007, 51, 1199–1208.

242. Damasceno, N.R.T.; Perez-Heras, A.; Serra, M.; Cofan, M.; Sala-Vila, A.; Salas-Salvado, J.; Ros, E. Crossover study of diets enriched with virgin olive oil, walnuts or almonds. Effects on lipids and other cardiovascular risk markers. Nutr. Metab. Cardiovasc. Dis. 2011, 21, S14–S20.

243. Covas, M.; Nyyssönen, K.; Poulsen, H. The effect of polyphenols in olive oil on heart disease risk factors. Ann. Intern. Med. 2006, 145, 333–341.

244. Weinbrenner, T.; Fito, M.; de la Torre, R.; Saez, G.T.; Rijken, P.; Tormos, C.; Coolen, S.; Albaladejo, M.F.; Abanades, S.; Schroder, H.; et al. Olive oils high in phenolic compounds modulate oxidative/antioxidative status in men. J. Nutr. 2004, 134, 2314–2321.

245. Marrugat, J.; Covas, M.I.; Fitó, M.; Schröder, H.; Miró-Casas, E.; Gimeno, E.; López-Sabater, M.C.; de la Torre, R.; Farré, M. Effects of differing phenolic content in dietary olive oils on lipids and LDL oxidation—A randomized controlled trial. Eur. J. Nutr. 2004, 43, 140–147.

246. Fitó, M.; Cladellas, M.; de la Torre, R.; Martí, J.; Muñoz, D.; Schröder, H.; Alcántara, M.; Pujadas-Bastardes, M.; Marrugat, J.; López-Sabater, M.C.; et al. Anti-inflammatory effect of virgin olive oil in stable coronary disease patients: A randomized, crossover, controlled trial. Eur. J. Clin. Nutr. 2008, 62, 570–574.

247. Fitó, M.; Cladellas, M.; de la Torre, R.; Martí, J.; Alcántara, M.; Pujadas-Bastardes, M.; Marrugat, J.; Bruguera, J.; López-Sabater, M.C.; Vila, J.; et al. Antioxidant effect of virgin olive oil in patients with stable coronary heart disease: A randomized, crossover, controlled, clinical trial. Atherosclerosis 2005,181, 149–158.

248. Bogani, P.; Galli, C.; Villa, M.; Visioli, F. Postprandial anti-inflammatory and antioxidant effects of extra virgin olive oil. Atherosclerosis 2007, 190, 181–186.

249. Rafehi, H.; Smith, A.J.; Balcerczyk, A.; Ziemann, M.; Ooi, J.; Loveridge, S.J.; Baker, E.K.; El-Osta, A.; Karagiannis, T.C. Investigation into the biological properties of the olive polyphenol, hydroxytyrosol: Mechanistic insights by genome-wide mRNA-Seq analysis. Genes Nutr. 2012, 7, 343–355.

250. Di Benedetto, R.; Varì, R.; Scazzocchio, B.; Filesi, C.; Santangelo, C.; Giovannini, C.; Matarrese, P.; D'Archivio, M.; Masella, R. Tyrosol, the major extra virgin olive oil compound, restored intracellular antioxidant defences in spite of its weak antioxidative effectiveness. Nutr. Metab. Cardiovasc. Dis. 2007,17, 535–545.

251. Salami, M.; Galli, C.; de Angelis, L.; Visioli, F. Formation of F2-isoprostanes in oxidize low density lipoprotein: Inhibitory effect of hydroxytyrosol. Pharmacol. Res. 1995, 31, 275–279.

252. Nakbi, A.; Dabbou, S.; Champion, S.; Fouchier, F.; Mehri, S.; Attia, N.; Leger, C.; Hammami, M. Modulation of the superoxide anion production and MMP-9 expression in PMA stimulated THP-1 cells by olive oil minor components: Tyrosol and hydroxytyrosol. Food Res. Int. 2011, 44, 575–581.

253. Masella, R.; Varì, R. Extra virgin olive oil biophenols inhibit cell-mediated oxidation of LDL by increasing the mRNA transcription of glutathione-related enzymes. J. Nutr. 2004, 134, 785–791.

254. Widmer, R.J.; Freund, M.A.; Flammer, A.J.; Sexton, J.; Lennon, R.; Romani, A.; Mulinacci, N.; Vinceri, F.F.; Lerman, L.O.; Lerman, A. Beneficial effects of polyphenol-rich olive oil in patients with early atherosclerosis. Eur. J. Nutr. 2013, 52, 1223–1231.

255. De la Cruz, J.P.; Villalobos, M.A.; Carmona, J.A.; Martin-Romero, M.; Smith-Agreda, J.M.; de la Cuesta, F.S. Antithrombotic potential of olive oil administration in rabbits with elevated cholesterol.Thromb. Res. 2000, 100, 305–315.

256. González-Santiago, M.; Martín-Bautista, E.; Carrero, J.J.; Fonollá, J.; Baró, L.; Bartolomé, M.V.; Gil-Loyzaga, P.; López-Huertas, E. One-month administration of hydroxytyrosol, a phenolic antioxidant present in olive oil, to hyperlipemic rabbits improves blood lipid profile, antioxidant status and reduces atherosclerosis development. Atherosclerosis 2006, 188, 35–42.

257. Petroni, A.; Blasevich, M.; Salami, M.; Papini, N.; Montedoro, G.F.; Galli, C. Inhibition of platelet aggregation and eicosanoid production by phenolic components of olive oil. Thromb. Res. 1995, 78, 151–160.

258. Faine, L. Effects of olive oil and its minor constituents on serum lipids, oxidative stress, and energy metabolism in cardiac muscle. Can. J. Physiol. Pharmacol. 2006, 84, 239–245.

259. Schmitt, C.A.; Handler, N.; Heiss, E.H.; Erker, T.; Dirsch, V.M. No evidence for modulation of endothelial nitric oxide synthase by the olive oil polyphenol hydroxytyrosol in human endothelial cells. Atherosclerosis 2007, 195, e58–e64.

260. Egeria, S.; Nadia, C.; Marika, M. Mediterranean diet polyphenols reduce inflammatory angiogenesis through MMP-9 and COX-2 inhibition in human vascular endothelial cells: A potentially protective.Arch. Biochem. Biophys. 2012, 527, 81–89.

261. Dell'Agli, M.; Fagnani, R.; Mitro, N.; Scurati, S.; Masciadri, M.; Mussoni, L.; Galli, G.V.; Bosisio, E.; Crestani, M.; de Fabiani, E.; et al. Minor components of olive oil modulate proatherogenic adhesion molecules involved in endothelial activation. J. Agric. Food Chem. 2006, 54, 3259–3264.

262. Manna, C.; Napoli, D.; Cacciapuoti, G.; Porcelli, M.; Zappia, V. Olive oil phenolic compounds inhibit homocysteine-induced endothelial cell adhesion regardless of their different antioxidant activity. J. Agric. Food Chem. 2009, 57, 3478–3482.

263. Carluccio, M.A.; Siculella, L.; Ancora, M.A.; Massaro, M.; Scoditti, E.; Storelli, C.; Visioli, F.; Distante, A.; de Caterina, R. Olive oil and red wine antioxidant polyphenols inhibit endothelial activation: Antiatherogenic properties of Mediterranean diet phytochemicals. Arterioscler. Thromb. Vasc. Biol.2003, 23, 622–629.

264. Abe, R.; Beckett, J.; Nixon, A.; Rochier, A.; Yamashita, N.; Sumpio, B. Olive oil polyphenol oleuropein inhibits smooth muscle cell proliferation. Eur. J. Vasc. Endovasc. Surg. 2011, 41, 814–820.

265. Manna, C.; Migliardi, V.; Golino, P.; Scognamiglio, A.; Galletti, P.; Chiariello, M.; Zappia, V. Oleuropein prevents oxidative myocardial injury induced by ischemia and reperfusion. J. Nutr. Biochem. 2004, 15, 461–466.

266. Camargo, A.; Delgado-Lista, J.; Garcia-Rios, A.; Cruz-Teno, C.; Yubero-Serrano, E.M.; Perez-Martinez, P.; Gutierrez-Mariscal, F.M.; Lora-Aguilar, P.; Rodriguez-Cantalejo, F.; Fuentes-Jimenez, F.; et al. Expression of proinflammatory, proatherogenic genes is reduced by the Mediterranean diet in elderly people. Br. J. Nutr. 2012, 108, 500–508.

267. Cicerale, S.; Lucas, L.; Keast, R. Biological activities of phenolic compounds present in virgin olive oil.Int. J. Mol. Sci. 2010, 11, 458–479.

268. Tasioula-Margari, M.; Okogeri, O. Simultaneous determination of phenolic compounds and tocopherols in virgin olive oil using HPLC and UV detection. Food Chem. 2001, 74, 377–383.

269. Gordon, M.H.; Paiva-Martins, F.; Almeida, M. Antioxidant activity of hydroxytyrosol acetate compared with that of other olive oil polyphenols. J. Agric. Food Chem. 2001, 49, 2480–2485.

270. Samuel, S.M.; Thirunavukkarasu, M.; Penumathsa, S.V.; Paul, D.; Maulik, N. Akt/FOXO3a/SIRT1-mediated cardioprotection by n-tyrosol against ischemic stress in rat in vivo model of myocardial infarction: Switching gears toward survival and longevity. J. Agric Food Chem. 2008, 56, 9692–9698.

271. Bayram, B.; Ozcelik, B.; Grimm, S.; Roeder, T.; Schrader, C.; Ernst, I.M.; Wagner, A.E.; Grune, T.; Frank, J.; Rimbach, G. A diet rich in olive oil phenolics reduces oxidative stress in the heart of SAMP8 mice by induction of Nrf2-dependent gene expression. Rejuvenation Res. 2012, 15, 71–81.

272. Miles, E.A.; Zoubouli, P.; Calder, P.C. Differential anti-inflammatory effects of phenolic compounds from extra virgin olive oil identified in human whole blood cultures. Nutrition 2005, 21, 389–394.

273. Beauchamp, G.K.; Keast, R.S.; Morel, D.; Lin, J.; Pika, J.; Han, Q.; Lee, C.H.; Smith, A.B.; Breslin, P.A. Phytochemistry: Ibuprofen-like activity in extra-virgin olive oil. Nature 2005, 437, 45–46.

274. Loued, S.; Berrougui, H.; Componova, P.; Ikhlef, S.; Helal, O.; Khalil, A. Extra-virgin olive oil consumption reduces the age-related decrease in HDL and paraoxonase 1 anti-inflammatory activities. Br. J. Nutr. 2013. in press.

275. Zrelli, H.; Matsuka, M.; Araki1, M.; Zarrouk, M.; Miyazaki, H. Hydroxytyrosol induces vascular smooth muscle cells apoptosis through NO production and PP2A activation with subsequent inactivation of Akt. Planta Med. 2011, 77, 1680–1686.

276. Visioli, F.; Caruso, D.; Grande, S.; Bosisio, R.; Villa, M.; Galli, G.; Sirtori, C.; Galli, C. Virgin Olive Oil Study (VOLOS): Vasoprotective potential of extra virgin olive oil in mildly dyslipidemic patients. Eur. J. Nutr. 2005, 44, 121–127.

277. Hennekens, C.H.; Buring, J.E.; Manson, J.E.; Stampfer, M.; Rosner, B.; Cook, N.R.; Belanger, C.; LaMotte, F.; Gaziano, J.M.; Ridker, P.M.; et al. Lack of effect of long-term supplementation with beta carotene on the incidence of malignant neoplasms and cardiovascular disease. N. Engl. J. Med. 1996,334, 1145–1149.

278. Christen, W. Design of Physicians' Health Study II—A randomized trial of beta-carotene, vitamins E and C, and multivitamins, in prevention of cancer, cardiovascular disease, and eye disease, and review of results of completed trials. Ann. Epidemiol. 2000, 10, 125–134.

279. Wong, R.H.X.; Howe, P.R.C.; Buckley, J.D.; Coates, A.M.; Kunz, I.; Berry, N.M. Acute resveratrol supplementation improves flow-mediated dilatation in overweight/obese individuals with mildly elevated blood pressure. Nutr. Metab. Cardiovasc. Dis. 2011, 21, 851–856.

280. Freedman, J.E.; Parker, C.; Li, L.; Perlman, J.A.; Frei, B.; Ivanov, V.; Deak, L.R.; Iafrati, M.D.; Folts, J.D. Select flavonoids and whole juice from purple grapes inhibit platelet function and enhance nitric oxide release. Circulation 2001, 103, 2792–2798.

281. Basu, A.; Du, M.; Leyva, M. Blueberries decrease cardiovascular risk factors in obese men and women with metabolic syndrome. J. Nutr. 2010, 140, 1582–1587.

282. Duffy, S.J.; Keaney, J.F., Jr.; Holbrook, M.; Gokce, N.; Swerdloff, P.L.; Frei, B.; Vita, J.A. Short-and long-term black tea consumption reverses endothelial dysfunction in patients with coronary artery disease. Circulation 2001, 104, 151–156.

283. Brown, A.L.; Lane, J.; Coverly, J.; Stocks, J.; Jackson, S.; Stephen, A.; Bluck, L.; Coward, A.; Hendrickx, H. Effects of dietary supplementation with the green tea polyphenol epigallocatechin-3-gallate on insulin resistance and associated metabolic risk factors: Randomized controlled trial. Br. J. Nutr. 2009,101, 886–984.

284. Van Mierlo, L.A.J.; Zock, P.L.; van der Knaap, H.C.M.; Draijer, R. Grape polyphenols do not affect vascular function in healthy men. J. Nutr. 2010, 140, 1769–1773.

285. Auclair, S.; Chironi, G.; Milenkovic, D.; Hollman, P.C.; Renard, C.M.; Mégnien, J.L.; Gariepy, J.; Paul, J.L.; Simon, A.; Scalbert, A. The regular consumption of a polyphenol-rich apple does not influence endothelial function: A randomised double-blind trial in hypercholesterolemic adults. Eur. J. Clin. Nutr. 2010, 64, 1158–1165.

286. Frank, J.; George, T. Daily consumption of an aqueous green tea extract supplement does not impair liver function or alter cardiovascular disease risk biomarkers in healthy men. J. Nutr. 2009, 139, 58–62.

287. Basu, A.; Du, M.; Sanchez, K.; Leyva, M.J.; Betts, N.M.; Blevins, S.; Wu, M.; Aston, C.E.; Lyons, T.J. Green tea minimally affects biomarkers of inflammation in obese subjects with metabolic syndrome.Nutrition 2011, 27, 206–213.

288. Trautwein, E.A.; Du, Y.; Meynen, E.; Yan, X.; Wen, Y.; Wang, H.; Molhuizen, H.O. Purified black tea theaflavins and theaflavins/catechin supplements did not affect serum lipids in healthy individuals with mildly to moderately elevated cholesterol concentrations. Eur. J. Nutr. 2010, 49, 27–35.

289. Mennen, L.I.; Walker, R.; Bennetau-Pelissero, C.; Scalbert, A. Risks and safety of polyphenol consumption. Am. J. Clin. Nutr. 2005, 81, 326S–329S.

290. Bravo, L. Polyphenols: Chemistry, dietary sources, metabolism, and nutritional significance. Nutr. Rev.1998, 56, 317–333.

291. Brune, M.; Rossander, L.; Hallberg, L. Iron absorption and phenolic compounds: Importance of different phenolic structures. Eur. J. Clin. Nutr. 1989, 43, 547–557.

292. Reddy, M.; Cook, J. Assessment of dietary determinants of nonheme-iron absorption in humans and rats. Am. J. Clin. Nutr. 1991, 54, 723–728.

293. Temme, E.H.; van Hoydonck, P.G. Tea consumption and iron status. Eur. J. Clin. Nutr. 2002, 56, 379–386.

294. Zijp, I.M.; Korver, O.; Tijburg, L.B. Effect of tea and other dietary factors on iron absorption. Crit. Rev. Food Sci. Nutr. 2000, 40, 371–398.

295. Sakihama, Y.; Cohen, M.F.; Grace, S.C.; Yamasaki, H. Plant phenolic antioxidant and prooxidant activities: Phenolics-induced oxidative damage mediated by metals in plants. Toxicology 2002, 177, 67–80.

296. Isbrucker, R.A.; Edwards, J.A.; Wolz, E.; Davidovich, A.; Bausch, J. Safety studies on epigallocatechin gallate (EGCG) preparations. Part 2: Dermal, acute and short-term toxicity studies. Food Chem. Toxicol.2006, 44, 636–650.

297. Hirose, M.; Hoshiya, T.; Mizoguchi, Y.; Nakamura, A.; Akagi, K.; Shirai, T. Green tea catechins enhance tumor development in the colon without effects in the lung or thyroid after pretreatment with 1,2-Dimethylhydrazine or 2,2′-dihydroxy-di-n-propylnitrosamine in male F344 rats. Cancer Lett.2001, 168, 23–29.

298. Van der Woude, H.; Gliszczyńska-Swigło, A.; Struijs, K.; Smeets, A.; Alink, G.M.; Rietjens, I.M.C.M. Biphasic modulation of cell proliferation by quercetin at concentrations physiologically relevant in humans. Cancer Lett. 2003, 200, 41–47.

299. Manach, C.; Williamson, G.; Morand, C.; Scalbert, A.; Rémésy, C. Bioavailability and bioefficacy of polyphenols in humans. I. Review of 97 bioavailability studies. Am. J. Clin. Nutr. 2005, 81, 230S–242S.

300. Kay, C.D. The future of flavonoid research. Br. J. Nutr. 2010, 104, S91–S95.

301. Wersching, H. An apple a day keeps stroke away? Consumption of white fruits and vegetables is associated with lower risk of stroke. Stroke 2011, 42, 3001–3002.

6

RECENT ADVANCES AND USES OF GRAPE FLAVONOIDS AS NUTRACEUTICALS

Vasil Georgiev *, Anthony Ananga and Violeta Tsolova

Center for Viticulture and Small Fruit Research, College of Agriculture and Food Sciences, Florida A & M University, 6505 Mahan Drive, Tallahassee, FL 32317, USA

ABSTRACT

Grape is one of the oldest fruit crops domesticated by humans. The numerous uses of grape in making wine, beverages, jelly, and other products, has made it one of the most economically important plants worldwide. The complex phytochemistry of the berry is characterized by a wide variety of compounds, most of which have been demonstrated to have therapeutic or health promoting properties. Among them, flavonoids are the most abundant and widely studied, and have enjoyed greater attention among grape researchers in the last century. Recent studies have shown that the beneficial health effects promoted by consumption of grape and grape products are attributed to the unique mix of polyphenolic compounds. As the largest group of grape polyphenols, flavonoids are the main candidates considered to have biological properties, including but not limited to antioxidant, anti-inflammatory, anti-cancer, antimicrobial, antiviral, cardioprotective, neuroprotective, and hepatoprotective activities. Here, we discuss the recent scientific advances supporting the beneficial health qualities of grape and grape-derived products, mechanisms of their biological activity, bioavailability, and their uses as nutraceuticals. The advantages of modern plant cell based biotechnology as an alternative method for production of grape nutraceuticals and improvement of their health qualities are also discussed.

Keywords: antioxidants; anti-inflammation; grapevine; polyphenols

1. INTRODUCTION

Grape (*Vitis* spp.) is one of the most economically important plant species due to its diverse uses in production of wine, grape juice and other food products [1]. It is cultivated in all continents in the temperate regions where sufficient rain, warm and dry summers as well as relatively mild winters are normal climatic patterns [2]. The qualities of grape products are characterized by their metabolic compositions. Flavonoids represent a widespread and common group of natural polyphenols produced by the phenylpropanoid pathway [3,4]. They confer UV-protection, determine flower coloration, attract pollinators, and act as tissue protectors in case of pathogen attack or oxidative damage [5]. In grapes, flavonoids are primarily located in the epidermal layer of berry skin and the seeds [6,7,8,9]. Flavonoids are the main groups of soluble phenolics in grapes as well as major contributors of the biological activities in products derived from grapes [10].

Recently, the strong beneficial health effect of grape flavonoids has been directly connected to the so called "French Paradox". The term refers to the epidemiological observation of comparatively low incidence of coronary heart disease in the population of the Mediterranean region, despite the presence of a local diet rich in saturated fats. The tradition of regular consumption of red wine which lowers the risk for development of cardiovascular diseases was reported as the main contributing factor [11]. Flavonoids in red wine are the most feasible phytochemicals, responsible for this phenomenon [12]. Flavonoids have cardioprotective, antioxidant, anti-inflammatory, anti-cancer and antimicrobial properties, and are one of the most potent nutraceuticals in food and phytopharmaceutical products [13,14,15,16,17,18]. Therefore, it is paramount to understand the principles of biological activity, bioavailability and metabolism of grape flavonoids in relation to human health.

2. BIOLOGICAL ACTIVITIES OF GRAPE PRODUCTS

Wine, the product of grape juice fermentation has played an important role in the development of human culture. The earliest chemical evidence for wine production was found in the Middle East in well-preserved ancient jars dated 5400–5000 BC [19]. The multitude of ancient and historical images of vines and grapes found as decorative elements on ancient coins, temples, ritual potteries, and mosaic sculptures clearly demonstrated the importance of grape and its products in ancient societies across the globe. For example, in the Balkans and the Eastern Mediterranean, grape and wine were considered divine and dedicated to various deities: "Zagreus" by Thracians, "Dionysus" by Greeks and "Bacchus" by the Romans [20,21,22]. The mystical powers of grape and wine in the social life and cultural traditions of ancient people were not futile. Modern science continues to decipher the benefits of grape as a rich source of valuable phytonutrients with remarkable positive effects on human health [1,23,24,25,26,27]. The unique combination of phytochemicals in grapes includes a variety of bioactive compounds such as simple phenolics, flavonoids, anthocyanins, stilbenes, proanthocyanidins, and vitamin E [1,3,25]. In excess of 500 compounds, including 160 esters, have been identified to be present in wines with active role in the formation of their organoleptic properties [1]. Simple phenolics in grapes are derivatives of hydroxycinnamic acid (p-coumaric, caffeic, sinapic and ferulic acids) and hydroxybenzoic acid (gallic, gentisic, protocatechuic and p-hydroxybenzoic acids) [1]. In wine, hydroxycinnamic acid derivatives are found as esters with tartaric acid, whereas the hydroxybenzoic acid derivatives are present in their free forms [1]. The North American Native grape*Muscadinia rotundifolia* (Michx.) Small, "Ison" var., was reported to have a higher gallic acid content (between 7 and 10 fold higher) than the European grape (*Vitis vinifera* L., "Chardonnay" and "Merlot" var., respectively) [28]. Gallic acid has been shown to possess various therapeutic properties, including antioxidant, anti-cancer, anti-inflammatory, antifungal and antiviral activities [29,30,31,32]. However, polyphenols including flavonoids, stilbenes and proanthocyanidins are the most important class of biologically active compounds in grapes. Grape is one of the richest sources of polyphenols among fruits. The flavonoids are the most abundant biologically active phytonutrients among the polyphenols found in grapes, possessing cardioprotective, neuroprotective, antimicrobial and antiaging properties [26,33,34,35,36]. Most of the flavonoids are found primarily in the outer epidermal cells (the grape skin), whereas about 60%–70% of total polyphenols are stored in grape seeds [1,25,37]. During processing of grape juice, only limited amounts of anthocyanins (~2%) are extracted with the cell sap [38]. However, when fermentation/maceration processes are involved, large amounts of polymeric products are obtained including proanthocyanidins, pyranoanthocyanins (vitisin A and vitisin B) and oligostilbenes (ε-viniferins and δ-viniferins). These polymeric compounds also increase the color stability and biological values of the resulting wines [39]. Nevertheless, more than 70% of grape polyphenols remain in the pomace (a byproduct of wine/grape juice processing), which becomes a valuable source of health promoting nutraceuticals [40]. Moreover, grape seeds may be separated from the pomace and used either for production of grape seed oil or as individual food supplements in the form of grape seed powder or grape seed extracts [41]. Additional flavonoids-rich products are also extracted from grape skins [42,43]. The North American grape species, such as *M. rotundifolia* (Michx.) Small and *V. labrusca* L. accumulate ellagic acid in their berries [44,45]. Recently, ellagic acid has attracted the increased attention because of its high antioxidant, anticarcinogenic, antimutagenic and hepatoprotective qualities [46]. The presence of ellagic acid significantly increase the nutraceutical value of food additives produced by the native North American grapes, compared to the similar products obtained by the processing of regular European grape species. Primary products and byproducts from the processing of fresh grapes used as supplements or in regular diets may provide significant health benefits for humans (Figure 1). Therefore, the wide range of pharmacological effects of grapes and grape products on human health is due to the fact that those additives are sources of unique combinations of nutraceuticals.

2.1. Flavonoids in Grapes

Flavonoids represent a large family of secondary metabolites and nearly 6000 structures have been identified in plants [47]. The diversity in their chemical structures contributes to their broad range of physiological and biological activities. The most common flavonoids found in grapes are anthocyanins (3-*O*-monoglucosides or 3,5-*O*-diglucosides of malvidin, cyanidin, peonidin, delphinidin, pelargonidin and petunidin **1–12**, as well as their acetyl-, p-coumaroyl- and/or caffeoyl-esters), flavonols (3-*O*-glycosides of quercetin **16**, kaempferol **17**, myricetin **18**, laricitrin, isorhamnetin **19** and syringetin), flavanols [(+)-catechin**13**, (−)-epicatechin **14**, (−)-epicatechin-3-*O*-gallate], dihydroflavonols (astilbin and engeletin) and proanthocyanidins **20** (Figure 2) [1,3,25,26,27,48]. Anthocyanins are found only in red grape varieties. They accumulate mainly in the berry skin, but in some varieties known as "teinturier" (or dyed), anthocyanin pigments are found to accumulate in the flesh of the berry [48,49]. It is important to note that there is a close correlation between anthocyanin biosynthesis and berry development: it starts at "veraison" when proanthocyanidin biosynthesis is concluded and reaches maximum level at berry "maturity" [50]. Each grape species and variety respectively has a unique set of anthocyanins [51]. European grapes produced only anthocyanidins 3-*O*-monoglucosides, whereas muscadine grapes produced only anthocyanidins 3,5-*O*-diglucosides [51].

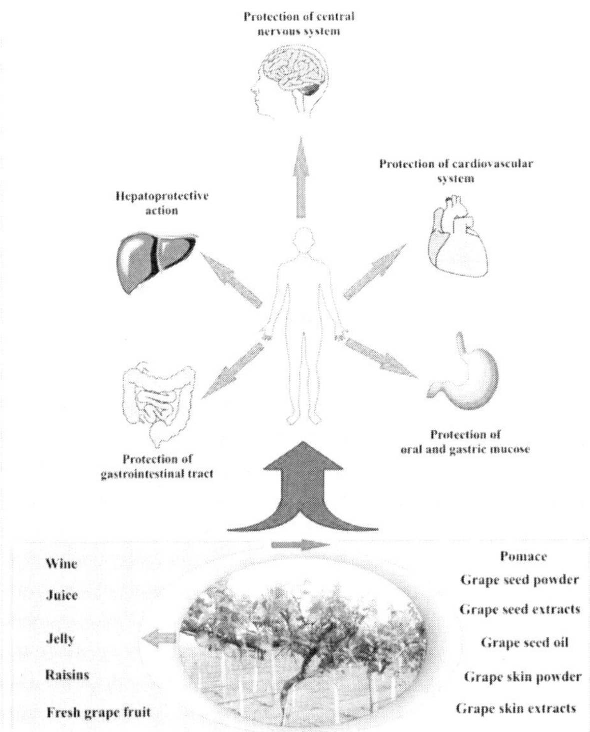

Figure 1. Primary grape products and byproducts and their beneficial effects on human body.

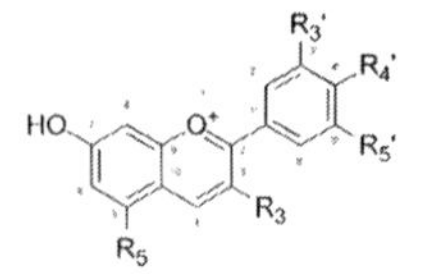

1	Pelargonidin 3-*O*-glucoside	R_3=glucose;	R_5=OH;	$R_{3'}$=H;	$R_{4'}$=OH;	$R_{5'}$=H
2	Pelargonidin 3,5-*O*-diglucoside	R_3=glucose;	R_5=glucose;	$R_{3'}$=H;	$R_{4'}$=OH;	$R_{5'}$=H
3	Cyanidin 3-*O*-glucoside	R_3=glucose;	R_5=OH;	$R_{3'}$=OH;	$R_{4'}$=OH;	$R_{5'}$=H
4	Cyanidin 3,5-*O*-diglucoside	R_3=glucose;	R_5=glucose;	$R_{3'}$=OH;	$R_{4'}$=OH;	$R_{5'}$=H
5	Delphinidin 3-*O*-glucoside	R_3=glucose;	R_5=OH;	$R_{3'}$=OH;	$R_{4'}$=OH;	$R_{5'}$=OH
6	Delphinidin 3,5-*O*-diglucoside	R_3=glucose;	R_5=glucose;	$R_{3'}$=OH;	$R_{4'}$=OH;	$R_{5'}$=OH
7	Peonidin 3-*O*-glucoside	R_3=glucose;	R_5=OH;	$R_{3'}$=OCH_3;	$R_{4'}$=OH;	$R_{5'}$=H
8	Peonidin 3,5-*O*-diglucoside	R_3=glucose;	R_5=glucose;	$R_{3'}$=OCH_3;	$R_{4'}$=OH;	$R_{5'}$=H
9	Petunidin 3-*O*-glucoside	R_3=glucose;	R_5=OH;	$R_{3'}$=OCH_3;	$R_{4'}$=OH;	$R_{5'}$=OH
10	Petunidin 3,5-*O*-diglucoside	R_3=glucose;	R_5=glucose;	$R_{3'}$=OCH_3;	$R_{4'}$=OH;	$R_{5'}$=OH
11	Malvidin 3-*O*-glucoside	R_3=glucose;	R_5=OH;	$R_{3'}$=OCH_3;	$R_{4'}$=OH;	$R_{5'}$=OCH_3
12	Malvidin 3,5-*O*-diglucoside	R_3=glucose;	R_5=glucose;	$R_{3'}$=OCH_3;	$R_{4'}$=OH;	$R_{5'}$=OCH_3

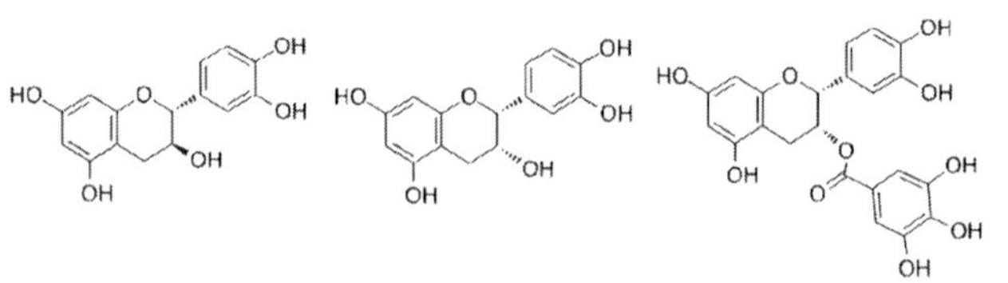

13 (+)-catechin **14** (-)-epicatechin **15** (-)-epicatechin-3-O-gallate

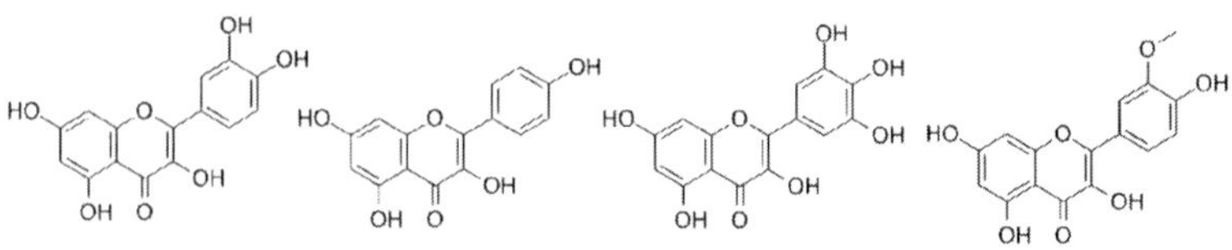

16 quercetin **17** kaempferol **18** myricetin **19** isorhamnetin

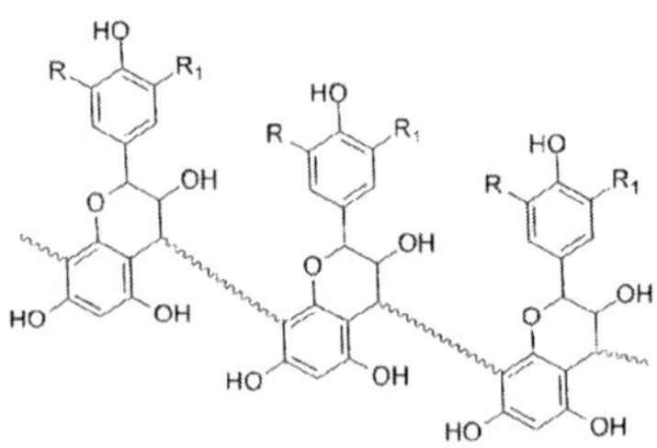

20 proanthocyanidins

Figure 2. Structures of some common grape flavonoids.

Flavanols are present in grapes mainly in the form of (+)-catechin **13**, (−)-epicatechin **14**, and proanthocyanidins **20**. They accumulate in the grape seeds, but are also found in the skin of the grape berries [52]. In white grape varieties flavanols represent 46% to 56% of total phenolics, whereas in red grapes they represent between 13% and 30% of total phenolic content [52]. As the second most abundant flavonoids in grapes, flavonols are present only as 3-*O*-glycosides in grape skins, but can be found also as aglycones (quercetin **16**, kaempferol **17**, myricetin **18**, isorhamnetin **19**) in wines and juices as a result of acid hydrolysis during processing and storage [53]. Quercetin, kaempferol and isorhamnetin derivatives are found in both red and white grapes, whereas myricetin derivatives are found only in red varieties [51,53]. The profile of flavonols strongly depends on grape cultivars, but in general quercetin-3-*O*-glucoside and quercetin-3-*O*-glucuronide are the predominant compounds present in most grapes [51]. In muscadine grapes, quercetin-3-*O*-rhamnoside and quercetin aglycone have been identified as the major flavonols [51]. The biological activities of flavonoids have been determined to strongly depend on several factors such as the degree of glycosylation, type of sugar residues and subsequent acyl esterification [54]. It is therefore possible to select different grape cultivars with unique flavonoid patterns having different health promoting effects on the human body.

2.2. Antioxidant Action

As a result of their aerobic metabolism, active cells produce toxic byproducts known as reactive oxygen species (ROS). ROS account for a wide range of aggressive free radicals produced by various metabolite pathways in living cells [55]. Under normal physiological conditions, ROS are considered to be important regulatory agents in the complex signaling network of cells. They play a major role in promoting cell growth and differentiation, adaptation to metabolic and physiological stresses, immune response as well as protection from pathogen invasion [55,56,57,58]. However, several factors may cause an over-accumulation of ROS by interrupting regular cellular processes and thus exposing tissues to conditions of oxidative stress (Figure 3).

When cells are exposed to oxidative stress they easily undergo oxidative damage that leads to a cascade of degenerative processes. Development of severe pathologies including neurodegenerative diseases, diabetes, cancer, liver diseases, cardiovascular diseases, and rapid aging are among the possible outcomes [57,58,59,60]. It is generally assumed that therapeutic treatment with antioxidants is the most effective way to control oxidative stress and to avoid occurrence of oxidative damage [57,60,61]. Various molecules by weight and structure including enzymes and hormones may have antioxidant activities in biological systems [62]. Antioxidants may neutralize oxidative stress in various ways including inhibition of free radical formation (preventive antioxidants), interrupting autoxidation chain reactions (chain breaking antioxidants), up-regulating and protecting cellular antioxidant defenses mechanisms (indirect antioxidants), neutralizing the action of metal pro-oxidant ions (metal chelators), inhibiting the action of pro-oxidative enzymes (enzyme inhibitors) and increasing the activities of other antioxidants (synergistic compounds) [63,64].

Flavonoids represent a large group of low molecular weight compounds with high antioxidant properties. Their specific chemical structure allows them to reduce oxidative stress through numerous mechanisms [34,65]. For example, it was reported that, *in vitro*, flavonoids could act both as preventive antioxidants and chain breaking antioxidants [scavenging superoxide, peroxyl, alkoxyl and hydroxyl radicals as well as preventing low-density lipoprotein (LDL) oxidation] [66]. On the other hand, flavonoids can also act as metal chelators (reducing ferric and cupric ions), and enzyme inhibitors (inhibiting the enzymes involved in ROS generation: xanthine oxidase; protein kinase C; cyclooxygenase; lipoxygenase; glutathione S-transferase; microsomal monooxygenase; mitochondrial succinoxidase and NADH oxidase) [66]. However,*in vivo* research has also demonstrated that flavonoids also may act as indirect antioxidants by up-regulating antioxidant defense system and increasing uric acid concentration in the plasma [63,64,66]. Therefore, as a result of their metabolic conversion in the human body, flavonoids generate large amounts of simple phenolic acids, which have significant effects in scavenging free radicals and improving the action of other antioxidants [66]. The consumption of grape-derived dietary flavonoids in the form of grape extracts and grape seed powders has been shown to effectively suppress oxidative stress and prevent oxidative damage*in vivo* [67,68,69]. Such activities are attributed to various functions of grape flavonoids as free radical scavengers and metal chelating compounds [67,68,69].

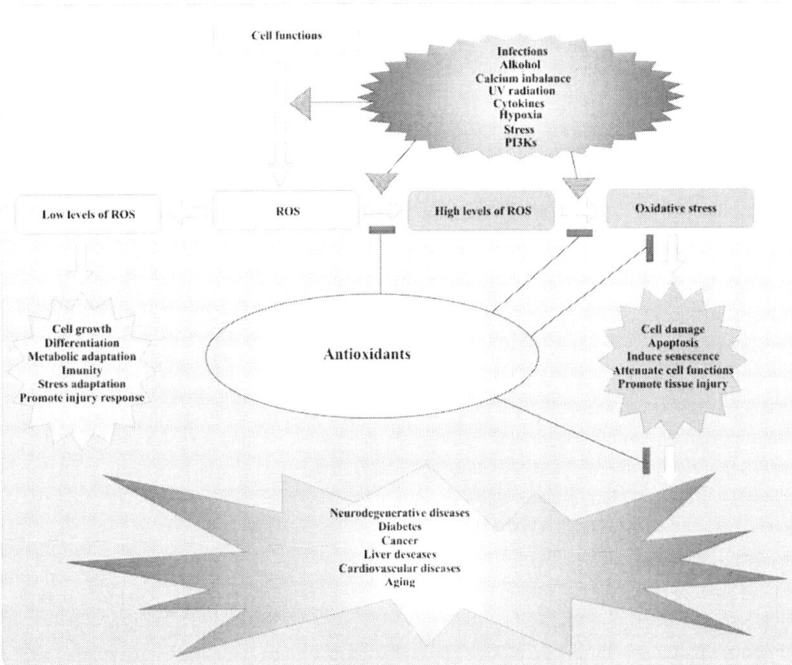

Figure 3. Reactive oxygen species (ROS) and their contribution to development of oxidative stress-related diseases. The presence of antioxidants may prevent diseases development by modulating damaging effects of ROS by suppressing multiple process steps.

2.3. Anti-Inflammatory Action

Inflammation is a protective response of tissues against cell injury, irritation, pathogen invasions, as well as mechanism for eliminating damaged and necrotic cells [70,71]. Several environmental stress factors may cause inflammation (Figure 4). Under normal physiological conditions, a short period of acute inflammation can overcome negative effects on injured tissue. However, if inflammation is prolonged, chronic inflammation can developed [70,72]. Chronic inflammation is considered to be the main mediator in the development of chronic diseases such as cancer, Alzheimer's, neurodegenerative diseases, cardiovascular diseases, diabetes, arthritis, autoimmune and pulmonary diseases [70,71,72,73,74,75]. Basic steps in progression of chronic inflammation are presented on Figure 4. When signal-dependent transcription factors [nuclear factor κB (NF-κB) and activating protein 1 (AP-1)] are activated, they induce the expression of genes involved in inflammatory response

[75]. Intensive production and secretion of pro-inflammatory cytokines and chemokines, once started, can form concentration gradients in affected tissues, which may lead to the amplification of the initial inflammatory response [70,72,75,76]. As a result, additional immune cells are recruited and increased levels of ROS are produced [70,75,76,77]. Under normal physiological conditions, anti-inflammatory cytokines act as immunoregulators to control the inflammatory reactions [70,77]. Deregulation of precise control mechanism of inflammation leads to chronic inflammation and promotion of chronic disease (Figure 4). Grape polyphenols have been shown to decrease chronic inflammation either by modulation of inflammatory pathways or by reducing ROS levels. As natural compounds, grape flavonoids and proanthocyanidins can target multiple pathways to overcome chronic inflammation, and thus are more effective compared to synthetic mono-targeted anti-inflammatory drugs [78]. Freeze-dried extract of wine from "Jacquez" grapes (*Vitis aestivalis-cinerea* × *Vitis vinifera*), which contains mainly flavonoids, anthocyanins, proanthocyanidins and hydroxycinnamic acid derivatives, showed higher anti-inflammatory activity when compared to the commercial non-steroidal anti-inflammatory drug (NSAID) indomethacin [79]. It has also been demonstrated that proanthocyanidins in grape seeds have high anti-inflammatory action, because they scavenge free radicals, prevent lipid peroxidation and inhibit formation of pro-inflammatory cytokines [80].

Proanthocyanidins extracted from the grape seeds have also been found to have an immune-modulatory role in inflammatory conditions that exert an overproduction of nitric oxide and prostaglandin E2 [81]. The suppression effect of extracts obtained by red and white grape pomaces on chronic inflammation induced by lipopolysaccharide and galactosamine, has been investigated *in vivo* [82]. The authors found that the extract of red grape pomace suppresses the activation of inflammatory transcription factor NF-κB and thus could be used as raw material for both extraction of new anti-inflammatory candidates or as an additive in processing functional foods [82].

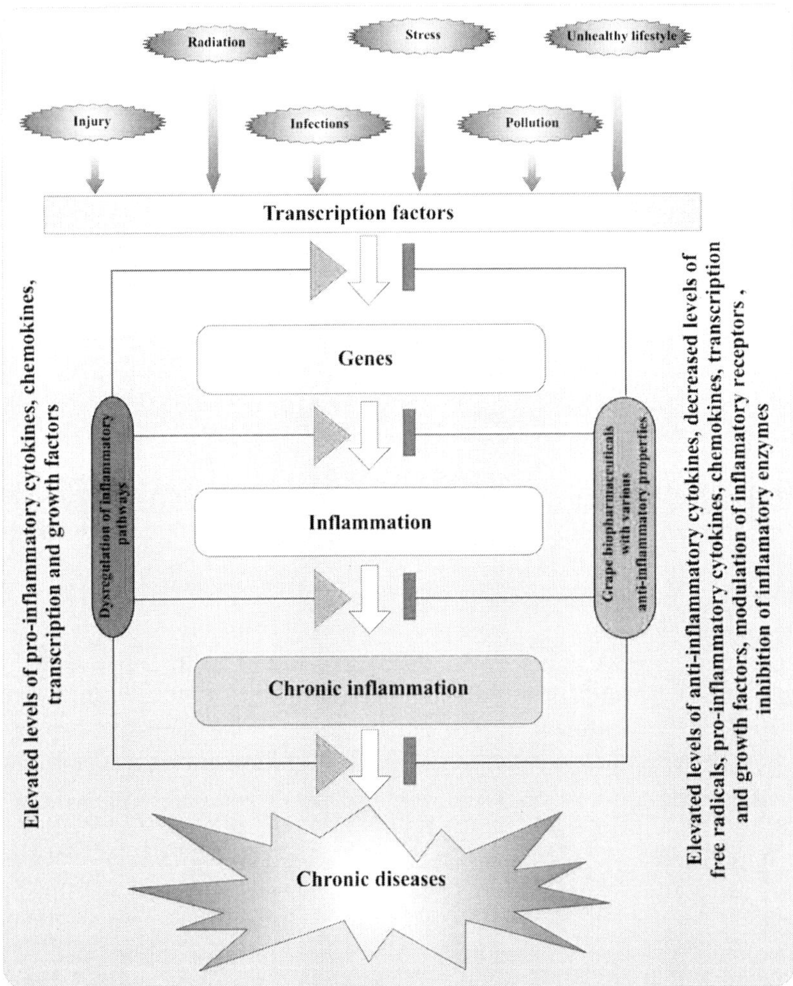

Figure 4. Principal way of development and modulation of chronic inflammation-related diseases.

2.4. Antimicrobial and Antiviral Activities

Antimicrobial activities of grape, wine and grape-derived byproducts have been widely discussed [26,83]. It has been demonstrated that grape seed extract of *V. vinifera* "Bangalore Blue Grapes" var. exhibits stronger antibacterial activity against Gram-positive bacteria compared to the response from Gram-negative bacteria [84]. Grape juice, skin and seed extracts from black table grapes "Ribier" var. have also been found to have a strong inhibitory effect against the growth of *Listeria monocytogenes* [85]. In addition, research has also shown that red colored (anthocyanin pigments) grape juice and skin extract have pH-dependent anti-listerial activity, while the seed extract showed pH-independent anti-listerial activity [85]. Strong anti-listerial activities have also been demonstrated for extracts of grape berries, seeds, pomace, and stems from red (*V. vinifera* "Mandilaria" and "Voidomato" var.) and white (*V. vinifera* "Asyrtiko" and "Aidani" var.) grape varieties. The main active compounds were catechine, epicatechine and epicatechine galate [86]. Recent research reported effective antiviral activity of grape skin extracts from fermented "Pinot Noir" var. and non-fermented "Pinot Gris" var. pomace against influenza virus [87]. Phytochemical analyses of the grape varieties from the study showed that the major phenolics in "Pinot Noir" var. extract were catechin and epicatechin, whereas rutin, catechin and epicatechin were predominant in extract of "Pinot Gris" var. [87]. However, no significant difference was observed between antiviral activities of both extracts, which suggested that they may be equally used as additives in different functional health promoting beverages [87]. Alcohol-free red and white wine extracts have been shown to have moderate antifungal activities on*Candida albicans* depending on their total phenolic contents [88]. Extracts from pomace, fermented seeds and skin of "Pinot Noir" var. were found to be more effective against *Candida albicans* than the ones from the "Pinot Meunier" var. [89]. Therefore, the observed antifungal activity of grape products made them attractive for commercial application, and some are being incorporated into skin care cosmetics. In addition to observed antimicrobial properties, grape flavonoids may play an important role in modulation of human gut microflora. Research has demonstrated that red wine grape extract (two parts of red wine extract and one part of grape juice extract) significantly reduced the ratio of Firmicutes: Bacteroidetes in an *in vitro*model simulator of the intestinal microbial ecosystem and thus could have beneficial effects in control of weight loss [90].

3. BIOAVAILABILITY AND ABSORPTION OF FLAVONOIDS

Studies investigating the bioavailability of anthocyanins that looked into the pharmacokinetics, absorption, metabolic fate and excretion have increased exponentially over the past decade in both human and animal models [91]. In the process of studying the bioavailability of anthocyanins, animals or volunteers are generally administered with anthocyanin-rich foods. For instance berries, juices, wines, extracts or pulps can be administered. After a certain period, plasma and urine are collected for analysis. In most studies focusing on anthocyanins, the resulting peak concentrations of pigments in plasma vary from the mid to extremely low levels [92]. Garcia-Alonso *et al.*, [93] reported an even lower amount of anthocyanins (0.05% of ingested dose), found in urine after the consumption of 12 g grape peel extract (equivalent to 183.9 mg total anthocyanins). However, even with low absorption capacity, grape polyphenols can have direct positive impact on gut mucosa [94]. Feeding experiments based on oral administration of wine to rats showed that poorly adsorbed grape polyphenols may decrease the oxidative damage exerted on DNA in caecal mucosal cells [94]. These studies suggest that some dietary flavonoids can exert a positive effect regardless of their poor absorption. However, it is important to realize that the most common flavonoids in the human diets are not necessarily the most active within the body, either because they have a lower intrinsic activity or because they are poorly absorbed from the intestine, highly metabolized, or rapidly eliminated [95]. In addition, the flavonoids that are found in blood and target organs and that result from digestive or hepatic activity may differ from the native substances in terms of biological activity [95]. Extensive knowledge of the bioavailability of flavonoids is thus essential if their health effects are to be understood. However, the beneficial activities of dietary flavonoids as antioxidants and/or anti-inflammatory agents could be under question in the human body, since these abilities are dependent on their structural properties, and currently very little is known about the bioavailability and further metabolism of those important nutraceuticals. Flavonoids are thought to be poorly absorbed because they occur in nature in highly hydrophilic glycosylated forms. However, only aglycones can effectively pass through the gut wall. It has been suggested that some species of colon microflora can hydrolyze flavonoid glycosides to their corresponding aglycones, although the microbial enzymes may also degrade the entire compound as well [96].

4. FACTORS AFFECTING BIOAVAILABILITY OF FLAVONOIDS

The diverse results in the area of bioavailability, including plasma and urine concentrations, as well as the availability of certain compounds can be attributed to factors affecting bioavailability of flavonoids. Some of the most important factors to consider are sources of flavonoids, specific chemical features of flavonoids, type of the food matrix, dosage, individual variation, analytical methodology, and detection minimum [92,97]. A recent study by Charron *et al.* [97], investigated the bioavalability of purple carrot juice anthocyanins, depending on the dosage, molecule acylation, and plant matrix. In their experiment, the highest concentration of anthocyanins in plasma was observed after consumption of 250 mL (323 mg total anthocyanins) carrot juice and it was found to decline in a dose-dependent manner, when lower doses (50 and 150 mL) were used. The authors found that the bioavailability of nonacylated anthocyanins was significantly higher, when compared to that of acylated anthocyanins. Moreover, the increased administration dose resulted in decrease in absorption efficiency and the authors suggested that saturation equilibrium of cyanidin-based anthocyanins was between 250 and 350 μM [97]. Therefore, increasing the dosage of consumed flavonoid compounds can result in improved plasma concentration but only until a saturation point is reached [98]. In addition to the above mentioned factors, sample preparation techniques and modifications of molecule structure can also contribute to the incensement on overall recovery of flavonoids as demonstrated by Woodward *et al.* [99].

5. GRAPE FLAVONOIDS AND HUMAN HEALTH

Currently, there are thousands of grape-derived products on the market including juices, wines, jam, jelly, raisins, and others. Recently, it was found that even byproducts, obtained as a result of grape processing (pomace, seeds, skins, seed oil) have high nutraceutical values and were commercialized in various forms of different powders, granulates, concentrated or dried extracts and other innovative means of packaging. Here some recent scientific facts, concerning the effects of these products on body health status are briefly discussed.

5.1. Brain Function

Consumption of flavonoid-rich grape products may have a significant beneficial effect on brain function and central nervous system [100]. Grape flavonoids, specifically anthocyanins, can prevent neurodegenerative processes both by inhibition of neuro-inflammation and by reducing oxidative stress. A clinical study demonstrated that 12 weeks supplementation with *Vitis labrusca* "Concord" var. grape juice in the diet may have neurocognitive benefits in older adults with early memory decline [101]. Consumption of "Concord" var. grape juice was also found to improve memory functions in older adults with mild memory decline [102]. Recently, it was demonstrated that polyphenol-rich grape seed extract has a significant capability of disrupting and disintegrating the ultrastructure of native paired helical filaments (a key neuropathological feature in Alzheimer's disease) [103]. The authors showed that resveratrol was ineffective in this process but rather catechin and epicatechin were involved [103].

5.2. Obesity and Diabetes

Metabolic syndrome–related diseases and obesity are the most prevalent nutrition-related issues in the United States [104]. Evidence suggests that polyphenols in grapes and grape products may reduce metabolic syndrome and prevent development of obesity and type 2 diabetes, by acting as multi-target modulators with antioxidant and anti-inflammatory effects [100,104]. Freeze-dried grape powder and grape powder extracts, obtained from red, green, and blue-purple seeded and seedless California grapes were tested for their effects on glucose tolerance and inflammation in obese mice [105]. The authors found that grape powder acutely improves glucose tolerance and chronically reduces inflammatory markers in obese mice [105]. They also reported that quercetin-3-*O*-glucoside was the compound with the highest bioavailability in grape powder extracts and can reduce several inflammatory markers in human adipocytes [105]. Animal model study showed that, in addition to the currently known anti-inflammatory and antioxidant activities, grape seed extract prevents metabolic syndrome, type 2 diabetes and obesity, also by modulating of metabolic endotoxemia and improving of gut barrier integrity [106].

5.3. Herpatoprotective Activity

Environmental factors such as pollutants, alcohol, viral infections, and aflatoxins, can promote development of liver disease [60]. Grape polyphenols have the ability to protect liver because of their anti-inflammatory and antioxidant properties [25]. Polyphenol-rich grape skin extract has been found to improve liver steatosis and to protect against diet-induced adiposity and hepatic steatosis [107]. These effects were probably due to the suppression of lipogenic enzymes in liver and adipose tissues and modulation of lipid metabolism by regulation of mRNA expression of enzymes, involved in regulation of lipogenesis and fatty acids oxidation [107]. Another study compared the protective effects of aqueous and ethanol seed extracts of red grapes against ethanol-induced cytotoxicity in the liver [60]. The research revealed that ethanol grape seed extracts was more effective against hepatotoxicity of alcohol, when compared to aqueous grape seeds extract. The authors attributed the observed effect to the nature and antioxidant activity of extract's constituents [60].

5.4. Cardiovascular Diseases

Several studies have shown that consumption of grape products may have beneficial effect on cardiovascular system by enhancing endothelial function, decreasing LDL oxidation, improving vascular function, altering blood lipids, and modulating inflammatory process [23,24,25,26,100]. It has also been demonstrated that consumption of flavonoid-rich purple grape juice may attenuate cardiovascular diseases and inhibit thrombosis [108]. Clinical study suggested that this effect is probably due to the suppression of platelet-dependent inflammation by significant decrease in levels of platelet-dependent superoxide and the inflammatory mediator sCD40L after consumption of purple grape juice [108]. Recently it was demonstrated that consumption of resveratrol-rich grape extract could exert additional vascular protective benefits in stable patients with coronary artery disease, when compared to the action of a conventional grape extract or a placebo [109]. A one year clinical study demonstrated that regular consumption of resveratrol-rich grape extract increased serum adiponectin, prevented incensement of plasminogen activator inhibitor type 1 (PAI-1) and inhibited atherothrombotic signals in peripheral blood mononuclear cells [109]. Recent research showed that consumption of grapes has anti-oxidative effect and increases the levels of anti-inflammatory factors in the absence of dyslipidemias in men with metabolic syndrome [110].

5.5. Cancer Prevention

Anticancer properties of grapes and grape products have been widely discussed in the scientific literature [1,25,26,111]. The remarkable anticancer effect of grape products is considered to be due to their unique mixture of polyphenolic compounds with various biological activities [111]. Flavonoids are the main group of active anticancer constituents in grape products, and are concentrated mainly in grape skins and seeds [111]. Researchers have shown that grape skin extract possesses chemotherapeutic efficacy against breast cancer with metastases in model system [112]. Recently, extracts of raisins from two grape varieties (*V. vinifera* "Currant" and "Sultana" var.) were investigated for their effect on human colon cancer cells [113]. The authors found that both extracts exhibited cancer preventive efficacy on colon cancer cells by having antioxidant and anti-inflammatory effects [113]. Treatment of human pancreatic cancer cells with grape seed proanthocyanidins significantly reduced cell viability and induced apoptosis in a dose- and time-dependent manner [114]. The authors demonstrated that grape seed proanthocyanidins can inhibit migration of human pancreatic cancer cell by inactivating the inflammatory transcription factor NF-κB [114].

6. PLANT CELL SUSPENSIONS AS ALTERNATIVE SOURCE OF GRAPE FLAVONOIDS

Plant cell cultures are generally considered as prospective alternatives for continuous production of phytochemicals under controlled conditions [115,116,117]. In the last few years, plant cell biotechnology of grapes and especially grape cell suspensions has enjoyed great attention from both science and industry [27]. Grape cell suspensions have been used to study the mechanism of secondary metabolite biosynthesis, for conducting functional genetic studies, somatic embryo development and *in vitro* production of valuable polyphenols [27,118,119,120,121,122]. Growth of grape cells in bioreactors for production of biologically active nutraceuticals exerts several advantages compared to conventional breeding (Figure 5). Strictly controlled environmental conditions during *in vitro* cultivation of grape cells minimize variation in yield and unpredictable metabolite composition that occurs with natural harvest. Production of nutraceutical-rich grape biomass can be done continuously throughout the year without concern about the seasons, soils and climate changes. Several optimization strategies may be involved for increasing the yields of the targeted phytochemicals, thus concentrations may exceed levels in the normal plant. For example, a non-resveratrol producing grapevine cell suspension of grape hybrid (*Vitis vinifera* "Chasselas" × *Vitis berlandieri*) elicited with 0.2 mM methyl jasmonate was found to initiate resveratrol production [123]. When the culture was scaled-up to a laboratory bioreactor, a total resveratrol yield of 230 mg/L was achieved. In addition, 90% of produced resveratrol (209 mg/L) was found to be secreted into the culture medium [123].

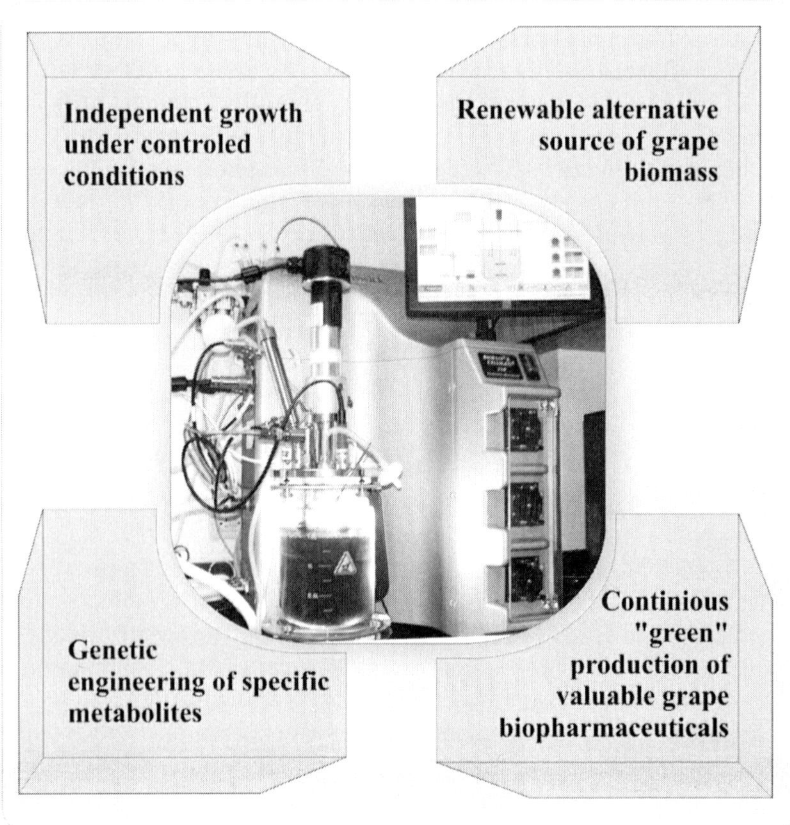

Figure 5. Advantages of *in vitro* grape cell suspension cultures as a source of nutraceuticals.

The ability of grape cells to secrete and accumulate secondary metabolites in culture medium is of high technological importance because this may significantly facilitate the downstream processing of target phytochemicals [116]. The development of reliable and sustainable sources of highly purified resveratrol is of special interest for the pharmaceutical industry because this compound may exert both estrogenic and anti-estrogenic effects *in vitro* and *in vivo* [124]. A recent study demonstrated that treatments with high concentrations of resveratrol may have cancer chemopreventive and therapeutic effects, the intake of resveratrol in low concentrations as a dietary supplement may also have promoting effect on mammary tumor growth and metastasis [125]. Thus, to achieve therapeutic effect and to eliminate the risk of side effects, resveratrol should be administrated only in high concentrations. Resveratrol-rich grape biomass, produced by *in vitro* cultivation of grape cells could be used as a potential natural additive to overcome this complication. In addition to the increased dose of resveratrol, the grape cells biomass can also provide the full unique mix of all naturally occurring nutrients found in field-growing grape, which usually have emphatic synergistic effect on its biological activity.

Flavonoid biosynthesis in grape cell suspensions is extremely sensitive to composition of nutrient medium. Studies using plant cell suspension of *V. vinifera* L. “Gamay Fréaux” var. Tenturier showed that two types of media (maintenance and production) should be used to support the best growth rate and to achieve the highest flavonoid production [126]. When cultivated on maintenance medium (low sucrose and high nitrate contents) the cells have maximum growth rate but extremely low levels of flavonoid accumulation [126]. When sucrose, ammonium, phosphate and magnesium concentrations in nutrient medium were increased (3, 2, 2 and 2 folds, respectively) the maximum yields of anthocyanins (1100 mg/L), proanthocyanidins (300 mg/L) and catechins (25 mg/L) were achieved [126]. Catechins [(+)-catechin, (−)-epicatechin and epicatechin 3-*O*-gallate], isolated from *V. vinifera* L. “Gamay Fréaux” var. cell suspensions were found to have cancer-chemopreventive effects by inhibiting cyclooxygenases (COX-1 and COX-2) activities, whereas the stilbenoids isolated from the same culture were more potent in inhibiting the development of 7,12-dimethylbenz[*a*]anthracene (DMBA)-induced preneoplastic lesions [127]. It is possible that common media manipulations may have significant effects on phytochemical patterns of *in vitro*growing grape cells. Adaptation of the well-established plant cell techniques may contribute to development of sustainable technology for production of improved grape cell biomass. It could be expected that such biomass will contribute to development of natural products with increased added value, since it contains the same unique mix of biologically active compounds compared to those found in regular growing grapes but in higher concentrations. However, the technology is still under investigation and more research and clinical studies are needed to strengthen the nutritional and beneficial health effects of *in vitro* produced grape cell biomass.

Another potential application of grape cell suspension is in production of marker compounds, used in *in vivo* study of bioavailability and metabolism of phytonutrients. Cell suspension culture of *Vitis* hybrid “Bailey Alicant A” [(*V. lincocumii* × *V. labrusca* × *V. vinifera*) × (*V. vinifera* × *V. vinifera*)] was used to produce radiolabeled anthocyanins, (+)-catechin and (–)-epicatechin by feeding with ^{14}C labeled sucrose during cultivation [128]. The production of radiolabeled flavonoids by grape cell suspension have great potential as a reliable source of labeled phytochemicals used for *in vivo* study of bioavailability, catabolism and accumulation of these chemicals in animals and humans. Further improvement of production yield of labeled flavonoids could significantly decrease the price and increase the availability of such rare and expensive isotopic markers.

Despite all the positive effects of plant cell technology, the cultivation of grape cells is still carried out in small scale within the laboratory. The slowdown in scale-up has mainly been caused by the relatively low yields and expensive equipment, which decrease the economic effectiveness of the entire process. Genetic engineering may be applied to achieve additional increase of grape cell culture productivity. Genetic manipulation of the flavonoid biosynthetic pathway is a powerful tool for increasing the yields of targeted products or redirecting cell metabolism to produce only the desired group of metabolites [3,27]. Moreover,*in vitro* cultivation of grape cells in an eco-friendly bio-safe environment is of great importance. Hence, the process ensures the complete isolation of genetically modified cells from the natural environment and eliminates the risk of cross-contaminations and transgene migration [117].

7. NUTRACEUTICAL PRODUCTS DERIVED BY GRAPES

Wine is the most popular and widely discussed nutritional grape product with proven beneficial health effects on human body. Moderate consumption of red wines in daily diet (often referred as "Mediterranean way of drinking") is considered to contribute for overall improvement of consumers' health, mainly due to the beneficial effects of quercetin and resveratrol [129]. However, wine also contains alcohol, which significantly restricts its mass consumption especially among underage and actively working individuals. Studies have shown that the consumption of red wine can increase antioxidant activity of plasma. However, over-consumption may lead to the increase of isoprostanes—an oxidative lipid damage marker [130]. The authors demonstrated that this effect may be avoided by consumption of dealcoholized red wine, which has the same flavonoid compounds (myricitin, quercetin and isorhamnetin) and in similar concentrations as in red wine, but is free of alcohol

[130]. The unique combination of grape polyphenols, including flavonoids, anthocyanins, proanthocyanins, and stilbenes, makes grape a promising source for the development of novel nutraceutical products. In the last few years, there has been a wide range of food additives and nutritional products originating from grapes, distributed in the worldwide market. Most of these commercialized products are obtained during processing of pomace from wine or grape juice production. This includes several grape skin or seed extracts, grape skin powder, dry seed powder (capsulated or bulk), pomace powder, and anthocyanin colorants. The diversity of these products, and their biological activities and health benefits are reviewed by Amarowicz and Weidner [131]. Recently, the biomass from grape cell suspension of *V. vinifera* L. "Gamay Fréaux" var. was commercialized by the Swiss company "Mibelle Biochemistry". The purpose of the commercialization was to develop a natural additive "PhytoCellTec™ Solar Vitis" for exclusive application in skin-care and other cosmetic products [132]. This is the first commercial grape product in the market, obtained by the methods of modern high-end plant biotechnology. According to the company, the product is rich in anthocyanins and its application may have beneficial effects on skin because of the presence of strong UV protectors and anti-aging ingredients.

8. CONCLUSIONS

Grape and grape products should be promoted in our daily diet not only as a nutrient, but as a healthy food as well. Currently, a growing number of researchers are focusing on the biological activities of grape and grape products as prospective sources of valuable nutraceuticals. Numerous studies have strongly suggested that the inclusion of grapes and grape products as supplements in our daily intake of foods may generate significant health benefits. However, to achieve beneficial therapeutic effects, most of these phytochemicals must be used in a strict dose-dependent manner. Bioavailability in *in vivo* conditions is a key issue to be resolved for establishing the level of therapeutic blood concentrations of grape flavonoids. Therefore, more studies are needed in this area. Future development of new renewable sources, such as *in vitro* cell systems that can continuously produce highly purified grape flavonoids is essential and can be broadly applicable.

ACKNOWLEDGMENTS

The authors are grateful to James Muchovej, Plant Physiology, Florida A&M University and Ernst Cebert, Plant Genetics and Breeding, Alabama A&M University for reviewing and editing this manuscript. The research has been done with the financial support of USDA/NIFA/AFRI Plant Biochemistry Program Grant #2009-03127 and USDA/NIFA/1890 Capacity Building Grant #2010-02388.

CONFLICTS OF INTEREST

The authors declare no conflict of interest.

REFERENCES

1. Ali, K.; Maltese, F.; Choi, Y.; Verpoorte, R. Metabolic constituents of grapevine and grape-derived products. Phytochem. Rev. 2010, 9, 357–378.
2. Vivier, M.A.; Pretorius, I.S. Genetic improvement of grapevine: Tailoring grape varieties for the third millennium—A review. S. Afr. J. Enol. Vitic. 2000, 21, 5–26.
3. Ananga, A.; Georgiev, V.; Tsolova, V. Manipulation and engineering of metabolic and biosynthetic pathway of plant polyphenols. Curr. Pharm. Des. 2013, 19, 6186–6206.
4. Vogt, T. Phenylpropanoid biosynthesis. Mol. Plant 2010, 3, 2–20.
5. Harborne, J.B.; Williams, C.A. Advances in flavonoid research since 1992. Phytochemistry 2000, 55, 481–504.
6. Waterhouse, A.L. Wine phenolics. Ann. N. Y. Acad. Sci 2002, 957, 21–36.
7. Bogs, J.; Jaffé, F.W.; Takos, A.M.; Walker, A.R.; Robinson, S.P. The grapevine transcription factorvvmybpa1 regulates proanthocyanidin synthesis during fruit development. Plant Physiol. 2007, 143, 1347–1361.
8. Dixon, R.A. Engineering of plant natural product pathways. Curr. Opin. Plant Biol. 2005, 8, 329–336.
9. Lepiniec, L.; Debeaujon, I.; Routaboul, J.M.; Baudry, A.; Pourcel, L.; Nesi, N.; Caboche, M. Genetics and biochemistry of seed flavonoids. Ann. Rev. Plant Biol. 2006, 57, 405–430.

10. Conde, C.; Silva, P.; Fontes, N.; Dias, A.C.; Tavares, R.M.; Sousa, M.J.; Agasse, A.; Delrot, S.; Gerós, H. Biochemical changes throughout grape berry development and fruit and wine quality. Food 2007, 1, 1–22.

11. Renaud, S.C.; Beswick, A.D.; Fehily, A.M.; Sharp, D.S.; Elwood, P.C. Alcohol and platelet aggregation: The caerphilly prospective heart disease study. Am. J. Clin. Nutr. 1992, 55, 1012–1017.

12. Formica, J.V.; Regelson, W. Review of the biology of quercetin and related bioflavonoids. Food Chem. Toxicol. 1995, 33, 1061–1080.

13. Lin, J.K.; Weng, M.S. Flavonoids as Nutraceuticals. In The Science of Favonoids; Grotewold, E., Ed.; Springer: Berlin, Germany, 2006; pp. 213–238.

14. De Groot, H.; Rauen, U. Tissue injury by reactive oxygen species and the protective effects of flavonoids. Fundam. Clin. Pharmacol. 1998, 12, 249–255.

15. Hertog, M.G.; Kromhout, D.; Aravanis, C.; Blackburn, H.; Buzina, R.; Fidanza, F.; Giampaoli, S.; Jansen, A.; Menotti, A.; Nedeljkovic, S.; et al. Flavonoid intake and long-term risk of coronary heart disease and cancer in the seven countries study. Arch. Intern. Med. 1995, 155, 381–386.

16. Knekt, P.; Jarvinen, R.; Reunanen, A.; Maatela, J. Flavonoid intake and coronary mortality in Finland: A cohort study. BMJ 1996, 312, 478–481.

17. Le Marchand, L. Cancer preventive effects of flavonoids—A review. Biomed. Pharmacother. 2002, 56, 296–301.

18. Khan, N.; Adhami, V.M.; Mukhtar, H. Apoptosis by dietary agents for prevention and treatment of prostate cancer. Endocr. Relat. Cancer 2010, 17, R39–R52.

19. McGovern, P.E.; Glusker, D.L.; Exner, L.J.; Voigt, M.M. Neolithic resinated wine. Nature 1996, 381, 480–481.

20. Riedel, H.; Saw, N.M.M.T.; Akumo, D.N.; Kütük, O.; Smetanska, I. Wine as Food and Medicine. InScientific, Health and Social Aspects of the Food Industry; Valdez, B., Ed.; InTech: Rijeka, Croatia, 2012; pp. 399–418.

21. This, P.; Lacombe, T.; Thomas, M.R. Historical origins and genetic diversity of wine grapes. Trends Genet. 2006, 22, 511–519.

22. Bertelli, A.A.A.; Das, D.K. Grapes, wines, resveratrol, and heart health. J. Cardiovasc. Pharmacol. 2009,54, 468–476.

23. Vislocky, L.M.; Fernandez, M.L. Grapes and grape products: Their role in health. Nutr. Today 2013, 48, 47–51.

24. Li, H.; Förstermann, U. Red wine and cardiovascular health. Circ. Res. 2012, 111, 959–961.

25. Nassiri-Asl, M.; Hosseinzadeh, H. Review of the pharmacological effects of Vitis vinifera (grape) and its bioactive compounds. Phytother. Res. 2009, 23, 1197–1204.

26. Xia, E.-Q.; Deng, G.-F.; Guo, Y.-J.; Li, H.-B. Biological activities of polyphenols from grapes. Int. J. Mol. Sci. 2010, 11, 622–646.

27. Ananga, A.; Georgiev, V.; Ochieng, J.; Phills, B.; Tsolova, V. Production of Anthocyanins in Grape Cell Cultures: A Potential Source of Raw Material for Pharmaceutical, Food, and Cosmetic Industries. InThe Mediterranean Genetic Code—Grapevine and Olive; Sladonja, B., Poljuha, D., Eds.; InTech: Rijeka, Croatia, 2012; pp. 247–287.

28. Yilmaz, Y.; Toledo, R.T. Major flavonoids in grape seeds and skins: Antioxidant capacity of catechin, epicatechin, and gallic acid. J. Agric. Food Chem. 2004, 52, 255–260.

29. Nguyen, D.M.; Seo, D.J.; Lee, H.B.; Kim, I.S.; Kim, K.Y.; Park, R.D.; Jung, W.J. Antifungal activity of gallic acid purified from Terminalia nigrovenulosa bark against Fusarium solani. Microb. Pathog. 2013, 56, 8–15.

30. Zhao, J.; Khan, I.A.; Fronczek, F.R. Gallic acid. Acta Crystallogr. Sect. E 2011, 67, 316–317.

31. Sameermahmood, Z.; Raji, L.; Saravanan, T.; Vaidya, A.; Mohan, V.; Balasubramanyam, M. Gallic acid protects rinm5f β-cells from glucolipotoxicity by its antiapoptotic and insulin-secretagogue actions.Phytother. Res. 2010, 24, S83–S94.

32. Rather, S.A.; Sarumathi, A.; Anbu, S.; Saravanan, N. Gallic acid protects against immobilization stress-induced changes in wistar rats. J. Stress Physiol. Biochem. 2013, 9, 136–147.

33. Raj, N.K.; Sripal, R.M.; Chaluvadi, M.R.; Krishna, D.R. Bioflavonoids classification, pharmacological, biochemical effects and therapeutic potential. Indian J. Pharmacol. 2001, 33, 2–16.

34. Heim, K.E.; Tagliaferro, A.R.; Bobilya, D.J. Flavonoid antioxidants: Chemistry, metabolism and structure-activity relationships. J. Nutr. Biochem. 2002, 13, 572–584.

35. Han, X.; Shen, T.; Lou, H. Dietary polyphenols and their biological significance. Int. J. Mol. Sci. 2007, 8, 950–988.

36. Alzand, K.I.; Mohamed, M.A. Flavonoids: Chemistry, biochemistry and antioxidant activity. J. Pharm. Res. 2012, 5, 4013–4012.

37. Tsao, R. Chemistry and biochemistry of dietary polyphenols. Nutrients 2010, 2, 1231–1246.

38. Capanoglu, E.; de Vos, R.C.H.; Hall, R.D.; Boyacioglu, D.; Beekwilder, J. Changes in polyphenol content during production of grape juice concentrate. Food Chem. 2013, 139, 521–526.

39. Sun, B.; Spranger, M.I. Review: Quantitative extraction and analysis of grape and wine proanthocyanidin and stilbenes. Ciência Téc. Vitiv. 2005, 20, 59–89.

40. Ratnasooriya, C.C.; Rupasinghe, H.P.V. Extraction of phenolic compounds from grapes and their pomace using β-cyclodextrin. Food Chem. 2012, 134, 625–631.

41. Chamorro, S.; Goñi, I.; Viveros, A.; Hervert-Hernández, D.; Brenes, A. Changes in polyphenolic content and antioxidant activity after thermal treatments of grape seed extract and grape pomace.Eur. Food Res. Technol. 2012, 234, 147–155.

42. Greenspan, P.; Bauer, J.D.; Pollock, S.H.; Gangemi, J.D.; Mayer, E.P.; Ghaffar, A.; Hargrove, J.L.; Hartle, D.K. Antiinflammatory properties of the muscadine grape (Vitis rotundifolia). J. Agric. Food Chem. 2005, 53, 8481–8484.

43. Jeong, Y.S.; Hong, J.H.; Cho, K.H.; Jung, H.K. Grape skin extract reduces adipogenesis- and lipogenesis-related gene expression in 3t3-l1 adipocytes through the peroxisome proliferator-activated receptor-γ signaling pathway. Nutr. Res. 2012, 32, 514–521.

44. Lee, J.-H.; Talcott, S.T. Ellagic acid and ellagitannins affect on sedimentation in muscadine juice and wine. J. Agric. Food Chem. 2002, 50, 3971–3976.

45. Ghafoor, K.; Al-Juhaimi, F.; Choi, Y.H. Effects of grape (Vitis labrusca B.) peel and seed extracts on phenolics, antioxidants and anthocyanins in grape juice. Pak. J. Bot. 2011, 43, 1581–1586.

46. Vattem, D.A.; Shetty, K. Biological functionality of ellagic acid: A review. J. Food Biochem. 2005, 29, 234–266.

47. Hichri, I.; Barrieu, F.; Bogs, J.; Kappel, C.; Delrot, S.; Lauvergeat, V. Recent advances in the transcriptional regulation of the flavonoid biosynthetic pathway. J. Exp. Bot. 2011, 62, 2465–2483.

48. He, F.; Mu, L.; Yan, G.-L.; Liang, N.-N.; Pan, Q.-H.; Wang, J.; Reeves, M.J.; Duan, C.-Q. Biosynthesis of anthocyanins and their regulation in colored grapes. Molecules 2010, 15, 9057–9091.

49. Rodríguez Montealegre, R.; Romero Peces, R.; Chacón Vozmediano, J.L.; Martínez Gascueña, J.; García Romero, E. Phenolic compounds in skins and seeds of ten grape Vitis vinifera varieties grown in a warm climate. J. Food Compos. Anal. 2006, 19, 687–693.

50. Zhang, Z.-Z.; Che, X.-N.; Pan, Q.-H.; Li, X.-X.; Duan, C.-Q. Transcriptional activation of flavan-3-ols biosynthesis in grape berries by UV irradiation depending on developmental stage. Plant Sci. 2013,208, 64–74.

51. Zhu, L.; Zhang, Y.; Lu, J. Phenolic contents and compositions in skins of red wine grape cultivars among various genetic backgrounds and originations. Int. J. Mol. Sci. 2012, 13, 3492–3510.

52. Cantos, E.; Espín, J.C.; Tomás-Barberán, F.A. Varietal differences among the polyphenol profiles of seven table grape cultivars studied by LC–DAD–MS–MS. J. Agric. Food Chem. 2002, 50, 5691–5696.

53. Castillo-Muñoz, N.; Gómez-Alonso, S.; García-Romero, E.; Hermosín-Gutiérrez, I. Flavonol profiles ofVitis vinifera red grapes and their single-cultivar wines. J. Agric. Food Chem. 2007, 55, 992–1002.

54. Cho, M.J.; Howard, L.R.; Prior, R.L.; Clark, J.R. Flavonoid glycosides and antioxidant capacity of various blackberry, blueberry and red grape genotypes determined by high-performance liquid chromatography/mass spectrometry. J. Sci. Food Agric. 2004, 84, 1771–1782.

55. Murphy, M.P.; Holmgren, A.; Larsson, N.G.; Halliwell, B.; Chang, C.J.; Kalyanaraman, B.; Rhee, S.G.; Thornalley, P.J.; Partridge, L.; Gems, D.; et al. Unraveling the biological roles of reactive oxygen species. Cell Metab. 2011, 13, 361–366.

56. Forman, H.J.; Maiorino, M.; Ursini, F. Signaling functions of reactive oxygen species. Biochemistry2010, 49, 835–842.

57. Sugamura, K.; Keaney, J.J.F. Reactive oxygen species in cardiovascular disease. Free Radic. Biol. Med.2011, 51, 978–992.

58. Panieri, E.; Gogvadze, V.; Norberg, E.; Venkatesh, R.; Orrenius, S.; Zhivotovsky, B. Reactive oxygen species generated in different compartments induce cell death, survival, or senescence. Free Radic. Biol. Med. 2013, 57, 176–187.

59. Sena, L.A.; Chandel, N.S. Physiological roles of mitochondrial reactive oxygen species. Mol. Cell 2012,48, 158–167.

60. Hassan, H.M.M. Hepatoprotective effect of red grape seed extracts against ethanol-induced cytotoxicity. Glob. J. Biotechnol. Biochem. 2012, 7, 30–37.

61. Heo, J.-H.; Lee, H.; Lee, K.-M. The possible role of antioxidant vitamin c in Alzheimer's disease treatment and prevention. Am. J. Alzheimer's Dis. Other Dement. 2013, 28, 120–125.

62. Prior, R.L.; Wu, X.; Schaich, K. Standardized methods for the determination of antioxidant capacity and phenolics in foods and dietary supplements. J. Agric. Food Chem. 2005, 53, 4290–4302.

63. Carocho, M.; Ferreira, I.C.F.R. A review on antioxidants, prooxidants and related controversy: Natural and synthetic compounds, screening and analysis methodologies and future perspectives. Food Chem. Toxicol. 2013, 51, 15–25.

64. Khlebnikov, A.I.; Schepetkin, I.A.; Domina, N.G.; Kirpotina, L.N.; Quinn, M.T. Improved quantitative structure–activity relationship models to predict antioxidant activity of flavonoids in chemical, enzymatic, and cellular systems. Bioorg. Med. Chem. 2007, 15, 1749–1770.

65. Procházková, D.; Boušová, I.; Wilhelmová, N. Antioxidant and prooxidant properties of flavonoids.Fitoterapia 2011, 82, 513–523.

66. Pietta, P.-G. Flavonoids as antioxidants. J. Nat. Prod. 2000, 63, 1035–1042.

67. Choi, S.-K.; Zhang, X.-H.; Seo, J.-S. Suppression of oxidative stress by grape seed supplementation in rats. Nutr. Res. Pract. 2012, 6, 3–8.

68. Lakshmi, B.V.S.; Sudhakar, M.; Aparna, M. Protective potential of black grapes against lead induced oxidative stress in rats. Environ. Toxicol. Pharmacol. 2013, 35, 361–368.

69. Scola, G.; Scheffel, T.; Gambato, G.; Freitas, S.; Dani, C.; Funchal, C.; Gomez, R.; Coitinho, A.; Salvador, M. Flavan-3-ol compounds prevent pentylenetetrazol-induced oxidative damage in rats without producing mutations and genotoxicity. Neurosci. Lett. 2013, 534, 145–149.

70. Aggarwal, B.B.; Shishodia, S.; Sandur, S.K.; Pandey, M.K.; Sethi, G. Inflammation and cancer: How hot is the link? Biochem. Pharmacol. 2006, 72, 1605–1621.

71. Dantzer, R.; O'Connor, J.C.; Freund, G.G.; Johnson, R.W.; Kelley, K.W. From inflammation to sickness and depression: When the immune system subjugates the brain. Nat. Rev. Neurosci. 2008, 9, 46–56.

72. Dinarello, C.A. Anti-inflammatory agents: Present and future. Cell 2010, 140, 935–950.

73. Sharma, M. Chemokines and their receptors: Orchestrating a fine balance between health and disease.Crit. Rev. Biotechnol. 2010, 30, 1–22.

74. Rubio-Perez, J.M.; Morillas-Ruiz, J.M. A review: Inflammatory process in Alzheimer's disease, role of cytokines. Sci. World J. 2012, 2012, 756357.

75. Tabas, I.; Glass, C.K. Anti-inflammatory therapy in chronic disease: Challenges and opportunities.Science 2013, 339, 166–172.

76. Dinarello, C.A. Proinflammatory cytokines. Chest 2000, 118, 503–508.

77. Opal, S.M.; DePalo, V.A. Anti-inflammatory cytokines. Chest 2000, 117, 1162–1172.

78. Sung, B.; Prasad, S.; Gupta, S.C.; Patchva, S.; Aggarwal, B.B. Regulation of Inflammation-Mediated Chronic Diseases by Botanicals. In Advances in Botanical Research: Recent trends in Medicinal Plants Research; Shyur, L.-F., Ed.; Academic Press: Oxford, UK, 2012; Volume 62, pp. 57–132.

79. Panico, A.M.; Cardile, V.; Avondo, S.; Garufi, F.; Gentile, B.; Puglia, C.; Bonina, F.; Santagati, N.A.; Ronsisvalle, G. The in vitro effect of a lyophilized extract of wine obtained from jacquez grapes on human chondrocytes. Phytomedicine 2006, 13, 522–526.

80. Li, W.G.; Zhang, X.Y.; Wu, Y.J.; Tian, X. Anti-inflammatory effect and mechanism of proanthocyanidins from grape seeds. Acta Pharmacol. Sin. 2001, 22, 1117–1120.

81. Terra, X.; Valls, J.; Vitrac, X.; Mérrillon, J.-M.; Arola, L.; Ardèvol, A.; Bladé, C.; Fernández-Larrea, J.; Pujadas, G.; Salvadó, J.; et al. Grape-seed procyanidins act as antiinflammatory agents in endotoxin-stimulated raw 264.7 macrophages by inhibiting nfkb signaling pathway. J. Agric. Food Chem. 2007, 55, 4357–4365.

82. Nishiumi, S.; Mukai, R.; Ichiyanagi, T.; Ashida, H. Suppression of lipopolysaccharide and galactosamine-induced hepatic inflammation by red grape pomace. J. Agric. Food Chem. 2012, 60, 9315–9320.

83. Perumalla, A.V.S.; Hettiarachchy, N.S. Green tea and grape seed extracts—Potential applications in food safety and quality. Food Res. Int. 2011, 44, 827–839.

84. Jayaprakasha, G.K.; Selvi, T.; Sakariah, K.K. Antibacterial and antioxidant activities of grape (Vitis vinifera) seed extracts. Food Res. Int. 2003, 36, 117–122.

85. Rhodes, P.L.; Mitchell, J.W.; Wilson, M.W.; Melton, L.D. Antilisterial activity of grape juice and grape extracts derived from Vitis vinifera variety ribier. Int. J. Food Microbiol. 2006, 107, 281–286.

86. Anastasiadi, M.; Chorianopoulos, N.G.; Nychas, G.-J.E.; Haroutounian, S.A. Antilisterial activities of polyphenol-rich extracts of grapes and vinification byproducts. J. Agric. Food Chem. 2009, 57, 457–463.

87. Bekhit, A.E.-D.A.; Cheng, V.J.; McConnell, M.; Zhao, J.H.; Sedcole, R.; Harrison, R. Antioxidant activities, sensory and anti-influenza activity of grape skin tea infusion. Food Chem. 2011, 129, 837–845.

88. Papadopoulou, C.; Soulti, K.; Roussis, I.G. Potential antimicrobial activity of red and white wine phenolic extracts against strains of Staphylococcus aureus, Escherichia coli and Candida albicans. Food Technol. Biotechnol. 2005, 43, 41–46.

89. Cheng, V.J.; Bekhit, A.E.-D.A.; McConnell, M.; Mros, S.; Zhao, J. Effect of extraction solvent, waste fraction and grape variety on the antimicrobial and antioxidant activities of extracts from wine residue from cool climate. Food Chem. 2012, 134, 474–482.

90. Kemperman, R.A.; Gross, G.; Mondot, S.; Possemiers, S.; Marzorati, M.; van de Wiele, T.; Doré, J.; Vaughan, E.E. Impact of polyphenols from black tea and red wine/grape juice on a gut model microbiome. Food Res. Int. 2013, 53, 659–669.

91. Lim, C.-G.; Koffas, M.A.G. Bioavailability and recent advances in the bioactivity of flavonoid and stilbene compounds. Curr. Org. Chem. 2010, 14, 1727–1751.

92. Galvano, F.; La Fauci, L.; Vitaglione, P.; Fogliano, V.; Vanella, L.; Felgines, C. Bioavailability, antioxidant and biological properties of the natural free-radical scavengers cyanidin and related glycosides. Ann. Ist. Super. Sanita 2007, 43, 382–393.

93. Garcia-Alonso, M.; Minihane, A.-M.; Rimbach, G.; Rivas-Gonzalo, J.C.; de Pascual-Teresa, S. Red wine anthocyanins are rapidly absorbed in humans and affect monocyte chemoattractant protein 1 levels and antioxidant capacity of plasma. J. Nutr. Biochem. 2009, 20, 521–529.

94. Scalbert, A.; Morand, C.; Manach, C.; Rémésy, C. Absorption and metabolism of polyphenols in the gut and impact on health. Biomed. Pharmacother. 2002, 56, 276–282.

95. Manach, C.; Scalbert, A.; Morand, C.; Rémésy, C.; Jiménez, L. Polyphenols: Food sources and bioavailability. Am. J. Clin. Nutr. 2004, 79, 727–747.

96. Bentz, A.B. A review of quercetin: Chemistry, antioxidant properties, and bioavailability. J. Young Investig. 2009. Available online: http://www.jyi.org/research/re.php?id=3416 (accessed on 1 October 2013).

97. Charron, C.S.; Kurilich, A.C.; Clevidence, B.A.; Simon, P.W.; Harrison, D.J.; Britz, S.J.; Baer, D.J.; Novotny, J.A. Bioavailability of anthocyanins from purple carrot juice: Effects of acylation and plant matrix. J. Agric. Food Chem. 2009, 57, 1226–1230.

98. Kurilich, A.C.; Clevidence, B.A.; Britz, S.J.; Simon, P.W.; Novotny, J.A. Plasma and urine responses are lower for acylated vs. nonacylated anthocyanins from raw and cooked purple carrots. J. Agric. Food Chem. 2005, 53, 6537–6542.

99. Woodward, G.; Kroon, P.; Cassidy, A.; Kay, C. Anthocyanin stability and recovery: Implications for the analysis of clinical and experimental samples. J. Agric. Food Chem. 2009, 57, 5271–5278.

100. Tsuda, T. Dietary anthocyanin-rich plants: Biochemical basis and recent progress in health benefits studies. Mol. Nutr. Food Res. 2012, 56, 159–170.

101. Krikorian, R.; Nash, T.A.; Shidler, M.D.; Shukitt-Hale, B.; Joseph, J.A. Concord grape juice supplementation improves memory function in older adults with mild cognitive impairment. Br. J. Nutr. 2010, 103, 730–734.

102. Krikorian, R.; Boespflug, E.L.; Fleck, D.E.; Stein, A.L.; Wightman, J.D.; Shidler, M.D.; Sadat-Hossieny, S. Concord grape juice supplementation and neurocognitive function in human aging. J. Agric. Food Chem. 2012, 60, 5736–5742.

103. Ksiezak-Reding, H.; Ho, L.; Santa-Maria, I.; Diaz-Ruiz, C.; Wang, J.; Pasinetti, G.M. Ultrastructural alterations of alzheimer's disease paired helical filaments by grape seed-derived polyphenols.Neurobiol. Aging 2012, 33, 1427–1439.

104. Chuang, C.C.; McIntosh, M.K. Potential mechanisms by which polyphenol-rich grapes prevent obesity-mediated inflammation and metabolic diseases. Ann. Rev. Nutr. 2011, 31, 155–176.

105. Chuang, C.-C.; Shen, W.; Chen, H.; Xie, G.; Jia, W.; Chung, S.; McIntosh, M.K. Differential effects of grape powder and its extract on glucose tolerance and chronic inflammation in high-fat-fed obese mice. J. Agric. Food Chem. 2012, 60, 12458–12468.

106. Goodrich, K.M.; Fundaro, G.; Griffin, L.E.; Grant, A.Q.; Hulver, M.W.; Ponder, M.A.; Neilson, A.P. Chronic administration of dietary grape seed extract increases colonic expression of gut tight junction protein occludin and reduces fecal calprotectin: A secondary analysis of healthy wistar furth rats.Nutr. Res. 2012, 32, 787–794.

107. Park, H.-J.; Jung, U.J.; Lee, M.-K.; Cho, S.-J.; Jung, H.-K.; Hong, J.H.; Park, Y.B.; Kim, S.R.; Shim, S.; Jung, J.; et al. Modulation of lipid metabolism by polyphenol-rich grape skin extract improves liver steatosis and adiposity in high fat fed mice. Mol. Nutr. Food Res. 2013, 57, 360–364.

108. Albers, A.R.; Varghese, S.; Vitseva, O.; Vita, J.A.; Freedman, J.E. The antiinflammatory effects of purple grape juice consumption in subjects with stable coronary artery disease. Arterioscler. Thromb. Vasc. Biol.2004, 24, e179–e180.

109. Tomé-Carneiro, J.; Gonzálvez, M.; Larrosa, M.; Yáñez-Gascón, M.; García-Almagro, F.; Ruiz-Ros, J.; Tomás-Barberán, F.; García-Conesa, M.; Espín, J. Grape resveratrol increases serum

adiponectin and downregulates inflammatory genes in peripheral blood mononuclear cells: A triple-blind, placebo-controlled, one-year clinical trial in patients with stable coronary artery disease. Cardiovasc. Drugs Ther. 2013, 27, 37–48.

110. Barona, J.; Blesso, C.N.; Andersen, C.J.; Park, Y.; Lee, J.; Fernandez, M.L. Grape consumption increases anti-inflammatory markers and upregulates peripheral nitric oxide synthase in the absence of dyslipidemias in men with metabolic syndrome. Nutrients 2012, 4, 1945–1957.

111. Zhou, K.; Raffoul, J.J. Potential anticancer properties of grape antioxidants. J. Oncol. 2012, 2012, 803294.

112. Sun, T.; Chen, Q.Y.; Wu, L.J.; Yao, X.M.; Sun, X.J. Antitumor and antimetastatic activities of grape skin polyphenols in a murine model of breast cancer. Food Chem. Toxicol. 2012, 50, 3462–3467.

113. Kountouri, A.M.; Gioxari, A.; Karvela, E.; Kaliora, A.C.; Karvelas, M.; Karathanos, V.T. Chemopreventive properties of raisins originating from Greece in colon cancer cells. Food Funct. 2013,4, 366–372.

114. Prasad, R.; Katiyar, S.K. Grape seed proanthocyanidins inhibit migration potential of pancreatic cancer cells by promoting mesenchymal-to-epithelial transition and targeting nf-κb. Cancer Lett. 2013,334, 118–126.

115. Georgiev, M.; Georgiev, V.; Penchev, P.; Antonova, D.; Pavlov, A.; Ilieva, M.; Popov, S. Volatile metabolic profiles of cell suspension cultures of Lavandula vera, Nicotiana tabacum and Helianthus annuus, cultivated under different regimes. Eng. Life Sci. 2010, 10, 148–157.

116. Cai, Z.; Kastell, A.; Knorr, D.; Smetanska, I. Exudation: An expanding technique for continuous production and release of secondary metabolites from plant cell suspension and hairy root cultures.Plant Cell Rep. 2012, 31, 461–477.

117. Wilson, S.A.; Roberts, S.C. Recent advances towards development and commercialization of plant cell culture processes for the synthesis of biomolecules. Plant Biotechnol. J. 2012, 10, 249–268.

118. Yin, Y.; Borges, G.; Sakuta, M.; Crozier, A.; Ashihara, H. Effect of phosphate deficiency on the content and biosynthesis of anthocyanins and the expression of related genes in

suspension-cultured grape (Vitis sp.) cells. Plant Physiol. Biochem. 2012, 55, 77–84.

119. Davis, G.; Ananga, A.; Krastanova, S.; Sutton, S.; Ochieng, J.W.; Leong, S.; Tsolova, V. Elevated gene expression in chalcone synthase enzyme suggests an increased production of flavonoids in skin and synchronized red cell cultures of north american native grape berries. DNA Cell Biol. 2012, 31, 939–945.

120. Colova (Tsolova), V.M.; Bordallo, P.N.; Phills, B.R.; Bausher, M. Synchronized somatic embryo development in embryogenic suspensions of grapevine Muscadinia rotundifolia (Michx.) small. Vitis2007, 46, 15–18.

121. Conn, S.; Curtin, C.; Bézier, A.; Franco, C.; Zhang, W. Purification, molecular cloning, and characterization of glutathione s-transferases (gsts) from pigmented Vitis vinifera l. Cell suspension cultures as putative anthocyanin transport proteins. J. Exp. Bot. 2008, 59, 3621–3634.

122. Cormier, F.; Brion, F.; Do, C.B.; Moresoli, C. Development of Process Strategies for Anthocyanin-Based Food Colorant Production Using Vitis vinifera Cell Cultures. In Plant Cell Culture Secondary Metabolism toward Industrial Application; DiCosmo, F., Misawa, M., Eds.; CRC Press LLC: Boca Raton, FL, USA, 1996; pp. 167–186.

123. Donnez, D.; Kim, K.-H.; Antoine, S.; Conreux, A.; de Luca, V.; Jeandet, P.; Clément, C.; Courot, E. Bioproduction of resveratrol and viniferins by an elicited grapevine cell culture in a 2 L stirred bioreactor. Process Biochem. 2011, 46, 1056–1062.

124. Bhat, K.P.L.; Lantvit, D.; Christov, K.; Mehta, R.G.; Moon, R.C.; Pezzuto, J.M. Estrogenic and antiestrogenic properties of resveratrol in mammary tumor models. Cancer Res. 2001, 61, 7456–7463.

125. Castillo-Pichardo, L.; Cubano, L.; Dharmawardhane, S. Dietary grape polyphenol resveratrol increases mammary tumor growth and metastasis in immunocompromised mice. BMC Complement. Altern. Med.2013, 13, 6.

126. Decendit, A.; Mérillon, J.M. Condensed tannin and anthocyanin production in Vitis vinifera cell suspension cultures. Plant Cell Rep. 1996, 15, 762–765.

127. Waffo-Téguo, P.; Hawthorne, M.E.; Cuendet, M.; Mérillon, J.-M.; Kinghorn, A.D.; Pezzuto, J.M.; Mehta, R.G. Potential cancer-

chemopreventive activities of wine stilbenoids and flavans extracted from grape (Vitis vinifera) cell cultures. Nutr. Cancer 2001, 40, 173–179.

128. Yousef, G.G.; Seigler, D.S.; Grusak, M.A.; Rogers, R.B.; Knight, C.T.G.; Kraft, T.F.B.; Erdman, J.W.; Lila, M.A. Biosynthesis and characterization of 14C-enriched flavonoid fractions from plant cell suspension cultures. J. Agric. Food Chem. 2004, 52, 1138–1145.

129. Carollo, C.; Caimi, G. Wine consumption in the mediterranean diet: Old concepts in a new sight. Food Nutr. Sci. 2012, 3, 1726–1733.

130. Schrieks, I.C.; van den Berg, R.; Sierksma, A.; Beulens, J.W.J.; Vaes, W.H.J.; Hendriks, H.F.J. Effect of red wine consumption on biomarkers of oxidative stress. Alcohol Alcohol. 2013, 48, 153–159.

131. Amarowitcz, R.; Weidner, S. Biological Activity of Grapevine Phenolic Compounds. In Grapevine Molecular Physiology & Biotechnology; Roubelakis-Angelakis, K.A., Ed.; Springer Science + Business Media: Dordrecht, The Netherlands, 2009; pp. 389–405.

132. PhytoCellTec™ Solar Vitis/Vitis Vinifera. Available online: www.phytocelltec.ch/pctvitisvinifera.php(accessed on 1 October 2013).

7

FLAVONOID BIOAVAILABILITY AND ATTEMPTS FOR BIOAVAILABILITY ENHANCEMENT

Surangi H. Thilakarathna and H. P. Vasantha Rupasinghe

Department of Environmental Sciences, Faculty of Agriculture, Dalhousie University, P.O. Box 550, Truro, NS B2N 5E3, Canada

ABSTRACT

Flavonoids are a group of phytochemicals that have shown numerous health effects and have therefore been studied extensively. Of the six common food flavonoid classes, flavonols are distributed ubiquitously among different plant foods whereas appreciable amounts of isoflavones are found in leguminous plant-based foods. Flavonoids have shown promising health promoting effects in human cell culture, experimental animal and human clinical studies. They have shown antioxidant, hypocholesterolemic, anti-inflammatory effects as well as ability to modulate cell signaling and gene expression related disease development. Low bioavailability of flavonoids has been a concern as it can limit or even hinder their health effects. Therefore, attempts to improve their bioavailability in order to improve the efficacy of flavonoids are being studied. Further investigations on bioavailability are warranted as it is a determining factor for flavonoid biological activity.

Keywords: flavonoids; bioavailability; diet; health; disease

1. INTRODUCTION

Consumption of fruits and vegetables has been shown to improve health and directly or indirectly reduce the risk of numerous chronic diseases [1]. Increasing one serving of fruit and vegetable intake per day could reduce the risk of coronary heart disease by 4% [2]. It is believed that the nutrients and non-nutrient bioactive compounds present in fruits and vegetables are responsible for these health benefits. Among numerous plant-based bioactive compounds, flavonoids have been studied extensively and have shown promising results improving various disease aspects. Flavonoids belong to the comprehensive category of polyphenols and six classes, namely flavan-3-ols (including proanthocyanidins), flavonols, anthocyanins, isoflavones, flavanones and flavones are found in plant foods.

Flavonoids exert beneficial effects on health directly and/or indirectly. Previous literature shows evidence that flavonoids (proanthocyanidins as an example) are antioxidants [3] and hypocholesterolemic compounds [4] as well as modulators of cell signaling and gene expression in different experimental models [5] and in human epidemiological studies [6]. Considering the distribution of flavonoids, some classes can be found in many foods whereas the presence of some classes is limited to certain foods. As an example, flavonols can be commonly found in fruits, vegetables and teas; however, isoflavones are almost exclusively located in leguminous plants [7]. Dietary sources of flavonoids and their intake can vary widely among populations as it depends on the availability of dietary sources, dietary practices and food habits of different demographic groups [6,8,9,10,11].

Although flavonoids have shown countless health benefits, their low bioavailability has been a concern. Phase 2 metabolism is known to affect the bioavailability of flavonoids in humans [12]. Usually, most flavonoids undergo sulfation, methylation and glucuronidation in the small intestine and liver [13] and conjugated metabolites can be found in plasma after flavonoid ingestion [14]. In general, metabolites of flavonoids show reduced bioactivity in comparison to parent compounds but there have been results that reported otherwise as well [15]. Despite the bioactivity expressed in different *in vitro* systems, bioavailability of flavonoids would be a determinant factor of their bioactivity *in vivo*. Therefore, enhancement of bioavailability would be of utmost importance in order to exert health effects, *in vivo*. In this regard, numerous attempts have been made to increase bioavailability such as: improving the intestinal absorption via use of absorption enhancers [16], novel delivery systems [17];

improving metabolic stability [18,19]; changing the site of absorption from large intestine to small intestine [20].

This review briefly discusses: flavonoids belonging to the six classes, some of the factors that determine their bioavailability, recent studies attempting to improve their bioavailability that in turn can improve their bioactivity *in vivo*.

2. FLAVONOIDS

Flavonoids are secondary metabolites in plants and fall under the broad category of polyphenols. Scientists have discovered more than 7000 flavonoids and the list of new discovered flavonoids keeps on growing [7]. Flavonoids consist of two aromatic carbon rings connected with a three-carbon bridge (Figure 1). Based on the "C" ring, there are six common food flavonoid classes: flavonols, flavan-3-ols (monomeric and condensed tannins), isoflavones, flavanones, flavones and anthocyanins. Most of the flavonoid compounds except flavan-3-ols (monomers and proanthocyanidins) exist as glycosides [6]. Different flavonoid compounds have shown numerous health promoting effects and have been studied extensively using different experimental model systems. The six classes of flavonoids, their intake and common dietary sources in four different populations are discussed briefly in this section. The common structures and some sources of the six flavonoid classes are shown in Table 1.

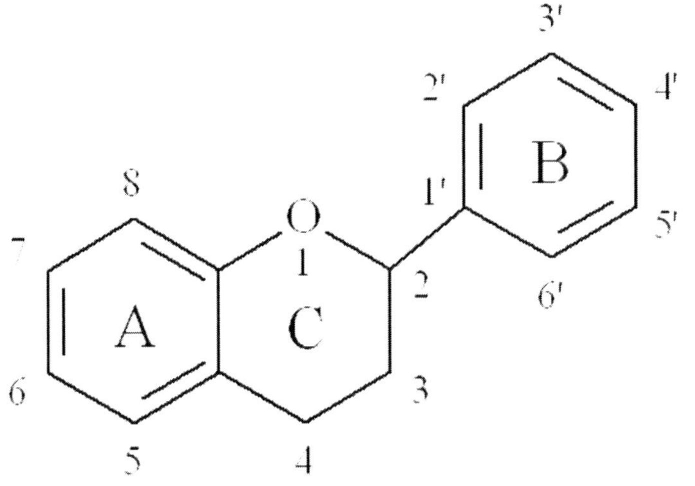

Figure 1. General chemical structure of flavonoids.

Table 1. Flavonoid classes, common compounds, their dietary sources and amounts *.

Flavonoid class (Common compounds)	Common food sources and amounts (mg/100 g edible portion)			
Flavan-3-ols	**Source**	**(i) [21]**	**(ii) [21]**	**(iii) [22]**
(i) (+)-Catechin, (ii) (−)-Epicatechin, (iii) Procyanidin B2 (dimer) an example; food values for all dimers present	Apples (Red Delicious, with skin) [1]	2.00	9.83	15.12
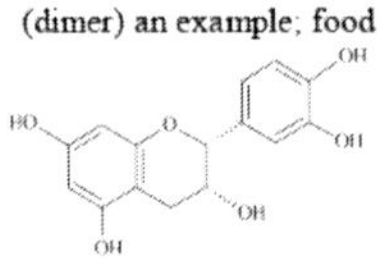 (i)	Apricots (raw) [1]	3.67	4.74	1.33
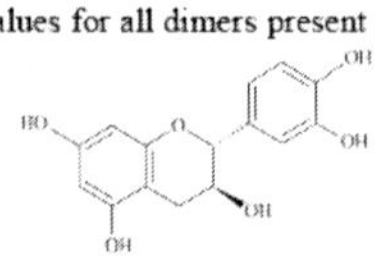 (ii)	Peaches (raw) [1]	4.92	2.34	12.24
	Pears (raw) [1]	0.27	3.76	2.73
	Strawberries (raw) [1]	6.65	1.56	5.26
	Black tea (brewed) [2]	1.51	2.13	3.74
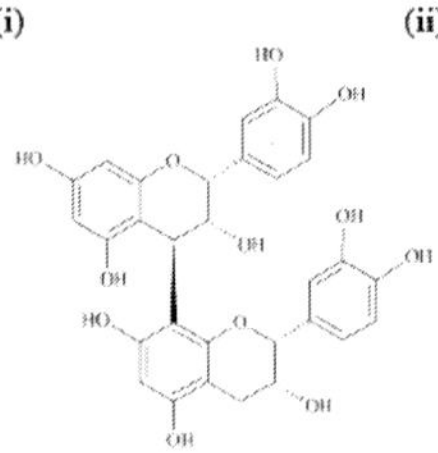 (iii)	Blueberries (highbush, raw) [3]	5.29	0.62	5.71
	Cranberries (raw) [3]	0.39	4.37	25.93
	Cocoa (dry powder) [4]	64.82	196.43	183.49
	Grapes (black/red) [5]	0.82	0.96	2.38
	Red wine (table) [5]	7.12	3.76	20.49
Flavonols	**Source [21]**	**(i)**	**(ii)**	**(iii)**
(i) Kaempferol,	Blueberries (highbush) [3]	1.66	1.26	7.67
(ii) Myricetin,	Garlic [6]	0.26	1.61	1.74
(iii) Quercetin-3-*O*-glucoside an example of a glucoside, food values are for quercetin	Onions [6]	0.63	0.03	21.40
	Kale [7]	46.80	0.00	22.58
	Broccoli [7]	7.84	0.06	3.26
	Spinach [8]	15.75	-	5.75
	Black tea (brewed) [2]	1.31	0.45	1.99
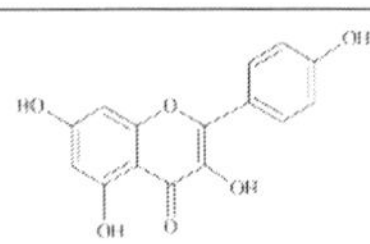 (i)	Red wine [5]	0.20	0.83	1.76
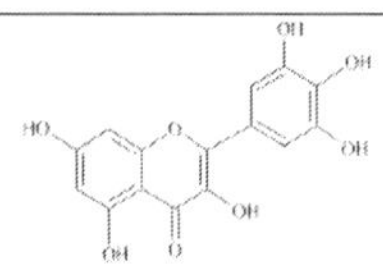 (ii)	Cherry tomatoes [9]	0.10	-	2.76
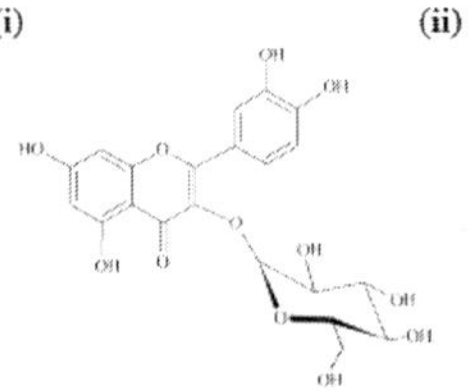 (iii)	Can be found ubiquitous in plant families.			

Anthocyanins

(i) Cyanidin-3-*O*-glucoside,
(ii) Delphinidin-3-*O*-glucoside,
(iii) Malvidin-3-*O*-glucoside,
(iv) Pelargonidin-3-*O*-glucoside.
Food values are for anthocyanidins (without the sugars)

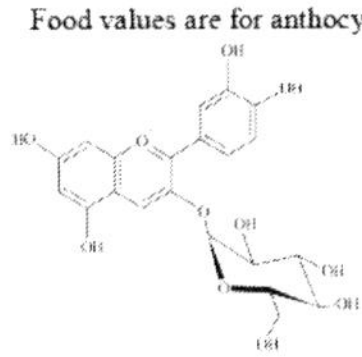
(i)

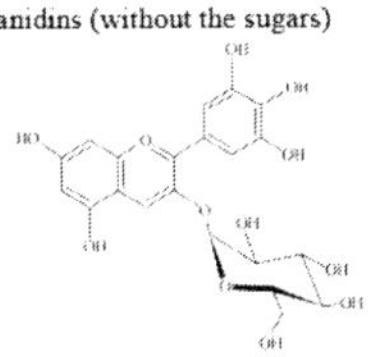
(ii)

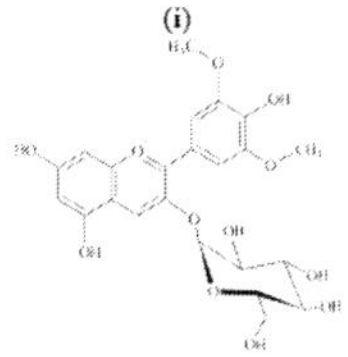
(iii)

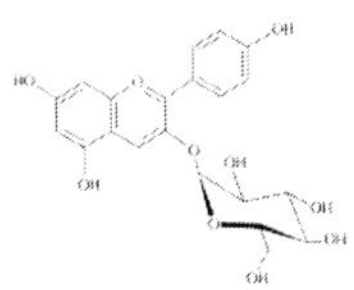
(iv)

Source [21]	(i)	(ii)	(iii)	(iv)
Apples [1]	1.27	0.00	0.00	0.00
Blueberries (lowbush) [3]	17.92	34.00	54.00	2.65
Red wine [5]	0.45	2.75	15.29	-
Strawberries [1]	1.63	0.31	0.01	25.69

Usually in any pink to purple fruit or vegetable; except the Chenopodiaceae family (beets, quinoa, spinach, Swiss chard, *etc.*).

Isoflavones

(i) Daidzein, (ii) Genistein, (iii) Glycitein

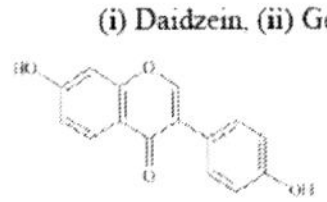
(i)

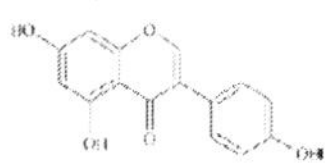
(ii)

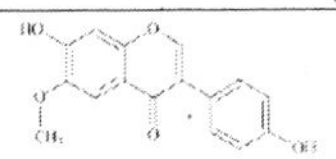
(iii)

Source [23]	(i)	(ii)	(iii)
Tofu (regular, raw) [10]	8.56	12.99	1.98
Tempeh [10]	22.66	36.15	3.82
Soybean (raw, mature seeds, USA) [10]	61.33	86.33	13.33
Peanuts (raw, all types) [10]	0.02	0.24	0.26
Beans (common, raw) [10]	0.29	0.30	0.00

In the Fabaceae (legume) family especially the genus Glycine (soy), but also in small amounts in other plants.

Flavanones

(i) Eriodictyol, (ii) Hesperetin, (iii) Naringenin

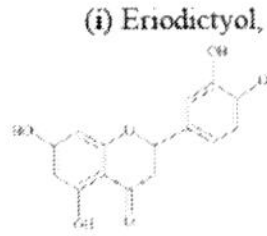
(i)

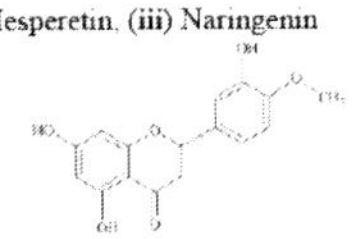
(ii)

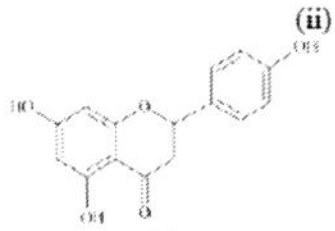
(iii)

Source [21]	(i)	(ii)	(iii)
Grapefruit (juice, white) [11]	0.65	2.35	18.23
Lemon (juice) [11]	4.88	14.47	1.38
Orange (juice) [11]	0.17	20.39	3.27
Peppermint [13]	30.92	9.52	-

Flavones

(i) Apigenin, (ii) Luteolin

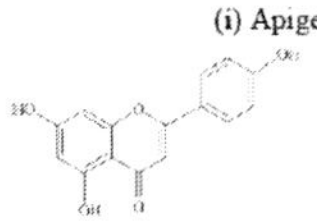
(i)

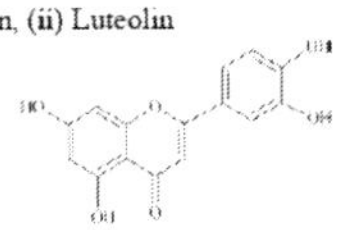
(ii)

Source [21]	(i)	(ii)
Celery [13]	2.85	1.05
Celery seed (spice) [13]	83.70	811.41
Parsley [13]	215.46	1.09
Green peppers [9]	0.00	4.71
Peppermint [12]	8.71	11.33

Common in leafy plants particularly Apiaceae family.

* Source: [21–23]. Plant families are given in italic superscripts: [1] Rosaceae; [2] Theaceae; [3] Ericaceae; [4] Malvaceae; [5] Vitaceae; [6] Alliaceae; [7] Brassicaceae; [8] Chenopodiaceae; [9] Solanaceae; [10] Fabaceae; [11] Rutaceae; [12] Lamiaceae; [13] Apiaceae.

2.1. Flavan-3-ols

2.1.1. Monomeric Flavan-3-ols: Catechin and Epicatechin

Flavan-3-ols are monomers and are the units for the oligomers and polymers known as proanthocyanidins or condensed tannins. Some examples of monomeric flavan-3-ols are catechin, epicatechin, gallocatechin, epigallocatechin, epigallocatechin gallate, *etc.* (Table 1). As reviewed by D'Archivio *et al.* [24], catechin and epicatechin are most commonly found in fruits (except citrus) whereas most other monomeric flavan-3-ols are commonly found in different teas (*Camellia sinensis*). Catechin and epicatechin are two flavan-3-ols most commonly found in apple peels [25,26] and about one half of the flavan-3-ols are monomeric in immature apples [27]. These compounds were found in lower concentrations in the flesh than in the skins of fruits [25]. Different types of berries, cherries, grapes, plums, apricots [28,29], red wine, chocolate and teas [24] are good sources.

Consumption of flavan-3-ols can vary among different populations due to different dietary sources. Average daily monomeric catechin and epicatechin intake of adult Australians were 9.36 mg and 16.64 mg respectively and black tea, green tea, apples and wine contributed the most [8]. In a Spanish population, average monomeric catechin and epicatechin intake per day was 13.05 ± 14.71 mg and 11.11 ± 9.63 mg, respectively and similar to the Australian population, wine, tea and apples contributed most to the flavan-3-ol intake [11]. According to a study on middle-aged Japanese women, 98% of the flavan-3-ol intake was from tea followed by apples which contributed to 1.9% of the daily intake [9].

2.1.2. Proanthocyanidins or Condensed Tannins

Proanthocyanidins are dimers, trimers, oligomers (4–10 units) or polymers (>10 units) of monomeric catechin or epicatechin units. Oligomeric and polymeric proanthocyanidin content is difficult to estimate due to their wide range of structures and molecular weights [30]. However, experimental evidence suggests that proanthocyanidins possess high antioxidant activity as these high molecular weight structures can easily complex with metal ions and proteins [31] and antioxidant activity increased with the degree of polymerization for compounds with (−)-epicatechin as the structural unit [31]. Contrastingly, a recent study revealed proanthocyanidins with lower molecular weight were better superoxide and hydroxyl radical scavengers and xanthine oxidase inhibitors [32].

These compounds occur in abundance in grapes, apples, various berries, tea, wine, beer, chocolate [24],*etc*. Immature fruits tend to contain more of these compounds than ripe fruits [33]. Procyanidin content is reported to be significantly higher in unripe apples than in ripe apples [33].

2.2. Flavonols

These compounds are nearly ubiquitous in foods [7]. Some food sources are apples, berries, red grapes [28,29], onions, red wine, teas, curly kale, leeks, broccoli, [24], *etc*. Some examples of flavonol compounds are isorhamnetin, kaempferol, myricetin, and quercetin. In apples, flavonols, especially quercetin glycosides are almost exclusively located in the apple peel [25,34]. Flavonols are present mostly in their conjugated forms, and apples contain a mixture of quercetin glycosides and traces of aglycone quercetin [26,27].

Mean quercetin, kaempferol and myricetin daily intake of Australian adults was 12.53 mg, 5.6 mg and 2.4 mg, respectively [8]. Black and green tea contributed most to the intake of the three compounds. Apples were also an important contributor for quercetin intake but not for other compounds. Quercetin and kaempferol contributed more to flavonol intake of Chinese adults [10] and Japanese middle-aged women [9]. In Spanish adults, quercetin accounted for 79.6% of flavonol intake and onions were the main dietary source contributing to 22.6% of the intake followed by lettuce, red wine and apples [11].

2.3. Anthocyanins

Anthocyanins are natural pigments in plants and exhibit a blue, purple or red color [24,30]. These compounds are abundant in purple berries, apples, cherries, red and purple grapes and pomegranates [35,36] as well as red wine and certain vegetables such as cabbage, onions and radishes [24]. Common food anthocyanins are cyanidin, delphinidin, malvidin, pelargonidin, peonidin and petunidin.

According to Somerset and Johannot [8], major dietary sources of anthocyanins in adult Australians were blueberries, cherries and wine. Wine contributed around 85%–95% of the daily intake of delphinidin, petunidin and malvidin [8]. In Spanish adults, red wine was the main contributor to anthocyanin intake (45.62%) and cyanidin (35.74%) and malvidin (35.99%) were the main compounds [11].

2.4. Isoflavones

Isoflavones are primarily found in leguminous plants and specifically soy and its products are excellent sources [7,35]. Compounds that belong to this class of flavonoids include biochanin A, daidzein, genistein, and glycitein. Isoflavones have phytoestrogenic activity and can bind to estrogen receptors [24]. Tofu (42.2%), natto (28.7%) and miso (16.3%) contributed more to the average daily isoflavone intake of middle-aged Japanese women [9] while non-fermented legume foods like soybean sprouts (71.96%), beans (17.46%) and chickpeas (7.96%) contributed more to the intake of Spanish adults [11]. Clearly from the above information, food habits have played a role in the isoflavone intake where Japanese populations consume more soy products (mostly fermented) and legumes and Spanish populations consume less.

2.5. Flavanones

Some examples of flavanones are eriodictyol, hesperetin, and naringenin. These compounds are commonly found in citrus fruits and to a lesser extent in tomatoes and mint [24,35]. Total hesperetin, naringenin and eriodictyol intake per day by Australian adults was 4.2 mg, 2.1 mg and 0.5 mg, respectively [8]. Comparatively, the daily intake of these three compounds were considerably higher in the Spanish adults where hesperetin, naringenin and eriodictyol daily intakes were 31.26 ± 29.85 mg, 18.29 ± 16.84 mg and 1.00 ± 1.36 mg, respectively [11]. Interestingly, the main dietary source for both populations was oranges.

2.6. Flavones

Flavones are the less common flavonoids [24] and can be found mainly in celery, green leafy herbs like parsley and chamomile [7,35,37]. Apigenin and luteolin are two compounds that belong to this class. Daily average apigenin and luteolin intake by adult Australians were 0.45 mg and 0.08 mg, respectively; parsley and celery were the main dietary sources of apigenin where, celery and English spinach were the main dietary sources of luteolin [8]. The daily average dietary intake of these two flavones was comparatively higher in Chinese adults. According to the data reported by Zhang *et al.* [10], daily average apigenin and luteolin intake of Chinese adults were 1.06 ± 0.56 mg and 3.82 ± 1.88 mg, respectively and their major dietary sources were eggplant and celery, respectively. In middle-aged Japanese women, Malabar spinach and green pepper contributed to 91.8% of the daily average flavone intake and parsley and celery contributed less than 4% [9]. Interestingly, red wine (32.18%) and oranges (24.25%) contributed more to the flavone intake of Spanish adults and the average daily flavone intake was 3.4 ± 2.92 mg [11].

3. BIOAVAILABILITY OF DIETARY FLAVONOIDS

3.1. Metabolism and Bioavailability

According to U.S. Food and Drug Administration (FDA), the definition of bioavailability is "the rate and extent to which the active ingredient or active moiety is absorbed from a drug product and becomes available at the site of action" [38]. This same principle can be applied to flavonoid compounds in food. As the definition implies, the rate of absorption and the availability at the site of action is of utmost importance for a bioactive to be effective within biological systems and thus be "bioavailable". Therefore, it is imperative to determine the amount of a specific nutrient or bioactive compound in a food or dietary supplement as well as its bioavailability. Despite the health claims of flavonoids, it is a known fact that the bioavailability of flavonoids is generally low and can vary drastically among different flavonoid classes as well as individual compounds in a particular class. Relative urinary excretion of anthocyanins and daidzin intake was 0.3% and 43% respectively which explains the variability in bioavailability of flavonoids [39]. When it comes to flavonoids with complex structures and larger molecular weights, bioavailability may be even lower [39,40]. (The content discussed under this and the following section is summarized in Table 2). Metabolism of flavonoids in general is illustrated in Figure 2. Flavonoids are substrates for conjugating and hydrolyzing enzymes in the small intestine, liver and colon and all are conjugated to *O*-glucuronides, sulfate esters and*O*-methyl esters and hardly any aglycones are present in the plasma [39]. Conjugation of flavonoids first occurs in the small intestine followed by the liver where they are further metabolized and the produced glucuronides and sulfate derivatives facilitate their excretion via urine and bile [39]. The compounds that are not absorbed in the intestine will reach the colon and be subjected to structural modifications by colonic microflora [41]. The flavonoid glucuronides that re-enter the enterohepatic circulation through bile excretion are hydrolyzed by the microbiota to aglycones [39,40]. Aglycones can further be catabolized to low molecular weight compounds that can readily be absorbed. The following paragraphs will discuss the bioavailability of compounds belonging to different flavonoid classes in brief.

As reviewed by Spencer *et al.* [42], monomeric flavan-3-ols are extensively metabolized to *O*-methylated forms and/or conjugated to glucuronides or sulphates during systemic absorption. Further, after reviewing different studies, the major bioactive forms of the monomeric flavan-3-ols as well as procyanidins are most likely metabolized to conjugates of epicatechin [42]. A study carried out on the absorption and metabolism of flavan-3-ols in humans after consuming a ready-to-drink tea (iced tea), confirmed the above statements where eight metabolites and conjugates of epicatechin were excreted in urine [41]. According to them, the major urinary excreted flavan-3-ol metabolites from iced tea were epigallocatechin-*O*-glucuronide and methyl-epicatechin-sulphate.

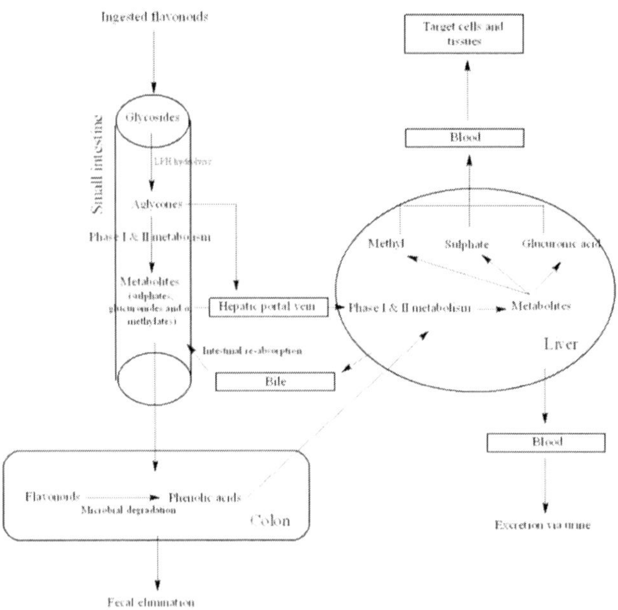

Figure 2. A simplified schematic of human flavonoid metabolism. Ingested flavonoids undergo extensive intestinal metabolism. Metabolites are then transported to the liver via hepatic portal vein and undergo further metabolism. The liver metabolites can be transported to targeted cells and tissues, excreted to bile and undergo enterohepatic re-circulation, or eliminated via urine and/or feces. The aglycones or flavonoid metabolites that reach the colon can undergo microbial degradation and reabsorption (LPH: lactase-phlorizin hydrolase; adapted from [43] with modifications).

Metabolism, rate and amount of dietary quercetin absorption in humans appear to depend primarily on the type and position of sugar moiety [44]. According to Graefe *et al.* [44], bioavailability of quercetin metabolites were five times higher when quercetin was administered as quercetin-4′-*O*-glucoside (C_{max}: 2.1 ± 1.6 μg/mL; t_{max}: 0.7 ± 0.3 h) instead of quercetin-3-*O*-rutinoside (C_{max}: 0.3 ± 0.3 μg/mL; t_{max}: 7.0 ± 2.9 h) and the site of absorption for these glycosides were different. Regardless of the type of quercetin glycoside administered, the potentially active quercetin metabolites (glucuronides) were identical in human plasma. Bioavailability of the ingested quercetin also depends on its dietary source. In a clinical study, consumption of onion powder (C_{max}: 273.2 ± 93.7 ng/mL; t_{max}: 2.0 ± 1.7 h; $t_{1/2}$: 14.8 ± 4.8 h) led to faster absorption, higher plasma concentrations and greater bioavailability compared to apple peel powder (C_{max}: 63.8 ± 22.4 ng/mL;t_{max}: 2.9 ± 2.0 h; $t_{1/2}$: 65.4 ± 80.0 h) [45]. Quercetin glycosides in onion powder were mainly quercetin-3,4′-*O*-glucoside and 4′-*O*-glucoside whereas in apple peels were quercetin-3-*O*-arabinoside, 3-*O*-galactoside, 3-*O*-glucoside and 3-*O*-rhamnoside [34].

It was reported that a significant proportion of intestinal metabolites formed from ingested anthocyanins were likely to be conjugates of protocatechuic acid and phloroglucinaldehyde (Figure 3) [46]. These compounds are the degradation products of anthocyanins. After a 4 h incubation of cyanidin and cyanidin-3-*O*-glucoside in a cell-free culture media, 96% of the cyanidin and 57% of the cyanidin-3-*O*-glucoside were degraded. In cultured human intestinal Caco-2 cell media, these degradation products (protocatechuic acid and phloroglucinaldehyde) were metabolized into their glucuronide and sulfate conjugates [46]. Degradation products and their metabolites are therefore part of anthocyanin bioactivity.

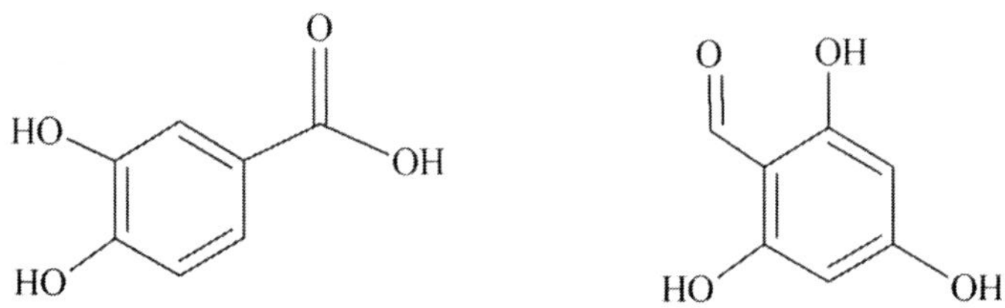

(i) Protocatechuic acid (ii) Phloroglucinaldehyde

Figure 3. Degradation products of anthocyanins. (i) Protocatechuic acid; (ii) Phloroglucinaldehyde.

Another recent study carried out on the bioavailability of an anthocyanin derivative, tried to address an aspect in anthocyanin metabolism that might have been overlooked. Fernandes *et al.* [47] studied the bioavailability of an anthocyanin derivative: flavan-3-ol-anthocyanin dimer [(+)-catechin-4,8-malvidin-3-glucoside], using Caco-2 cells to assess the transepithelial transport with comparison to (+)-catechin, malvidin-3-glucoside and procyanidin B3 (dimer). All the tested compounds crossed the Caco-2 cell model barrier and the catechin-malvidin dimer showed significantly less absorption efficiency compared to catechin or malvidin. Transport efficiency of the catechin-malvidin dimer was higher compared to procyanidin B3 dimer; the presence of the anthocyanin and its glucose moiety in the flavan-3-ol-anthocyanin dimer was thought to be responsible for this increased efficiency. Interestingly, no metabolites of the catechin-malvidin dimer were detected after 2 h incubation and only the breakdown of parent compounds was detected. Findings of this recent study suggested that the absorption of anthocyanins can take place as anthocyanin derivatives and certain derivatives, *i.e.*, the catechin-malvidin dimer, are metabolically more resistant than their parent compounds.

A study carried out on the bioavailability of genistein (aglycone) and its glycoside genistin, confirmed that the bioavailability of the aglycone was higher compared to its glycoside form [48]. Major amounts of genistein and its metabolites were recovered from the small intestinal luminal contents and feces. The experiment was carried out on unanesthetized rats and after ingestion of the compounds, blood was collected using a permanently inserted cannula into the portal vein. The isoflavone profile from the portal vein plasma provided an insight into deglycosylation of isoflavones in the small intestine before undergoing hepatic metabolism.

Oral administration of citrus flavanone aglycones, hesperetin and naringenin to human subjects showed a rapid absorption but low bioavailability according to cumulative urinary recovery data [49]. Compounds appeared to undergo extensive first-pass metabolism partly by intestinal bacteria and degraded into phenolic compounds. Hesperetin and naringenin concentrations were observed in plasma 20 min after dosing and reached a peak in 4.0 and 3.5 h, respectively. C_{max} for hesperetin and naringenin were 825.78 ± 410.63 and 2009.51 ± 770.82 ng/mL, respectively.

3.2. Factors Affecting Bioavailability

Numerous factors affect the bioavailability of ingested dietary flavonoids. Some factors are discussed briefly under this section. When it comes to flavonoid absorption, chemical structure in terms of molecular weight, glycosylation and esterification play a pivotal role [40].

3.2.1. Molecular Weight

Molecular weight is an important factor that greatly affects the absorption and thus bioavailability of certain flavonoids. One example would be the polymeric proanthocyanidins for which, their larger molecular weight, absorption would practically be impossible [40]. The unaltered proanthocyanidins will reach the colon, get catabolized by microorganisms and the resulting microbial metabolites be absorbed into the circulatory systems and excreted via urine [50]. Colonic breakdown products of proanthocyanidins were suggested to be the actual active compounds that exert biological activity. Contrastingly, Shoji and coworkers [51] concluded that oligomeric apple proanthocyanidins (dimer to pentamer) were absorbed in the digestive tract of rats and free procyanidins were present in their plasma. As reported, free proanthocyanidin levels in rat plasma peeked 2 h after administration and decreased subsequently up to 24 h. Furthermore, proanthocyanidin concentration took much longer to peek when compared to other flavan-3-ols and polyphenols. Therefore, oligomeric procyanidins were assumed to be absorbed in the small intestine and were not degraded to lower molecular weight compounds other than the intact procyanidins 2 h after administration [51]. On the other hand, *in vitro* results have shown that polymeric proanthocyanidins were degraded by the colonic microflora into lower molecular weight compounds and these results have yet to be confirmed *in vivo*.

3.2.2. Glycosylation

Absorption of flavonoids can vary drastically among different classes as well as among different conjugates of the same compound in a particular class. Absorption of some flavonoid glycosides can be very rapid, some can be very slow, and thus affect the bioavailability. Bioavailability of apple quercetin glycosides was 30% of that from onions [52]. The associated sugar moiety had a great influence on absorption; quercetin glucosides was absorbed 10 times faster and the plasma concentration peaked 20 times higher than quercetin rutinosides in humans [53]. It was suggested that glucosides were absorbed in the small intestine whereas quercetin rutinosides may be absorbed in the colon after deglycosylation. The daily plasma level of quercetin was predicted to be substantially less than 1 μM [54]. Catechins are rapidly absorbed and thus the small intestine is the probable site of absorption. The type of catechin monomer was not a factor determining absorption but dimerization reduced bioavailability [54]. Although anthocyanins are rapidly absorbed, their bioavailability was the lowest compared to other flavonoids [54]. These compounds are not easily hydrolyzed to their aglycones [54]. Although most glycosylated flavonoids need to be hydrolyzed to their aglycones for absorption, anthocyanins were absorbed and detected in the circulation without sugars or with their sugars intact [55].

3.2.3. Metabolic Conversion

Once ingested, the flavonoids interact with human conjugating enzymes in the enterocytes as well as in the liver. Metabolic conversion is known as a major factor affecting flavonoid bioavailability. Quercetin aglycone or its glycosides are generally not found in plasma but its glucuronic acid, sulfate or methyl conjugates were exclusively present in plasma [56,57]. Sulfation, methylation and glucuronidation occur in the enterocytes and liver [13] and, generally, most of the flavonoids undergo these metabolic conversions. Contradictory reports have been published on the bioactivity of flavonoid metabolites. Quercetin-3-*O*-glucuronic acid, quercetin-3-sulphate and isorhamnetin-3-glucuronic acid demonstrated LDL oxidation inhibition *in vitro* at physiological concentrations (100 nM) that was not different from the activity of their parent compound, quercetin or its glycosides [15]. Catechin is found exclusively in the plasma as methyl, sulfate and glucuronic acid conjugates and generally has a shorter half-life [12]. Epicatechin was metabolized mainly to sulfate conjugates and not glucuronidated by the liver, small intestine or large intestine [25].

3.2.4. Interaction with Colonic Microflora

Interaction of the flavonoid compounds with colonic microflora was reported to influence their bioavailability. As reviewed by Del Rio *et al.* [42], a significant amount of the ingested flavonoids were not absorbed in the small intestine. They reached the large intestine and were degraded by colonic microflora into simple phenolic acids that were absorbed into the circulatory system [58]. These colonic catabolites were known to express biological activities and potential health properties relevant to flavonoids, although the ingested flavonoids primarily were not absorbed in the small intestine. Proanthocyanidins were known to be catabolized to phenylacetic acid, mono- and dihydroxyphenylacetic acids, mono- and dihydroxyphenylpropionic acids, and hydroxybenzoic acid; anthocyanins were catabolized mainly to protocatechuic acid [58]. As reviewed by Williamson and Clifford [50], a key step in the catabolism of flavonoids is the fission of the A-ring and loss of carbon C_5 to C_8 as oxaloacetate which is eventually metabolized to carbon dioxide.

After consuming orange juice containing 168 μM of hesperetin-7-*O*-rutinoside, two hesperetin-*O*-glucuronides appeared in the human plasma with a peak concentration of 922 nmol/L at 4.4 h [59]. Cleavage of the rutinose moiety was suggested to occur due to enzymes of the colonic microflora and was indicative of absorption in the large intestine rather than small intestine [59]. Interesting findings were reported in a study where tomato juice containing rutin (quercetin-3-*O*-rutinoside) was consumed by healthy volunteers and subjects with an ileostomy [60]. In healthy subjects, low concentrations of quercetin-3-*O*-glucuronide and isorhamnetin-3-*O*-glucuronide appeared in the plasma 4 h after ingestion and nine metabolites appeared in urine. In ileostomists, no metabolites were detected in the plasma or urine and around 86% of the rutin was recovered in the ileal fluid. Further, phenolic acid catabolites of rutin appeared in the urine of healthy subjects which accounted for 22% of the rutin intake.

Metabolism of isoflavones is a complicated process which involves the gut microflora. Regarding metabolism, the rate of conjugation is known to be high and therefore, isoflavone aglycones are scarcely present in the circulation after ingestion of isoflavones [61]. Equol is a metabolite formed specifically after daidzein consumption and production of equol from diadzein is greatly influenced by the gut microflora [61,62]. This process also shows a greater inter-individual variation owing to the compositional variation in the gut microflora among different individuals [63,64]. Interestingly, all adult humans cannot produce equol and thus, two subpopulations can be identified based on equol production. The inability to produce equol could be due to the absence of bacterial species that involve in equol production or lack of the appropriate enzyme in the gut microflora [62]. Equol can be responsible for the clinical effectiveness of isoflavones as its bioactivity was reported to be stronger than daidzein [65].

3.3. Efforts to Improve Bioavailability

Dietary flavonoids have shown promising anti-atherosclerotic effects in different experimental models (*in vitro*, *ex vivo* and *in vivo*) but contradictory results are often reported in human clinical trials. Low bioavailability of these bioactives in humans plays a key role in these findings. To improve the bioavailability of a bioactive, one has to have a thorough understanding of the metabolism of the bioactive(s) of concern. Some metabolic process areas concerned with improving bioavailability are: increasing the intestinal absorption [16], improving metabolic stability [18,19], changing the site of absorption (from colon to small intestine) [20], *etc*. To achieve these goals microencapsulation, nano-delivery systems, microemulsions, enzymatic methylation of flavonoids were among some of the techniques explored. Under this section, some of the methods used to improve the bioavailability of selected flavonoid compounds are discussed briefly.

3.3.1. Improving the Intestinal Absorption

Borneol/methanol eutectic mixtures have been used as intestinal absorption enhancers of drugs and a similar mixture was used to improve daidzein absorption in a recent study. The borneol/methanol mixture enhanced bioavailability of daidzein by improving its solubility and permeability [16]. The combination of borneol/methanol eutectic mixture with a micro-emulsion, further improved bioavailability of daidzein. Micro-emulsions are lipid-based delivery systems that have greater solubilization, thermodynamic stability and permeability enhancement induced by a surfactant [66]. The micro-emulsion used in the study contained a surfactant (Cremophor RH40, PEG400) and acted as an absorption promoter of the water insoluble daidzein [16]. The study reported similar findings for *in vitro* and rat experiments.

Solid dispersion of daidzein at different daidzein polyvinylpyrrolidone ratios was tested in order to improve aqueous solubility and bioavailability of daidzein [67]. Daidzein solubility in the solid dispersion was eight times more than the free drug in water. Authors stated that the rate-limiting step in daidzein absorption may be the dissolution process and using polyvinylpyrrolidone dispersion as an oral preparation can improve the bioavailability of daidzein.

Table 2. Summary of the metabolism and bioavailability of flavonoid classes discussed.

Flavonoid class	Molecular Weight	Glycosylation	Metabolic conversion	Colonic microflora
General	Decreases bioavailability	Generally removed	Major factor in bioavailability; can take place in small intestine, liver and colon; usually to glucuronides but also sulphation and methylation [39]; facilitates urinary and biliary excretion [39].	Influence availability; catabolize compounds to low molecular weight compounds that are readily absorbed [58].
Flavan-3-ols (monomeric)			Major bioactive forms: conjugates of epicatechin [41]; catechin: methyl, sulfate and glucuronic acid conjugates; epicatechin: mainly to sulfate conjugates, no glucuronidation [41].	
Proanthocyanidins	Decreases bioavailability [40].		Major bioactive forms: conjugates of epicatechin [41]; oligomeric procyanidins can absorb in small intestine [51].	Influences polymeric proanthocyanidin degradation [50].
Flavonols		Sugars and their position affects bioavailability [44].	Potentially active metabolites: glucuronides [44].	Facilitates glucuronidation [60].
Anthocyanins	Anthocyanin derivatives (flavan-3-ol-anthocyanin dimer) can potentially be absorbed with less efficiency [47].	Sometimes found with sugars intact in circulation [55].	Major intestinal metabolites: glucuronide and sulfate conjugates of protocatechuic acid and phloroglucinaldehyde [46]; anthocyanin derivatives metabolically more resistant than parent compounds [47].	
Isoflavones		Aglycone more bioavailable; possible deglycosylation prior hepatic metabolism [48].		Metabolize daidzein to equol [58].
Flavanones		Rapid absorption, low bioavailability [49].		Extensive first-pass metabolism partly by intestinal bacteria degraded into phenolic compounds [49].

A nano-delivery system was designed and used to improve the oral bioavailability and intestinal absorption of daidzein. A daidzein-lecithin complex that self-assembled to form micelles with lecithin and sodium bile (nanometer sized particles) significantly improved intestinal absorption [17]. This particular daidzein-lecithin complex had stability during assembly of the micelles and the micelles themselves had good stability over time. In the pharmacokinetic study, the daidzein-lecithin self-assembled micelles distributed mainly in the stomach and proximal intestine after oral administration to rats and the intestinal bioavailability significantly improved compared to the free daidzein suspension [17].

Absorption of an isoflavone extract was improved by complexing with β-cyclodextrin in an *in vitro* system [68]. The aqueous solubility was reported to be 26 times greater than the solubility of the isoflavone extract itself. Oral administration of the extract complexed with β-cyclodextrin (isoflavone glycoside basis) to Sprague-Dawley rats showed enhanced bioavailability of daidzein, genistin and glycitin.

3.3.2. Changing the Site of Absorption

Another approach to improve bioavailability of dietary flavonoids would be to change the site of absorption from large intestine to small intestine. As discussed before, most of the flavonoids pass through the small intestine, reach the colon, and get extensively metabolized into phenolic acids by the colonic microflora. In the hesperidin molecule, rutinose (6-O-α-L-rhamnosyl-D-glucose) is attached at the 7th position of the A ring and are known to be a determinant factor for absorption as glycosides with rhamnose were poorly absorbed compared to hesperetin or hesperetin glucoside [20]. Enzymatic conversion of hesperidin into hesperetin-7-glucoside in orange juice using hesperidinase, improved plasma bioavailability of total hesperetin and reduced the time taken to reach maximum plasma concentration in human subjects when compared to subjects consuming untreated orange juice. The cleavage of the rhamnose moiety changed the absorption site and as a result, bioavailability was improved.

3.3.3. Improving the Metabolic Stability

Blocking the free hydroxyl groups in flavones by capping with methyl groups was tested as an approach to prevent conjugation and improve metabolic resistance and thereby, bioavailability [18]. The two methylated-flavones, 5,7-dimethoxyflavone and 3′,4′-

dimethoxyflavone were metabolically very stable compared to a non-methylated form galangin (3,5,7-trihydroxyflavone) which was easily glucuronidated in the liver S9 fraction [69]. As reviewed by Walle [18], this approach greatly improved metabolic stability of flavones *in vitro* and improved bioavailability and tissue distribution of methylated flavones in rats. Genistein and kaempferol along with their monomethylated forms (biochanin A and kaempferide, respectively) were examined for their affinity to human serum albumin and ovalbumin [19]. Serum albumins are the main transport proteins for many xenobiotics. Methylation of flavonoids improved affinity to these proteins by 2–16 times and improved transporting ability. Improved hydrophobicity of flavonoids may be responsible for increasing their binding ability [19].

As an attempt to increase the circulatory and organ levels of quercetin, several ester derivatives of quercetin were formulated to bypass the phase II metabolism during absorption [70]. Quercetin ester derivatives were synthesized and transepithelial transport across monolayers of three cell lines (canine MDCK-1, -2 and human Caco-2) were tested. Certain esters crossed some monolayers (MDCK and some Caco-2 clones) without phase II metabolism whereas for certain Caco-2 clones, complete deacylation occurred followed by metabolism of quercetin. Since elimination of residual acyl groups are expected *in vivo*, this method may increase the systemic levels of quercetin.

3.3.4. Effect of the Food Matrix

Another approach to improve bioavailability of bioactive flavonoids is food ingredient supplementation. For this attempt to be successful, different food ingredients have to be tested with the particular bioactive/s of concern. Bioavailability of green tea catechins were significantly improved in mice by supplementing with steamed rice [71]. Steamed rice supplementation increased the bioavailability of non-gallated catechins, especially epigallocatechin. The authors predicted proline-rich proteins in the rice endosperm are capable of binding gallated catechins like epigallocatechingallate and convert them into non-gallated catechins like epigallocatechin by tannase, thus enhancing epigallocatechin bioavailability.

Carbohydrate composition of the food matrix was suggested to be an important determinant of the total flavonol absorption in the small intestine [72]. Consumption of flavonols along with maltitol decreased the flavonol absorption in the small intestine compared to flavonol consumption with sucrose without changing the catechol-*O*-

methyltransferase activity. Furthermore, when flavan-3-ol content was low, influence of the food matrix was greater.

In a randomized, single-blinded, diet-controlled, cross-over study, six healthy females (aged 22–28) consumed 130 mg quercetin equivalents from either quercetin-enriched cereal bars or quercetin powder filled capsules. Systemic availability in terms of plasma concentration-time curves was five times higher and the maximum concentration was six times higher after quercetin-enriched cereal bar ingestion [73].

4. CONCLUSIONS

In conclusion, though flavonoids have shown promising health properties under experimental conditions, low bioavailability of some flavonoids needs to be enhanced for full exploitation of their therapeutic benefits in prevention and treatment of diseases. Therefore, continuing investigation is required to enhance the bioavailability and subsequent efficacy of certain flavonoids using consumer-friendly technologies.

CONFLICTS OF INTEREST

The authors declare no conflict of interest.

REFERENCES

1. Boeing, H.; Bechthold, A.; Bub, A. Critical review: Vegetables and fruit in the prevention of chronic diseases. Eur. J. Nutr. 2012, 51, 637–663.
2. Joshipura, K.J.; Hu, F.B.; Manson, J.E.; Stampfer, M.J.; Rimm, E.B.; Speizer, F.E.; Colditz, G.; Ascherio, A.; Rosner, B.; Spiegelman, D.; et al. The effect of fruit and vegetable intake on risk for coronary heart disease. Ann. Intern. Med. 2001, 134, 1106–1114.
3. Lourenço, C.F.; Gago, B.; Barbosa, R.M.; de Freitas, V.; Laranjinha, J. LDL isolated from plasma-loaded red wine proanthocyanidins resist lipid oxidation and tocopherol depletion. J. Agric. Food Chem. 2008,56, 3798–3804.
4. Thilakarathna, S.H.; Wang, Y.; Rupasinghe, H.P.V.; Ghanam, K. Apple peel flavonoid- and triterpene-enriched extracts

differentially affect cholesterol homeostasis in hamsters. J. Funct. Foods 2013, 4, 963–971.

5. Noll, C.; Hamelet, J.; Matulewicz, E.; Paul, J.L.; Delabar, J.M.; Janel, N. Effects of red wine polyphenolic compounds on paraoxonase-1 and lectin-like oxidized low-density lipoprotein receptor-1 in hyperhomocysteinemic mice. J. Nutr. Biochem. 2009, 20, 586–596.

6. Peterson, J.J.; Dwyer, J.T.; Jacques, P.F.; McCullough, M.L. Associations between flavonoids and cardiovascular disease incidence or mortality in European and US populations. Nutr. Rev. 2012, 70, 491–508.

7. Beecher, G.R. Overview of dietary flavonoids: Nomenclature, occurrence and intake. J. Nutr. 2003, 3, 3248S–3254S.

8. Somerset, S.M.; Johannot, L. Dietary flavonoid sources in Australian adults. Nutr. Cancer 2008, 60, 442–449.

9. Otaki, N.; Kimira, M.; Katsumata, S.; Uehara, M.; Watanabe, S.; Suzuki, K. Distribution and major sources of flavonoid intakes in the middle-aged Japanese women. J. Clin. Biochem. Nutr. 2009, 44, 231–238.

10. Zhang, Y.; Li, Y.; Cao, C.; Cao, J.; Chen, W.; Zhang, Y.; Wang, C.; Wang, J.; Zhang, X.; Zhao, X. Dietary flavonol and flavone intakes and their major food sources in Chinese adults. Nutr. Cancer 2010, 62, 1120–1127.

11. Zamora-Ros, R.; Andres-Lacueva, C.; Lamuela-Raventós, R.M.; Berenguer, T.; Jakszyn, P.; Barricarte, A.; Ardanaz, E.; Amiano, P.; Dorronsoro, M.; Larrañaga, N.; et al. Estimation of dietary sources and flavonoid intake in a Spanish adult population (EPIC-Spain). J. Am. Diet. Assoc. 2010, 110, 390–398.

12. Manach, C.; Williamson, G.; Morand, C.; Scalbert, A.; Rémésy, C. Bioavailability and bioefficacy of polyphenols in humans. I. Review of 97 bioavailability studies. Am. J. Clin. Nutr. 2005, 81, 230S–242S.

13. Mullen, W.; Edwards, C.A.; Crozier, A. Absorption, excretion and metabolite profiling of methyl-, glucuronyl-, glucosyl- and sulpho-conjugates of quercetin in human plasma and urine after ingestion of onions. Br. J. Nutr. 2006, 96, 107–116.

14. Rupasinghe, H.P.V.; Ronalds, C.M.; Rathgeber, B.; Robinson, R. Absorption and tissue distribution of dietary quercetin in broiler chickens. J. Sci. Food Agric. 2010, 90, 1172–1178.

15. Thilakarathna, S.H.; Rupasinghe, H.P.; Needs, P.W. Apple peel bioactive rich extracts effectively inhibit in vitro human LDL cholesterol oxidation. Food Chem. 2013, 138, 463–470.

16. Shen, Q.; Li, X.; Li, W.; Zhao, X. Enhanced intestinal absorption of daidzein by borneol/menthol eutectic mixture and microemulsion. AAPS Pharm. Sci. Tech. 2011, 12, 1044–1049.

17. Zhang, Z.; Huang, Y.; Gao, F.; Gao, Z.; Bu, H.; Gu, W.; Li, Y. A self-assembled nanodelivery system enhances the oral bioavailability of daidzein: In vitro characteristics and in vivo performance.Nanomedicine (London) 2011, 6, 1365–1379.

18. Walle, T. Methylation of dietary flavones greatly improves their hepatic metabolic stability and intestinal absorption. Mol. Pharm. 2007, 4, 826–832.

19. Cao, H.; Jing, X.; Wu, D.; Shi, Y. Methylation of genistein and kaempferol improves their affinities for proteins. Int. J. Food Sci. Nutr. 2013.

20. Nielsen, I.L.; Chee, W.S.; Poulsen, L.; Offord-Cavin, E.; Rasmussen, S.E.; Frederiksen, H.; Enslen, M.; Barron, D.; Horcajada, M.N.; Williamson, G. Bioavailability is improved by enzymatic modification of the citrus flavonoid hesperidin in humans: A randomized, double-blind, crossover trial. J. Nutr. 2006,136, 404–408.

21. U.S. Department of Agriculture, Agricultural Research Service. USDA National Nutrient Database for the Flavonoid Content of Selected Foods, Release 3.0. 2011. Available online: http://www.ars.usda.gov/SP2UserFiles/Place/12354500/Data/Flav/Flav_R03.pdf (accessed on 2 June 2013).

22. U.S. Department of Agriculture, Agricultural Research Service. USDA National Nutrient Database for the Proanthocyanidin Content of Selected Foods. 2004. Available online: http://www.ars.usda.gov/SP2UserFiles/Place/12354500/Data/PA/PA.pdf (accessed on 2 June 2013).

23. U.S. Department of Agriculture, Agricultural Research Service. USDA National Nutrient Database for the Isoflavone Content of Selected Foods, Release 2.0. 2008. Available online: http://www.ars.usda.gov/SP2UserFiles/Place/12354500/Data/isoflav/Isoflav_R2.pdf (accessed on 2 June 2013).

24. D'Archivio, M.; Filesi, C.; Di Benedetto, R.; Gargiulo, R.; Giovannini, C.; Masella, R. Polyphenols, dietary sources and bioavailability. Ann. Ist. Super. Sanita 2007, 43, 348–361.

25. Boyer, J.; Liu, R.H. Apple phytochemicals and their health benefits. Nutr. J. 2004, 3, 5.

26. Huber, G.M.; Rupasinghe, H.P.V. Phenolic profiles and antioxidant properties of apple skin extracts. J. Food Sci. 2009, 74, 693–699.

27. Vrhovsek, U.; Rigo, A.; Tonon, D.; Mattivi, F. Quantitation of polyphenols in different apple varieties.J. Agric. Food Chem. 2004, 52, 6532–6538.

28. Ratnasooriya, C.; Rupasinghe, H.P.V.; Jamieson, A. Juice quality and polyphenol concentration of fresh fruits and pomace of selected Nov Scotia-grown grape cultivars. Can. J. Plant Sci. 2010, 90, 193–205.

29. Lotito, S.; Frei, B. Consumption of flavonoid-rich foods and increased plasma antioxidant capacity in humans: Cause, consequence, or epiphenomenon? Free Radi. Biol. Med. 2006, 41, 1727–1746.

30. Wojdylo, A.; Oszmianski, J.; Laskowski, P. Polyphenolic compounds and antioxidant activity of new and old apple varieties. J. Agric. Food Chem. 2008, 56, 6520–6530.

31. Da Silva, P.A.; Laranjinha, J.A.; de Freitas, V.A. Antioxidant protection of low density lipoprotein by proanthocyanidins: Structure/activity relationships. Biochem. Pharmacol. 2003, 66, 947–954.

32. Arimboor, R.; Arumughan, C. Effect of polymerization on antioxidant and xanthine oxidase inhibitory potential of sea buckthorn (H. rhamnoides) proanthocyanidins. J. Food Sci. 2012, 77, C1036–C1041.

33. Ohnishi-Kameyama, M.; Yanagida, A.; Kanda, T.; Nagata, T. Identification of catechin oligomers from apple (Malus pumila cv. Fuji) in matrix-assisted laser desorption/ionization time-of-flight mass spectrometry and fast-atom bombardment mass spectrometry. Rapid Commun. Mass Spectrom 1997, 11, 31–36.

34. Rupasinghe, H.P.V.; Erkan, N.; Yasmin, A. Antioxidant protection of eicosapentaenoic acid and fish oil oxidation by polyphenolic-enriched apple skin extract. J. Agric. Food Chem. 2010, 58, 1233–1239.

35. Manach, C.; Scalbert, A.; Morand, C.; Rémésy, C.; Jiménez, L. Polyphenols: Food sources and bioavailability. Am. J. Clin. Nutr. 2004, 79, 727–747.

36. De Pascual-Teresa, S.; Moreno, D.A.; Garcia-Viguera, C. Flavanols and anthocyanins in cardiovascular health: A review of current evidence. Int. J. Mol. Sci. 2010, 11, 1679–1703.

37. Srivastava, J.K.; Gupta, S. Extraction, characterization, stability and biological activity of flavonoids isolated from chamomile flowers. Mol. Cell. Pharmacol. 2009, 1, 138.

38. Food and Drug Administration. Code of federal regulations, Title 21—Food and Drugs, Volume 5, Chapter 1—Food and Drug Administration, Department of Health and Human Services, Subchapter D—Drugs for Human Use, Part 320—Bioavailability and Bioequivalence Requirements. 2012. Available online: http://www.accessdata.fda.gov/scripts/cdrh/cfdocs/cfCFR/CFRSearch.cfm?fr=320.1&SearchTerm=bioavailability (accessed on 2 June 2013).

39. Landete, J.M. Updated knowledge about polyphenols: Functions, bioavailability, metabolism, and health. Crit. Rev. Food Sci. Nutr. 2012, 52, 936–948.

40. Scalbert, A.; Morand, C.; Manach, C.; Remesy, C. Absorption and metabolism of polyphenols in the gut and impact on health. Biomed. Pharmacother. 2002, 56, 276–282.

41. Del Rio, D.; Calani, L.; Scazzina, F.; Jechiu, L.; Cordero, C.; Brighenti, F. Bioavailability of catechins from ready-to-drink tea. Nutrition 2010, 26, 528–533.

42. Spencer, J.P.; Schroeter, H.; Rechner, A.R.; Rice-Evans, C. Bioavailability of flavan-3-ols and procyanidins: Gastrointestinal tract influences and their relevance to bioactive forms in vivo. Antioxid. Redox Signal. 2001, 3, 1023–1039.

43. Rupasinghe, H.P.V.; Thilakarathna, S.; Nair, S. Polyphenols of Apples and Their Potential Health Benefits. In Polyphenols: Chemistry, Dietary Sources and Health Benefits; Sun, J., Prasad, K.N., Ismail, A., Yang, B., You, X., Eds.; Nova Science Publishers Inc.: New York, NY, USA, 2013; pp. 333–368.

44. Graefe, E.U.; Wittig, J.; Mueller, S.; Riethling, A.K.; Uehleke, B.; Drewelow, B.; Pforte, H.; Jacobasch, G.; Derendorf, H.; Veit, M. Pharmacokinetics and bioavailability of quercetin glycosides in humans. J. Clin. Pharmacol. 2001, 41, 492–499.

45. Lee, J.; Mitchell, A.E. Pharmacokinetics of quercetin absorption from apples and onions in healthy humans. J. Agric. Food Chem. 2012, 60, 3874–3881.

46. Kay, C.D.; Kroon, P.A.; Cassidy, A. The bioactivity of dietary anthocyanins is likely to be mediated by their degradation products. Mol. Nutr. Food Res. 2009, 53, S92–S101.

47. Fernandes, I.; Nave, F.; Gonçalves, R.; de Freitas, V.; Mateus, N. On the bioavailability of flavanols and anthocyanins: Flavanol-anthocyanin dimers. Food Chem. 2012, 135, 812–818.

48. Steensma, A.; Faassen-Peters, M.A.; Noteborn, H.P.; Rietjens, I.M. Bioavailability of genistein and its glycoside genistin as measured in the portal vein of freely moving unanesthetized rats. J. Agric. Food Chem. 2006, 54, 8006–8012.

49. Kanaze, F.I.; Bounartzi, M.I.; Georgarakis, M.; Niopas, I. Pharmacokinetics of the citrus flavanone aglycones hesperetin and naringenin after single oral administration in human subjects. Eur. J. Clin. Nutr. 2007, 61, 472–477.

50. Williamson, G.; Clifford, M.N. Colonic metabolites of berry polyphenols: The missing link to biological activity? Br. J. Nutr. 2010, 104, S48–S66.

51. Shoji, T.; Masumoto, S.; Moriichi, N. Apple proanthocyanidin oligomers absorption in rats after oral administration: Analysis of proanthocyanidins in plasma using the porter method and high-performance liquid chromatography/tandem mass spectrometry. J. Agric. Food Chem. 2006, 54, 884–892.

52. Hollman, P.C.H.; van Trijp, J.M.P.; Buysman, M.N.C.P.; van der Gaag, M.S.; Mengelers, M.J.B.; de Vries, J.H.M.; Katan, M.B. Relative bioavailability of the antioxidant quercetin from various foods in man. FEBS Lett. 1997, 418, 152–156.

53. Hollman, P.C.H.; Buijsman, M.N.C.P.; van Gameren, Y.; Cnossen, P.J.; de Vries, J.H.M.; Katan, M.B. The sugar moiety is a major determinant of the absorption of dietary flavonoid glycosides in man.Free Radic. Res. 1999, 31, 569–573.

54. Walle, T. Serial review: Flavonoids and isoflavones (phytoestrogens): Absorption, metabolism, and bioactivity. Free Radic. Biol. Med. 2004, 36, 829–837.

55. Nurmi, T.; Mursu, J.; Heinonen, M.; Nurmi, A.; Hiltunen, R.; Voutilainen, S. Metabolism of berry anthocyanins to phenolic acids in humans. J. Agric. Food Chem. 2009, 57, 2274–2281.

56. Williamson, G.; Manach, C. Bioavailability and bioefficacy of polyphenols in humans. II. Review of 93 intervention studies. Am. J. Clin. Nutr. 2005, 81, 243S–255S.

57. Ishizawa, K.; Yoshizumi, M.; Kawai, Y. Pharmacology in health food: Metabolism of quercetin in vivoand its protective effect against arteriosclerosis. J. Pharmacol. Sci. 2011, 115, 466–470.

58. Moco, S.; Martin, F.P.; Rezzi, S. Metabolomics view on gut microbiome modulation by polyphenol-rich foods. J. Proteome Res. 2012, 11, 4781–4790.

59. Mullen, W.; Archeveque, M.A.; Edwards, C.A.; Matsumoto, H.; Crozier, A. Bioavailability and metabolism of orange juice flavanones in humans: Impact of a full-fat yogurt. J. Agric. Food Chem.2008, 56, 11157–11164.

60. Jaganath, I.B.; Mullen, W.; Edwards, C.A.; Crozier, A. The relative contribution of the small and large intestine to the absorption and metabolism of rutin in man. Free Radic. Res. 2006, 40, 1035–1046.

61. Rowland, I.; Faughnan, M.; Hoey, L.; Wahala, K.; Williamson, G.; Cassidy, A. Bioavailability of phyto-oestrogens. Br. J. Nutr. 2003, 89, S45–S58.

62. Cassidy, A. Dietary phyto-oestrogens: Molecular mechanisms, bioavailability and importance to menopausal health. Nutr. Res. Rev. 2005, 18, 183–201.

63. Rowland, I.R.; Wiseman, H.; Sanders, T.A.; Adlercreutz, H.; Bowey, E.A. Interindividual variation in metabolism of soy isoflavones and lignans: Influence of habitual diet on equol production by the gut microflora. Nutr. Cancer 2000, 36, 27–32.

64. Rafii, F.; Davis, C.; Park, M.; Heinze, T.M.; Beger, R.D. Variations in metabolism of the soy isoflavonoid daidzein by human intestinal microfloras from different individuals. Arch. Microbiol.2003, 180, 11–16.

65. Setchell, K.D.; Brown, N.M.; Lydeking-Olsen, E. The clinical importance of the metabolite equol-a clue to the effectiveness of soy and its isoflavones. J. Nutr. 2002, 132, 3577–3584.

66. Constantinides, P.P. Lipid microemulsions for improving drug dissolution and oral absorption: Physical and biopharmaceutical aspects. Pharm. Res. 1995, 12, 1561–1572.

67. Feng, B.L.; Li, H.W.; Zhou, M.Y.; Lu, W. Dispersion of daidzein with polyvinylpyrrolidone effects on dissolution rate and bioavailability. Zhong Yao Cai 2011, 34, 605–610.

68. Lee, S.H.; Kim, Y.H.; Yu, H.J. Enhanced bioavailability of soy isoflavones by complexation with beta-cyclodextrin in rats. Biosci. Biotechnol. Biochem. 2007, 71, 2927–2933.

69. Wen, X.; Walle, T. Methylation protects dietary flavonoids from rapid hepatic metabolism. Xenobiotica2006, 36, 387–397.

70. Biasutto, L.; Marotta, E.; de Marchi, U.; Zoratti, M.; Paradisi, C. Ester-based precursors to increase the bioavailability of quercetin. J. Med. Chem. 2007, 50, 241–253.

71. Monobe, M.; Ema, K.; Tokuda, Y.; Maeda-Yamamoto, M. Increased plasma concentration of epigallocatechin in mice after orally administering a green tea (Camellia sinensis L.) extract supplemented by steamed rice. Biosci. Biotechnol. Biochem. 2011, 75, 152–154.

72. Rodriguez-Mateos, A.; Oruna-Concha, M.J.; Kwik-Uribe, C.; Vidal, A.; Spencer, J.P. Influence of sugar type on the bioavailability of cocoa flavanols. Br. J. Nutr. 2012, 108, 2243–2250.

73. Egert, S.; Wolffram, S.; Schulze, B. Enriched cereal bars are more effective in increasing plasma quercetin compared with quercetin from powder-filled hard capsules. Br. J. Nutr. 2012, 107, 539–546.

8

UNDENATURED TYPE II COLLAGEN (UC-II®) FOR JOINT SUPPORT: A RANDOMIZED, DOUBLE-BLIND, PLACEBO-CONTROLLED STUDY IN HEALTHY VOLUNTEERS

James P Lugo[1] , Zainulabedin M Saiyed[1] , Francis C Lau[1] , Jhanna Pamela L Molina[2] , Michael N Pakdaman[2] , Arya Nick Shamie[3] and Jay K Udani2,[4]*

[1]InterHealth Nutraceuticals, Benicia, CA 94510, USA.

[2]Medicus Research LLC, 28720 Roadside Drive, Suite 310, Agoura Hills, CA 91301, USA.

[3]UCLA Medical Center, Santa Monica, CA 90401, USA.

[4]Northridge Hospital Integrative Medicine Program, Northridge, CA 91325, USA.

ABSTRACT

Background

UC-II contains a patented form of undenatured type II collagen derived from chicken sternum. Previous preclinical and clinical studies support the safety and efficacy of UC-II in modulating joint discomfort in osteoarthritis and rheumatoid arthritis. The purpose of this study was to assess the efficacy and tolerability of UC-II in moderating joint function and joint pain due to strenuous exercise in healthy subjects.

Methods

This randomized, double-blind, placebo-controlled study was conducted in healthy subjects who had no prior history of arthritic disease or joint pain at rest but experienced joint discomfort with physical activity. Fifty-five subjects who reported knee pain after participating in a standardized stepmill performance test were randomized to receive placebo (n = 28) or the UC-II (40 mg daily, n = 27) product for 120 days. Joint function was assessed by changes in degree of knee flexion and knee extension as well as measuring the time to experiencing and recovering from joint pain following strenuous stepmill exertion.

Results

After 120 days of supplementation, subjects in the UC-II group exhibited a statistically significant improvement in average knee extension compared to placebo (81.0 ± 1.3º vs 74.0 ± 2.2º; p = 0.011) and to baseline (81.0 ± 1.3º vs 73.2 ± 1.9º; p = 0.002). The UC-II cohort also demonstrated a statistically significant change in average knee extension at day 90 (78.8 ± 1.9º vs 73.2 ± 1.9º; p = 0.045) versus baseline. No significant change in knee extension was observed in the placebo group at any time. It was also noted that the UC-II group exercised longer before experiencing any initial joint discomfort at day 120 (2.8 ± 0.5 min, p = 0.019), compared to baseline (1.4 ± 0.2 min). By contrast, no significant changes were seen in the placebo group. No product related adverse events were observed during the study. At study conclusion, five individuals in the UC-II cohort reported no pain during or after the stepmill protocol (p = 0.031, within visit) as compared to one subject in the placebo group.

Conclusions

Daily supplementation with 40 mg of UC-II was well tolerated and led to improved knee joint extension in healthy subjects. UC-II also demonstrated the potential to lengthen the period of pain free strenuous exertion and alleviate the joint pain that occasionally arises from such activities.

Keywords : UC-II Undenatured type II collagen Joint function Knee extension Stepmill Joint pain

INTRODUCTION

The impact of strenuous exercise on knee joints may cause localized pain and stiffness, which are hallmark features of pathologic inflammatory disease [1]. It has been shown that when dogs undergo a strenuous running regimen, significant losses in articular cartilage and glycosaminoglycans occur [2]. Such studies suggest that strenuous exercise may activate some of the same physiological processes that occur in arthritic disease [2, 3, 4]. In fact, *in vitro*studies have shown that many of the cytokines implicated in the onset and progression of both rheumatoid arthritis (RA) and osteoarthritis (OA) also appear to regulate the remodeling of the normal knee extracellular matrix (ECM) following strenuous exertion [5].

When normal chondrocytes undergo strenuous mechanical stimulation under static conditions, their physiology shifts towards ECM breakdown, as indicated by the upregulation of several metalloproteinases (MMPs), such as MMP-13 as well as tumor necrosis factor (TNF)-α, interleukin (IL)-1β, IL-6, and various aggrecanases [5, 6]. This *in vitro* catabolic response is mediated by changes in the phosphorylation, expression, or translocation of several transcription factors to the cell nucleus such as NF-κB, p38 MAPK, Akt, and ERK [7, 8]. By contrast, normal chondrocytes produce the anti-inflammatory cytokine IL-4 when mechanically stimulated under moderate and dynamic conditions [9]. The secretion of this autocrine molecule not only helps in shifting chondrocyte metabolism towards the synthesis of aggrecan and type II collagen, it also downregulates production of nitric oxide (NO) and various MMPs and aggrecanases [10, 11, 12]. This conclusion is corroborated by the finding that pretreatment of strenuously compressed normal chondrocytes with IL-4 attenuates their catabolic response [11]. This suggests that IL-4 plays a key role in downregulating remodeling functions, restoring articular cartilage homeostasis, as well as decreasing chondrocyte apoptosis following strenuous mechanical loading [12, 13].

Mechanically stressed chondrocytes also produce a number of other molecules known to participate in inflammatory responses, including prostoglandin E2, NO, and vascular endothelial growth factor [14]. These are proinflammatory molecules that, in conjunction with TNF-α, IL-6 and IL-1β, result in a localized, and transitory inflammatory-like response that is part of the normal repair process occurring in knee joints, serves to moderate remodeling events [3]. Ostrowski et al. [15] showed that healthy individuals express up to 27-fold greater concentrations of the anti-inflammatory cytokine IL-10 in blood following a marathon run when compared to IL-10 blood levels at rest. This finding is not surprising given that these same individuals also show marked increases in the proinflammatory cytokines TNF-α, IL-1β, and IL-6. It therefore appears that in healthy subjects undergoing strenuous exertion, the induction of proinflammatory cytokines is offset by the synthesis of anti-inflammatory agents as part of the recovery process. This view is supported by the observation that IL-10 reduces the catabolic impact of IL-1β and TNF-α on cartilage explants from healthy volunteers, and this effect is enhanced by combining IL-10 with IL-4 [13].

Another protein released by dynamically compressed chondrocytes is transforming growth factor (TGF)-β [16, 17, 18]. This factor is secreted by many cell types and is known to interfere with the cell cycle and arrest differentiation [19]. With regard to chondrocytes, TGF-β induces cell proliferation *in vitro* and slows terminal differentiation into hypertrophic cells [20]. Numerous studies have shown that TGF-β reverses the *in vitro* catabolic effect of various proinflammatory cytokines on normal chondrocytes as well as chondrocytes harvested from RA and OA donors [21, 22, 23].

The overall findings discussed above point to a new, unifying view of joint physiology. It suggests that many of the biological processes occurring in knee joints affected by RA and OA also participate in the maintenance of healthy knees [1, 4, 5]. It therefore seems appropriate to test the efficacy of natural supplements or ingredients, which have been shown to moderate joint pain in RA and OA, as possible candidates for treating the joint discomfort that occasionally results from strenuous exercise in healthy individuals.

UC-II is a natural ingredient which contains a glycosylated, undenatured type-II collagen [24]. Previous studies have shown that small doses of UC-II modulate joint health in both OA and RA [24, 25, 26]. Tong et al. [27], using an *in vivo* model of collagen induced arthritis (CIA), demonstrated that ingesting microgram quantities of undenatured type II collagen significantly reduces circulating levels of inflammatory cytokines, potentially serving to decrease both the incidence and the severity of arthritis [28]. The ability to alter immunity via the ingestion of a food, or an antigen, is called oral tolerance. This is an ongoing normal physiological process that protects the alimentary tract against untoward immunological damage [29, 30]. Research into its mechanism of action has revealed that several distinct types of T regulator cells mediate this phenomenon by releasing IL-10 and TGF-β [30]. It has also been shown that this effect is transitory in nature requiring that the food, or antigen, be consumed continuously in order to maintain the tolerogenic state [30]. Given these findings, plus our current understanding of the role of various cytokines in normal joint physiology, it was hypothesized that supplementation with UC-II might relieve joint discomfort and restore joint function in healthy subjects.

The aim of this randomized, double blind, placebo-controlled study was to assess the impact of UC-II on knee function in otherwise healthy subjects with no prior history of arthritic disease who experienced knee pain upon strenuous physical exertion. The primary efficacy variable for assessing knee function included measurements of flexibility using range of motion (ROM) goniometry.

METHODS

Investigational product

The investigational study product UC-II is derived from chicken sternum. It is manufactured using a patented, low-temperature process to preserve its native structure. For the clinical study, 40 mg of UC-II material (Lot 1109006), which provides 10.4 ± 1.3 mg of native type-II collagen, was encapsulated in an opaque capsule with excipients. Placebo was dispensed in an identical capsule containing only excipients (microcrystalline cellulose, magnesium stearate and silicon dioxide). Both study materials were prepared in a good manufacturing practice (GMP)-certified facility and provided by InterHealth Nutraceuticals, Inc. (Benicia, CA). Subjects were instructed to take one capsule daily with water before bedtime.

Recruitment of subjects

One hundred and six subjects were screened for eligibility using the inclusion–exclusion criteria defined in Table 1. Only healthy adults who presented with no knee joint pain at rest and no diagnosable markers indicative of active arthritic disease, as outlined by the American College of Rheumatology (ACR) guidelines [31, 32], were admitted into the study. To accomplish this, all potential subjects were screened by a board certified clinician. Subjects presenting with any knee pain at rest and at least 3 of 6 clinical classification criteria, which included age greater than 50 years, morning stiffness in the joint lasting 30 minutes or less, crepitus on knee joint manipulation, body tenderness, bony enlargements, knee swelling or presence of excess fluid, and palpable warmth, were excluded. Potential subjects reporting the occasional use of NSAIDs, other pain relief medication, or anti-inflammatory supplements underwent a 2-week washout period before randomization.

Table 1. Inclusion–exclusion criteria

Inclusion

- Subject must be ≥30 and ≤65 years of age
- Body mass index (BMI) must be ≥18 and ≤35 kg/m^2
- Knee joint criteria: (1) no knee joint discomfort at rest; (2) must achieve a knee joint discomfort score of at least 5 on an 11-point Likert scale within 10 minutes of initiating the stepmill protocol
- Maintain existing food and physical activity patterns throughout the study period
- Judged by Investigator to be in general good health on the basis of medical history
- Subject understands the study procedures and provides signed informed consent to participate in the study and authorizes the release of relevant health information to the study investigator
- Females of child bearing age must agree to use approved birth control methods during the study

Exclusion

- Subjects with any indicators of arthritis, joint disorders, or history of immune system or autoimmune disorders
- Daily use of NSAIDs; however, daily use of 81 mg of aspirin for cardioprotection is allowed
- Daily use of anti-inflammatory or omega-3-fatty acid dietary supplements or using supplements to maintain joint health 30 days prior to screening
- Subjects with a history of knee or hip joint replacement surgery, or any hip or back pain which interferes with ambulation
- Use of any immunosuppressive drugs in the last 12 months (including steroids or biologics)
- Glucocorticoid injection or hyaluronic acid injection in affected knee within 3 months prior to enrollment

- History of surgery or significant injury to the target joint within 6 months prior to study enrollment, or an anticipated need for surgical or invasive procedure that will be performed during the study
- Subjects with a chronic pain syndrome and in the judgment of the Investigator is unlikely to respond to any therapy
- Participation in a clinical study with exposure to any non-registered drug product within 30 days prior
- Subjects who have any physical disability which could interfere with their ability to perform the functional performance measures included in this protocol
- Any significant GI condition that would potentially interfere with the evaluation of the study product
- Clinically significant renal, hepatic, endocrine (including diabetes mellitus), cardiac, pulmonary, pancreatic, neurologic, hematologic, or biliary disorder
- Subjects with vascular condition which interferes with ambulation
- Known allergy or sensitivity to herbal products, soy or eggs
- Vegetarian or Vegan
- History or presence of cancer in the prior two years, except for non-melanoma skin cancer.
- Individual has a condition the Investigator believes would interfere with his or her ability to provide informed consent, comply with the study protocol, which might confound the interpretation of the study results or put the person at undue risk
- Untreated or unstable hypothyroidism, an active eating disorder, or evidence of any neurological disorders
- Recent history of (within 12 months) or strong potential for alcohol or substance abuse
- Females who are pregnant, lactating, or unwilling to use adequate contraception during the study

Subjects were required to undergo a 10 minute period of performance testing using a standardized stepmill test developed and validated by Medicus Research (Udani JK, unpublished observation). It involved exercising at level 4 on a StepMill® model 7000PT (StairMaster® Health & Fitness Products, Inc., Kirkland, WA) until one or both knees achieved a discomfort level of 5 on an 11 point (0–10) Likert scale [33]. This pain threshold had to be achieved within a 10 minute period otherwise the subject was excluded. Once the requisite pain level was achieved the subject was asked to continue stepping for an additional two minutes in order to record the maximum pain level achieved before disembarking from the stepmill. The following knee discomfort measures were recorded from the start of the stepmill test: (1) time to onset of initial joint pain; (2) time to onset of maximum joint pain; (3) time to initial improvement in knee joint pain; (4) time to complete recovery from knee joint pain. Subjects who experienced a pain score of 5 (or greater) within one minute of starting the stress test were excluded. Out of 106 screened candidates, 55 subjects were enrolled in the study. Each subject voluntarily signed the IRB-approved informed consent form. After enrollment, the subjects were randomly assigned to either the placebo or the UC-II group.

Study design and trial site

This randomized, double blind, placebo-controlled study was conducted at the Staywell Research clinical site located in Northridge, CA. Medicus Research (Agoura Hills, CA) was the contract research organization (CRO) of record. The study protocol was approved by Copernicus Group IRB (Cary, NC) on April 25th 2012. The study followed the principles outlined in the Declaration of Helsinki (version 1996).

Randomization and blinding

Simple randomization was employed using a software algorithm based on the atmospheric noise method (http://www.random.org). Sequential assignment was used to determine group allocation. Once allocated, the assignment was documented and placed in individually numbered envelopes to maintain blinding. Subjects, clinical staff, plus data analysis and management staff remained blinded throughout the study.

Study schedule

The study duration was 17 weeks with a total of 7 visits that included screening, baseline, days 7, 30, 60, 90 and 120 (final visit). Table 2 summarizes the study visits and activities. Figure 1 depicts the sequence of study procedures that subjects underwent during each visit. All subjects completed a medical history questionnaire at baseline and compliance reports during follow-up evaluations at 7, 30, 60, 90 and 120 days. Subjects were assessed for anthropometric measures, vital signs, knee range of motion (flexion and extension), six-minute timed walk, as well as the onset and recovery from pain using the Udani Stepmill Procedure. A Fitbit (San Francisco, CA) device was used to measure daily distance walked, steps taken and an average step length for study participants. Subjects were also asked to complete the KOOS survey as well as the Stanford exercise scales.

Table 2. Protocol summary

Protocol activities	V1 Day −7 Screen	V2 Day 0 Baseline	V3 Day 7	V4 Day 30	V5 Day 60	V6 Day 90	V7 Day 120 End
Informed consent	x						
Inclusion/Exclusion	x						
Medical history and physical exam	x						
Vital signs/anthropometric measures	x	x	x	x	x	x	x
Urine pregnancy test	x	x					
Administer and review scales/questionnaires/diaries	x	x	x	x	x	x	x
Stressor (Udani Stepmill protocol)	x	x	x	x	x	x	x
Functional measures (6-min timed walk)	x	x	x	x	x	x	x
Goniometry (range of motion)		x	x	x	x	x	x
Review concomitant therapies	x	x	x	x	x	x	x
Intercurrent medical issues review		x	x	x	x	x	x
Compliance assessment (including phone calls)		x	x	x	x	x	x
Randomization		x					
Study supplement preparation & dispensing		x	x	x	x	x	

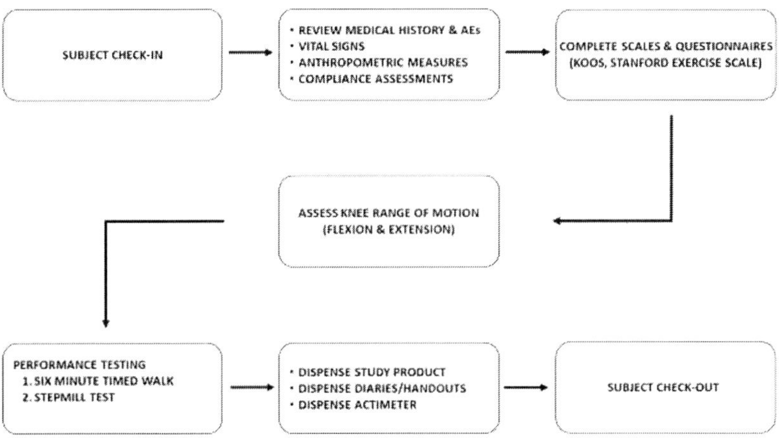

Figure 1. Sequence of study procedures at a typical clinic visit.

Knee range of motion measurements

Knee extension was measured by goniometry. Briefly, subjects were instructed to sit in an upright position on a table edge with their backs straight (knee position defined as 90°). The axis of a goniometer was placed at the intersection of the thigh and shank at the knee joint. Subjects were asked to bring their knees to full extension without changing the position of the pelvis and lumbar spine. The extended knee joint angle was measured and recorded. For knee flexion measurement, subjects were asked to actively flex their knees while lying in a prone position with their shins off the end of the table. The range of knee flexion motion was then measured and documented.

Timed joint discomfort measurements

Briefly, a stopwatch was started when subjects began climbing the stepmill. Time to onset of pain was recorded at the first sign of pain in the target knee. The baselines at each time point were normalized to account for dropouts. Percent change in time to complete recovery from pain was measured as follows: a new stopwatch was started when the subjects disembarked from the stepmill and the time to complete recovery from pain was recorded. The baselines at each time point were normalized to account for dropouts then compared against the reference interval which was defined as the percentage change between the study baseline and day 7.

KOOS knee survey & Stanford exercise scales

The KOOS survey is a validated instrument consisting of 42 questions that are classified into sub-scales such as symptoms, stiffness, pain, daily activities, recreational activities and quality of life [34]. It measures the subjects' opinion about their knees and their ability to perform daily activities during the past week. The Stanford exercise behavior scale comprises 6 questions designed to assess exercise behaviors during the previous week [35].

Six minute timed walk

Subjects were instructed to walk up and down a hallway for 6 minutes as rapidly as possible without causing any pain. A measuring wheel (RoadRunner Wheel, Keson Industries, Aurora, IL) was used to measure distance travelled in 6 minutes.

Rescue medication

No rescue medications were allowed during the course of the study. At all study visits, subjects were given a list of the 43 prohibited medications and supplements (Table 3). Changes in overall medication history, or the use of these substances, were then recorded by the study coordinator. Subjects found to have used any of these prohibited substances were excluded from further participation in the study as per protocol.

Table 3. Representative list of prohibited medications* by category

Category	Medications
Joint supplements (Omega-3, Omega-6 plus others)	Alpha-Linolenic acid
	Docosapentaenoic acid
	Docosahexaenoic acid
	Eicosatrienoic acid
	Eicosatetraenoic acid
	Eicosapentaenoic acid
	Hexadecatrienoic acid
	Heneicosapentaenoic acid
	Stearidonic acid
	Tetracosapentaenoic acid
	Tetracosahexaenoic acid
	Glucosamine (all forms)
	Chondroitin (all forms)
	Other herbal ingredients
NSAIDs (OTC and prescription)	Aspirin
	Diflunisal
	Diclofenac
	Celecoxib
	Etodolac
	Fenoprofen
	Flurbiprofen
	Ibuprofen
	Indomethacin
	Ketoprofen
	Meclofenamate
	Mefenamic acid
	Meloxicam
	Nabumetone
	Naproxen
	Oxaprozin
	Piroxicam
	Rofecoxib
	Sulindac
	Tolmetin
	Valdecoxib

*Selected from a list of 43 prohibited medications and supplements.

Statistics

Outcome variables were assessed for conformance to the normal distribution and transformed as required. Within group significance was analyzed by non-parametric Sign test or by non-parametric Wilcoxon Signed Rank test, while Wilcoxon Mann–Whitney test was used to analyze between groups significance. The Fisher Exact test was used to evaluate the complete loss of pain between study cohorts whereas the binomial test was used to assess the likelihood of complete loss of pain at each visit. P-values equal to or less than 0.05 were considered statistically significant. All analyses were done on a per protocol basis using SPSS, v19 (IBM, Armonk, NY). Results were presented as mean ± SEM.

RESULTS

Baseline demographics

A total of 55 individuals met the eligibility criteria and were randomized to the placebo (n = 28) or to the UC-II (n = 27) group. Baseline demographic characteristics for subjects in both groups were similar with respect to age, gender, height, weight and BMI (Table 4). A total of nine subjects, three in UC-II group and six in placebo group, were lost to follow-up. The results presented herein encompass 46 total subjects, 22 subjects in the placebo group plus 24 subjects in the UC-II group. It should be noted that the average age of the study participants was approximately 46 years which is about 16 years younger than the average age observed in many OA studies [36, 37, 38].

Table 4. Demographic and baseline characteristics of enrolled subjects

Characteristics	UC-II	Placebo
Total number of subjects	27	28
Number of males	11	12
Number of females	16	16
Age (years)	46.1 ± 1.5	46.6 ± 1.8
Weight (kg)	75.5 ± 2.9	77.5 ± 3.1
Height (cm)	167.1 ± 2.0	168.4 ± 2.0
BMI (kg/m^2)	26.8 ± 0.8	27.1 ± 0.7

Values are expressed as Mean ± SEM.

Knee extension and flexion

Figure 2 summarizes the average knee extension changes over time for subjects supplemented with either UC-II or placebo. The UC-II supplemented cohort presented with a statistically significant greater increase in the ability to extend the knee at day 120 as compared to the placebo group (81.0 ± 1.3º vs 74.0 ± 2.2º, $p = 0.011$) and to baseline (81.0 ± 1.3º vs 73.2 ± 1.9º, $p = 0.002$). The UC-II group also demonstrated a significant increase in knee extension at day 90 (78.8 ± 1.9º vs 73.2 ± 1.9º, $p = 0.045$) compared to baseline only. An intent to treat (ITT) analysis of these data also demonstrated a statistically significant net increase in knee extension at day 120 versus placebo (80.0 ± 1.3º vs 73.7 ± 1.8º, $p = 0.006$). No statistically significant changes were observed in the placebo group at any time during this study. With respect to knee flexion, no significant changes were noted in either study group ($p > 0.05$). The power associated with the former per protocol statistical analyses was 80%.

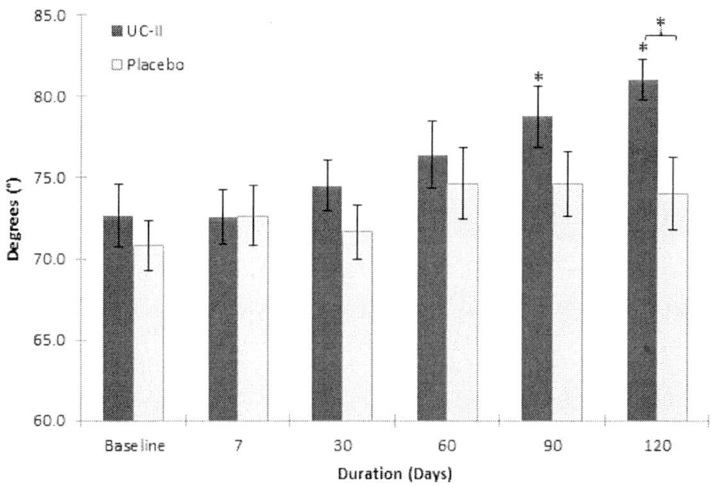

Figure 2. Knee extension as measured by goniometry. Values are presented as Mean ± SEM. *$p \leq 0.05$ indicates a statistically significant difference versus baseline or placebo. Number of completers: n = 24 in UC-II group (n = 3 dropouts); n = 20 in placebo group (n = 6 dropouts; n = 2 did not participate in ROM assessment).

Time to onset of initial joint pain

Supplementation with UC-II resulted in statistically significant increases in the time to onset of initial joint pain at day 90 (2.75 ± 0.5 min, p = 0.041) and at day 120 (2.8 ± 0.5 min, p = 0.019) versus a baseline of 1.4 min for each visit. No statistically significant differences were noted for either the placebo group or between groups (Figure 3).

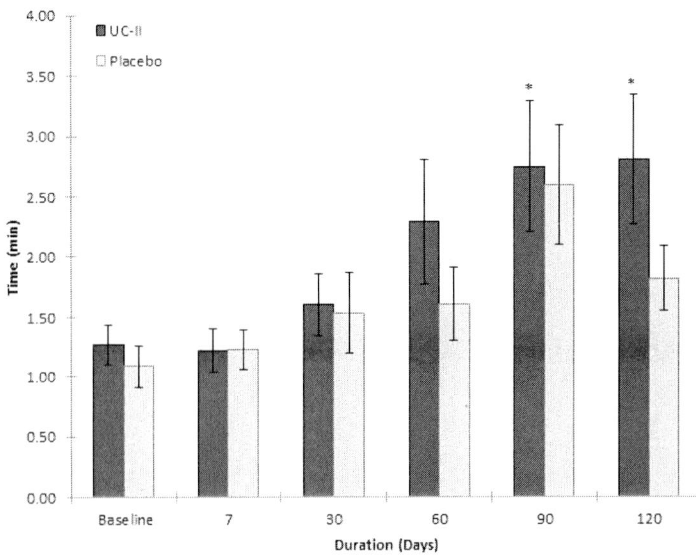

Figure 3. Impact of stepmill procedure on the onset of pain. Values are presented as Mean ± SEM. *p ≤ 0.05 indicates a statistically significant difference from baseline. Number of completers: n = 19 in UC-II group (n = 3 dropouts; n = 5 did not have pain); n = 20 in placebo group (n = 6 dropouts; n = 1 did not have pain; n = 1 did not use stepmill).

Five individuals in the UC-II group and one in the placebo group reported no onset of pain by the end of study (see below and Table 5). Given this unexpected finding, an additional analysis was undertaken which included these individuals in the time to onset of initial pain analysis. The 10 minute limit of the stepmill procedure was used as the lower limit to pain onset. Under these conservative assumptions, supplementation with UC-II yielded statistically significant increases in time to onset of pain at day 90 (3.65 ± 0.7 min, p = 0.011) and day 120 (4.31 ± 0.7 min, p = 0.002) versus a baseline of 1.4 min for each visit. The between-group comparison at day 120 approached the statistical level of significance favoring the UC-II cohort ($p = 0.051$).

Table 5. Subjects reporting complete loss of knee pain on stepmill test

Visit	UC-II			Placebo		
	No. of pain free subjects (%)	Continuity of pain loss#	P value (Binomial test)	No. of pain free subjects (%)	Continuity of pain loss#	P value (Binomial test)
Baseline	0.0 (0)	0	NA	0.0 (0)	0	NA
Day 7	0.0 (0)	0	NA	0.0 (0	0	NA
Day 30	1.0 (4)	1N	0.5	0.0 (0)	0	NA
Day 60	3.0 (13)	1R, 2N	0.125	0.0 (0)	0	NA
Day 90	3.0 (13)	2R, 1N	0.125	1 (5)	1N	0.5
Day 120	5.0 (21)	3R, 2N	0.031†	1 (5)	1R	0.5

Values denote number of subjects while parenthesis provides the percent of total subjects who did not have any pain on stepmill. Continuity indicates the number of subjects in whom the absence of pain was maintained across visits. †Significant at $p \leq 0.05$ based on independent binomial testing of each visit using the null hypothesis that the probability of a subject experiencing no joint pain is equal to zero. There was no statistical difference between groups. #*R* Repeat subject (i.e. same subject who reported no pain in previous visit), *N* New subject who reports no pain for the first time.

Values denote number of subjects while parenthesis provides the percent of total subjects who did not have any pain on stepmill. Continuity indicates the number of subjects in whom the absence of pain was maintained across visits. †Significant at $p \leq 0.05$ based on independent binomial testing of each visit using the null hypothesis that the probability of a subject experiencing no joint pain is equal to zero. There was no statistical difference between groups. #*R* Repeat subject (i.e. same subject who reported no pain in previous visit), *N* New subject who reports no pain for the first time.

Time to onset of maximum joint pain

A statistically significant difference between groups was noted at day 60 (6.39 ± 0.5 min vs 4.78 ± 0.5 min; $p = 0.025$) favoring the UC-II cohort. This significance did not persist during the remainder of the study suggesting that this was a random occurrence.

Time to initial improvement in knee joint pain

The time to offset of joint pain was recorded immediately upon the subject stepping off the stepmill. Both groups began to recover from pain with the same rate resulting in no significant differences between groups in the time to initial offset of joint pain ($p > 0.05$).

Time to complete recovery from knee joint pain

The time to complete recovery from joint pain showed significant reductions at days 60, 90 and 120 compared to baseline for both the UC-II group as well as the placebo group (Figure 4). Percent changes in times were calculated after normalizing the baselines against the reference range of baseline to day 7. The UC-II group exhibited average reductions of 31.9 ± 11.7% (p = 0.041), 51.1 ± 6.1% (p = 0.004) and 51.9 ± 6.0% (p = 0.011) at days 60, 90 and 120, respectively. By contrast, the reductions for the same time points for the placebo cohort, 21.9 ± 10.2% (p = 0.017), 22.2 ± 15.5% (p = 0.007) and 30.0 ± 11.8% (p = 0.012), were of lower magnitude but nonetheless statistically significant versus baseline. None of these between group differences achieved statistical significance.

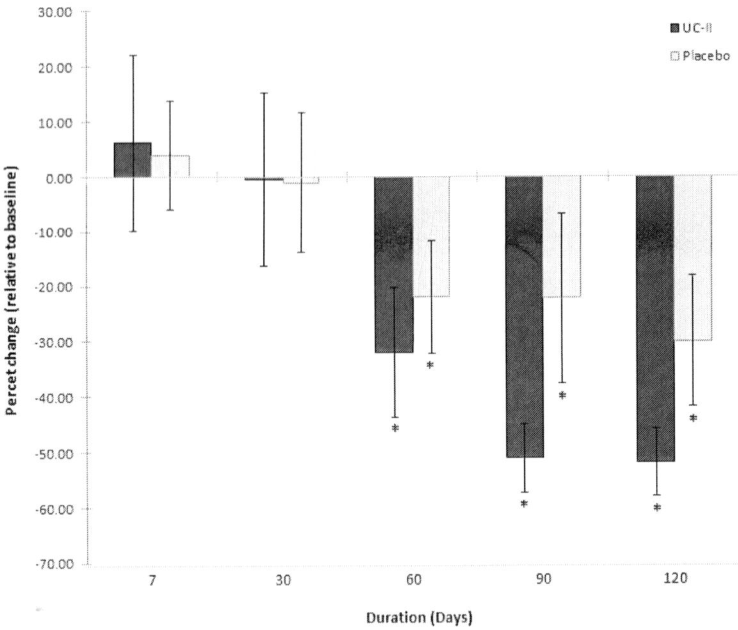

Figure 4. Percent change in time to complete recovery from pain. Values are presented as Mean ± SEM. *p ≤ 0.05 indicates a statistically significant difference from baseline. Number of completers: n = 18 in UC-II group (n = 3 dropouts; n = 5 did not have pain; n = 1 time to complete recovery from pain was not achieved); n = 20 in placebo group (n = 6 dropouts; n = 1 did not have pain; n = 1 did not use stepmill).

Time to complete loss of knee joint pain

During the course of this study it was noted that a number of subjects in both the placebo and the supplemented cohorts no longer reported any pain during the stepmill protocol. For the UC-II group, 5 subjects (21%) no longer reported pain by day 120, whereas only 1 subject (5%) in placebo group reported complete loss of pain (Table 5). This effect did not reach statistical significance between groups but there was an evident trend in the data towards a greater number of subjects losing pain in the UC-II cohort ($p = 0.126$). A binomial analysis for complete loss of pain at each visit demonstrated a statistical significance for the UC-II group by day 120 ($p = 0.031$). It is important to note that the complete loss of knee pain was not a random event. The pattern among the subjects indicates that loss of knee pain appeared to be a persistent phenomenon that spanned multiple visits (Table 5). A detailed review of the clinical report forms showed that none of these individuals consumed pain relief medication prior to their visits.

Six-minute timed walk & Daily number of steps

No significant differences were observed between the study groups for the six-minute time walk or the daily number of steps taken ($p > 0.05$). The distance walked in six-minutes by the UC-II (range = 505 to 522 meters) and the placebo (range = 461 to 502 meters) groups were within the reference range previously reported [39] for healthy adults (399 to 778 meters, males; 310 to 664 meters, females). Similarly, the average step length calculated from Fitbit data for both study groups (0.69 to 0.71 meters) also agreed with previously published results for normal adults [40].

KOOS knee survey & Stanford exercise scales

No significant differences were seen between the study groups for either the KOOS survey or the Stanford exercise scale ($p > 0.05$).

Use of analgesics and NSAIDs

Review of the clinical report forms showed that no subject in either study cohort consumed any of the 43 prohibited medicines or supplements during the study.

Safety assessments

A total of eight adverse events, equally dispersed between both groups, were noted (Table 6). None of the adverse events was considered to be associated with UC-II supplementation. All events resolved spontaneously without the need for further intervention. No subject withdrew from the study due to an adverse event. Finally, no differences were observed in vital signs after seventeen weeks of supplementation, and no serious adverse events were reported in this study.

Table 6. Summary of analysis of adverse events (AEs) in all subjects

Study groups	Adverse event (Body system)	Number of AEs
UC-II	Upper respiratory infection (Pulmonary)	3
	Food poisoning (Gastrointestinal)	1
Total number of AEs		**4**
Total number of subjects reporting AEs: n		**4/27**
Placebo	Bilateral ankle edema (Musculoskeletal)	1
	Right ankle fracture (Musculoskeletal)	1
	Sinusitis (Ears/Nose/Throat)	1
	Skin infection right ankle (Dermatological)	1
Total number of AEs		**4**
Total number of subjects reporting AEs: n		**2/28**

DISCUSSION

In this study, the UC-II supplement, consisting of undenatured type II collagen, was investigated for its ability to improve joint function in healthy subjects who develop joint pain while undergoing strenuous exercise. The rationale behind this approach centered on the hypothesis that strenuous exercise might uncover transient joint changes due to daily physical activities that are not attributable to a diagnosable disease. In the same way that nominally elevated blood levels of lipids, glucose plus high blood pressure and obesity can be predictive of future progression to diabetes and heart disease [41], the development of joint pain upon strenuous exercise may be indicative of possible future joint problems.

At study conclusion, we found that subjects ingesting the UC-II supplement experienced a significantly greater forward ROM in their knees versus baseline and placebo as measured by knee extension goniometry. Knee extension is necessary for daily function and sport activities. Loss of knee extension has been shown to negatively impact the function of the lower extremity [42, 43]. For example, loss of knee extension can cause altered gait patterns affecting ankles and the hip which could result in difficulty with running and jumping [42, 43]. Studies have further shown that a permanent loss of 3-5º of extension can significantly impact patient satisfaction and the development of early arthritis [44].

By contrast, when knee flexion, another measure of knee function, was assessed via goniometry, no differences in clinical outcomes were observed between the two study cohorts. From a structure-function perspective this outcome is not surprising. During the earliest characterized phases of OA there is an apparent preferential loss of knee extension over knee flexion, and this loss has been shown to correlate with WOMAC pain scores [45, 46]. In addition, MRI imaging of the early osteoarthritic knee has shown that initial changes in knee structure appear to center on articular cartilage erosions (fibrillations) about the patella and other weight bearing regions of the knee [47]. Such changes might favor a loss in knee ROM that preferentially affects extension over flexion. The pathophysiology of the early osteoarthritic knee, we believe, provides insight regarding the effect of daily physical activities on the healthy knee insofar as it helps explain the discordance in clinical outcomes between knee extension and flexion.

Both the time to onset of initial joint pain as well as time to full recovery were measured in this study. For each of these measures the clinical outcomes favored the UC-II supplemented cohort versus their baseline status. The ability of UC-II to modulate knee extension may relate to its ability to moderate knee joint pain. Crowley et al. [26] and Trentham et al. [25] demonstrated that UC-II effectively enhances joint comfort and flexibility thereby improving the quality of life (QoL) in both OA and RA subjects, respectively. This effect may be attributable to the finding that microgram quantities of undenatured type II collagen moderate CIA in both the rat and the mouse via the induction of T regulator cells [27, 28, 48]. The induction of these T regulators takes place within gut associated lymphatic tissues (GALT), including mesenteric lymph nodes, in response to the consumption of undenatured type II collagen [27].

Studies have shown that these regulatory cells produce IL-10 and TGF-β [30, 49]. A special class of $CD103^{+}$ dendritic cells, found almost exclusively in the GALT, facilitates this process [48, 50]. Once activated, T regulator cells appear to downregulate a wide range of immunologic and proinflammatory activities resulting in the moderation of the arthritic response initiated by undenatured type II collagen [27]. The phenomenon of oral tolerance has also been demonstrated in humans, and appears to involve a similar set of T regulators [30, 51, 52, 53].

The above description of how UC-II might modulate joint function is most easily understood in the context of RA given that the CIA animal model resembles this disease most closely [27, 28,54]. However, the case for T regulators and immune cytokines having a moderating effect on healthy or OA knee joint function appears less apparent. This view has changed in recent years due to a growing body of evidence suggesting that both OA and normal chondrocyte biology appears to be regulated by some of the same cytokines and chemokines that regulate inflammation [5, 6, 55]. For example, Mannelli and coworkers [56] recently reported that feeding microgram amounts of native type II collagen (porcine) prevents monoiodoacetate-induced articular cartilage damage in this rat model of osteoarthritis, as measured by pain thresholds and by circulating levels of cross linked c-telopeptides derived from type II collagen. This finding corroborates the efficacy of undenatured type II collagen in improving joint comfort in osteoarthritic conditions [26].

In the present study, we show for the first time that UC-II can improve joint function in healthy subjects undergoing strenuous physical exercise. This observation, when considered in context with normal chondrocyte physiology, suggests that activated T regulator cells, specific for undenatured type II collagen, home to an overstressed knee joint where their release of the anti-inflammatory cytokines, IL-10 and TGF-β reverse the catabolic changes caused by strenuous exertion [13, 21, 57]. In addition, the IL-10 and TGF-β produced by these T regulators may tilt the T_H balance in the knee joint towards T_H2 [30, 58] responses which preferentially result in IL-4 production further fostering a shift in chondrocyte metabolism towards ECM replenishment.

Several additional tests were used in this study to assess overall joint function, QoL, and physical activity. The additional parameters and tests measured included a six minute timed walk plus the Stanford exercise scale and KOOS survey. With respect to the KOOS survey, both cohorts were statistically significant versus baseline for symptoms, pain, daily function, recreational activities and QoL but were not significant from each other. This is not an unexpected finding given that this study was carried out with healthy subjects who do not present with any joint issues at rest. It is only when the knee is stressed via the stepmill do subjects report any joint discomfort. Under these conditions, and as indicated above, the UC-II group appears to experience less joint discomfort and greater joint flexibility. No difference in clinical outcomes between groups was seen in the six minute timed walk, the daily distance walked, or the Stanford exercise scale questionnaire. Once again we are not surprised by these results given that these tests and questionnaires are designed and clinically validated to assess the severity of arthritic disease in unhealthy populations.

No clinical biomarkers associated with arthritic diseases were assessed in this study. Healthy subjects would not be expected to present with significant alterations in their inflammatory biomarker profile as they lack clinical disease [59]. In addition, it should be noted that the joint discomfort measured in this study is acute pain induced by a stressor rather than due to an ongoing inflammatory event. Therefore, any elevation in inflammation markers that might occur in these healthy subjects may simply be due to the physiological impact of strenuous exercise.

There are two study limitations to consider when reviewing these results. The first, time to onset of initial pain, was limited to a 10-minute interval. The current study design did not address the possibility that subjects might cease to experience pain on the stepmill. Future studies should allow for an extension of the exertion interval in order to gauge how much longer a subject can exercise before reporting pain. In this way better defined parameters can be placed upon the degree to which UC-II supplementation results in the cessation of joint pain due to strenuous exercise in healthy subjects.

The second limitation that merits consideration is the possibility that study subjects may have early signs of arthritis that do not meet the ACR criteria. This possible limitation was addressed by performing an extensive medical examination for signs and symptoms of OA and by excluding volunteers who experienced pain levels of 5 or greater within one minute of using the stepmill.

UC-II is a unique ingredient that supports healthy joints. Previous studies have focused on the efficacy of this ingredient in OA subjects. By including healthy subjects in this study, and using non-disease endpoints as a measure of efficacy, it is believed that the benefits that derive from UC-II usage now extends to include healthy individuals. Further, this ingredient appears to be safe for human consumption based on an extensive series of *in vivo* and *in vitro* toxicological studies as well as the absence of any adverse events in this and in previous human studies [24,26, 60]. In conclusion, daily supplementation with 40 mg of UC-II supports joint function and flexibility in healthy subjects as demonstrated by greater knee extension and has the potential both to alleviate the joint pain that occasionally arises from strenuous exercise as well as to lengthen periods of pain free exertion.

DECLARATIONS

Acknowledgements

Medicus Research thanks InterHealth Nutraceuticals, Inc., Benicia, California, for supporting this clinical trial and for providing the treatment and placebo products. We thank the entire Staywell clinical staff for their tireless efforts and dedication to the health and welfare of the subjects. The study design and the protocol preparation was the result of a collaborative effort between InterHealth Nutraceuticals, Inc., Benicia, California and Medicus Research LLC, Agoura Hills, CA, the Contract Research Organization (CRO) chosen to manage the clinical and other logistics of this study.

Funding

InterHealth Nutraceuticals, Inc., Benicia, California.

Competing interests

Medicus Research received research grants from InterHealth Nutraceuticals, Inc., Benicia, California. Dr. Udani has provided consulting services to InterHealth Nutraceuticals, Inc. Drs. JPL, ZMS, and FCL are employees of InterHealth Nutraceuticals, Inc. Medicus Research does not endorse any brand or product nor does it have any financial interests with any supplement manufacturer or distributor.

Authors' contributions

JKU was the principal investigator and together with JPL, JKU, ZMS, FCL JPM, MNP and ANS contributed to the writing, data analyses and data interpretation that are a part of this manuscript. All the authors read and approved the final draft of the manuscript.

REFERENCES

1. Shek PN, Shephard RJ: Physical exercise as a human model of limited inflammatory response. Can J Physiol Pharmacol. 1998, 76: 589-597.
2. Kiviranta I, Tammi M, Jurvelin J: Articular cartilage thickness and glycosaminoglycan distribution in the canine knee joint after strenuous running exercise. Clin Orthop Relat Res. 1992, 283: 302-308.
3. Guilak F: Biomechanical factors in osteoarthritis. Best Pract Res Clin Rheumatol. 2011, 25: 815-823.
4. Kawamura S, Lotito K, Rodeo SA: Biomechanics and healing response of the meniscus. Oper Tech Sports Med. 2003, 11: 68-76.
5. Ramage L, Nuki G, Salter DM: Signalling cascades in mechanotransduction: cell-matrix interactions and mechanical loading. Scand J Med Sci Sports. 2009, 19: 457-469.
6. Honda K, Ohno S, Tanimoto K: The effects of high magnitude cyclic tensile load on cartilage matrix metabolism in cultured chondrocytes. Eur J Cell Biol. 2000, 79: 601-609.
7. Agarwal S, Deschner J, Long P: Role of NF-kappaB transcription factors in antiinflammatory and proinflammatory actions of mechanical signals. Arthritis Rheum. 2004, 50: 3541-3548.
8. Berg V, Sveinbjornsson B, Bendiksen S: Human articular chondrocytes express chemR23 and chemerin; chemR23 promotes inflammatory signalling upon binding the ligand chemerin(21–157). Arthritis Res Ther. 2010, 12: R228-
9. Millward-Sadler SJ, Wright MO, Lee H: Integrin-regulated secretion of interleukin 4: a novel pathway of mechanotransduction in human articular chondrocytes. J Cell Biol. 1999, 145: 183-189.
10. Millward-Sadler SJ, Wright MO, Davies LW: Mechanotransduction via integrins and interleukin-4 results in altered aggrecan and matrix metalloproteinase 3 gene expression in normal, but not osteoarthritic, human articular chondrocytes. Arthritis Rheum. 2000, 43: 2091-2099.
11. Doi H, Nishida K, Yorimitsu M: Interleukin-4 downregulates the cyclic tensile stress-induced matrix metalloproteinases-13 and

cathepsin B expression by rat normal chondrocytes. Acta Med Okayama. 2008, 62: 119-126.

12. Yorimitsu M, Nishida K, Shimizu A: Intra-articular injection of interleukin-4 decreases nitric oxide production by chondrocytes and ameliorates subsequent destruction of cartilage in instability-induced osteoarthritis in rat knee joints. Osteoarthritis Cartilage. 2008, 16: 764-771.

13. van Meegeren ME, Roosendaal G, Jansen NW: IL-4 alone and in combination with IL-10 protects against blood-induced cartilage damage. Osteoarthritis Cartilage. 2012, 20: 764-772.

14. Pufe T, Lemke A, Kurz B: Mechanical overload induces VEGF in cartilage discs via hypoxia-inducible factor. Am J Pathol. 2004, 164: 185-192.

15. Ostrowski K, Rohde T, Asp S: Pro- and anti-inflammatory cytokine balance in strenuous exercise in humans. J Physiol. 1999, 515 (Pt 1): 287-291.

16. Allen JL, Cooke ME, Alliston T: ECM stiffness primes the TGFbeta pathway to promote chondrocyte differentiation. Mol Biol Cell. 2012, 23: 3731-3742.

17. Bougault C, Aubert-Foucher E, Paumier A: Dynamic compression of chondrocyte-agarose constructs reveals new candidate mechanosensitive genes. PLoS One. 2012, 7

18. Li TF, O'Keefe RJ, Chen D: TGF-beta signaling in chondrocytes. Front Biosci. 2005, 10: 681-688.

19. Donovan J, Slingerland J: Transforming growth factor-beta and breast cancer: cell cycle arrest by transforming growth factor-beta and its disruption in cancer. Breast Cancer Res. 2000, 2: 116-124.

20. Rosier RN, O'Keefe RJ, Crabb ID: Transforming growth factor beta: an autocrine regulator of chondrocytes. Connect Tissue Res. 1989, 20: 295-301.

21. Roman-Blas JA, Stokes DG, Jimenez SA: Modulation of TGF-beta signaling by proinflammatory cytokines in articular chondrocytes. Osteoarthritis Cartilage. 2007, 15: 1367-1377.

22. Loeser RF: Aging and osteoarthritis: the role of chondrocyte senescence and aging changes in the cartilage matrix. Osteoarthritis Cartilage. 2009, 17: 971-979.

23. van Beuningen HM, van der Kraan PM, Arntz OJ: Protection from interleukin 1 induced destruction of articular cartilage by transforming growth factor beta: Studies in anatomically intact cartilage in vitro and in vivo. Ann Rheum Dis. 1993, 52: 185-191.

24. Bagchi D, Misner B, Bagchi M: Effects of orally administered undenatured type II collagen against arthritic inflammatory diseases: a mechanistic exploration. Int J Clin Pharmacol Res. 2002, 22: 101-110.

25. Trentham DE, Dynesius-Trentham RA, Orav EJ: Effects of oral administration of type II collagen on rheumatoid arthritis. Science. 1993, 261: 1727-1730.

26. Crowley DC, Lau FC, Sharma P: Safety and efficacy of undenatured type II collagen in the treatment of osteoarthritis of the knee: a clinical trial. Int J Med Sci. 2009, 6: 312-321.

27. Tong T, Zhao W, Wu YQ: Chicken type II collagen induced immune balance of main subtype of helper T cells in mesenteric lymph node lymphocytes in rats with collagen-induced arthritis. Inflamm Res. 2010, 59: 369-377.

28. Nagler-Anderson C, Bober LA, Robinson ME: Suppression of type II collagen-induced arthritis by intragastric administration of soluble type II collagen. Proc Natl Acad Sci USA. 1986, 83: 7443-7446.

29. Brandtzaeg P: 'ABC' of mucosal immunology. Nestle Nutr Workshop Ser Pediatr Program. 2009, 64: 23-38. discussion 38–43, 251–7

30. Weiner HL, da Cunha AP, Quintana F: Oral tolerance. Immunol Rev. 2011, 241: 241-259.

31. Aletaha D, Neogi T, Silman AJ: 2010 Rheumatoid arthritis classification criteria: an american college of rheumatology/european league against rheumatism collaborative initiative. Arthritis Rheum. 2010, 62: 2569-2581.

32. Altman R, Asch E, Bloch D: Development of criteria for the classification and reporting of osteoarthritis. Classification of osteoarthritis of the knee. Diagnostic and therapeutic criteria committee of the american rheumatism association. Arthritis Rheum. 1986, 29: 1039-1049.

33. Likert R: A technique for the measurement of attitudes. Arch Psychol. 1932, 22: 1-55.

34. Roos EM, Roos HP, Ekdahl C: Knee injury and osteoarthritis outcome score (KOOS)–validation of a swedish version. Scand J Med Sci Sports. 1998, 8: 439-448.

35. Lorig K, Stewart A, Ritter P: Outcome measures for health education and other health care interventions. Outcome measures for health education and other health care interventions. 1996, Thousand Oaks, CA: SAGE Publications, Inc.

36. Hawkey C, Laine L, Simon T: Comparison of the effect of rofecoxib (a cyclooxygenase 2 inhibitor), ibuprofen, and placebo on the gastroduodenal mucosa of patients with osteoarthritis: a randomized, double-blind, placebo-controlled trial. The rofecoxib osteoarthritis endoscopy multinational study group. Arthritis Rheum. 2000, 43: 370-377.

37. Pincus T, Koch GG, Sokka T: A randomized, double-blind, crossover clinical trial of diclofenac plus misoprostol versus acetaminophen in patients with osteoarthritis of the hip or knee. Arthritis Rheum. 2001, 44: 1587-1598.

38. Petrella RJ, DiSilvestro MD, Hildebrand C: Effects of hyaluronate sodium on pain and physical functioning in osteoarthritis of the knee: a randomized, double-blind, placebo-controlled clinical trial. Arch Intern Med. 2002, 162: 292-298.

39. Enright PL, Sherrill DL: Reference equations for the six-minute walk in healthy adults. Am J Respir Crit Care Med. 1998, 158: 1384-1387.

40. Perry J: Gait analysis: normal and pathological function. 1992, Thorofare: SLACK Inc.

41. Viera AJ: Predisease: when does it make sense?. Epidemiol Rev. 2011, 33: 122-134.

42. Norkin CC, Levangie PK: Joint structure & function: a comprehensive analysis. 1992, Philadelphia: F.A. Davis

43. Shah N: Increasing knee range of motion using a unique sustained method. N Am J Sports Phys Ther. 2008, 3: 110-113.

44. Shelbourne KD, Biggs A, Gray T: Deconditioned knee: the effectiveness of a rehabilitation program that restores normal knee motion to improve symptoms and function. N Am J Sports Phys Ther. 2007, 2: 81-89.

45. Serrao PR, Gramani-Say K, Lessi GC: Knee extensor torque of men with early degrees of osteoarthritis is associated with pain, stiffness and function. Rev Bras Fisioter. 2012, 16: 289-294.

46. Heiden TL, Lloyd DG, Ackland TR: Knee extension and flexion weakness in people with knee osteoarthritis: Is antagonist cocontraction a factor?. J Orthop Sports Phys Ther. 2009, 39: 807-815.

47. Karachalios T, Zibis A, Papanagiotou P: MR imaging findings in early osteoarthritis of the knee. Eur J Radiol. 2004, 50 (3): 37-40.

48. Park MJ, Park KS, Park HS: A distinct tolerogenic subset of splenic IDO(+)CD11b(+) dendritic cells from orally tolerized mice is responsible for induction of systemic immune tolerance and suppression of collagen-induced arthritis. Cell Immunol. 2012, 278: 45-54.

49. Li MO, Flavell RA: TGF-beta: a master of all T cell trades. Cell. 2008, 134: 392-404.

50. Coombes JL, Siddiqui KR, Arancibia-Carcamo CV: A functionally specialized population of mucosal CD103+ DCs induces Foxp3+ regulatory T cells via a TGF-beta and retinoic acid-dependent mechanism. J Exp Med. 2007, 204: 1757-1764.

51. Ilan Y, Zigmond E, Lalazar G: Oral administration of OKT3 monoclonal antibody to human subjects induces a dose-dependent immunologic effect in T cells and dendritic cells. J Clin Immunol. 2010, 30: 167-177.

52. Caminiti L, Passalacqua G, Barberi S: A new protocol for specific oral tolerance induction in children with IgE-mediated cow's milk allergy. Allergy Asthma Proc. 2009, 30: 443-448.

53. Ben Ahmed M, Belhadj Hmida N, Moes N: IL-15 renders conventional lymphocytes resistant to suppressive functions of regulatory T cells through activation of the phosphatidylinositol 3-kinase pathway. J Immunol. 2009, 182: 6763-6770.

54. Courtenay JS, Dallman MJ, Dayan AD: Immunisation against heterologous type II collagen induces arthritis in mice. Nature. 1980, 283: 666-668.

55. Pelletier JP, Martel-Pelletier J, Abramson SB: Osteoarthritis, an inflammatory disease: potential implication for the selection of new therapeutic targets. Arthritis Rheum. 2001, 44: 1237-1247.

56. Di Cesare Mannelli L, Micheli L, Zanardelli M: Low dose native type II collagen prevents pain in a rat osteoarthritis model. BMC Musculoskelet Disord. 2013, 14: 228

57. Muller RD, John T, Kohl B: IL-10 overexpression differentially affects cartilage matrix gene expression in response to TNF-alpha in human articular chondrocytes in vitro. Cytokine. 2008, 44: 377-385.

58. Zouali M: Immunological tolerance: mechanisms. 2001, eLS: John Wiley & Sons, Ltd

59. Chu CR, Williams AA, Coyle CH: Early diagnosis to enable early treatment of pre-osteoarthritis. Arthritis Res Ther. 2012, 14: 212-

60. Marone PA, Lau FC, Gupta RC: Safety and toxicological evaluation of undenatured type II collagen. Toxicol Mech Methods. 2010, 20: 175-189.

9

DIETARY POLYPHENOLS AS POTENTIAL NUTRACEUTICALS IN MANAGEMENT OF DIABETES: A REVIEW

Zahra Bahadoran[1] , Parvin Mirmiran[2*] and Fereidoun Azizi[3]

[1]Nutrition and Endocrine Research Center, and Obesity Research Center, Research Institute for Endocrine Sciences, Shahid Beheshti University of Medical Sciences, No 24 Parvaneh St, Yemen St, Chamran Exp, 19395-4763 Tehran, Iran.

[2]Department of Clinical Nutrition and Dietetics, Faculty of Nutrition Sciences and Food Technology, National Nutrition and Food Technology Research Institute, Shahid Beheshti University of Medical Sciences, No 46 Arghavan-e-gharbi St, Farahzadi Blv, Shahrak-e-Ghods, 19395-4741 Tehran, Iran.

[3]Endocrine Research Center, Research Institute for Endocrine Sciences, Shahid Beheshti University of Medical Sciences, No 24 Parvaneh St, Yemen St, Chamran Exp, 19395-4763 Tehran, Iran

ABSTRACT

In recent years, there is growing evidence that plant-foods polyphenols, due to their biological properties, may be unique nutraceuticals and supplementary treatments for various aspects of type 2 diabetes mellitus. In this article we have reviewed the potential efficacies of polyphenols, including phenolic acids, flavonoids, stilbenes, lignans and polymeric lignans, on metabolic disorders and complications induced by diabetes. Based on several *in vitro*, animal models and some human studies, dietary plant polyphenols and polyphenol-rich products modulate carbohydrate and lipid metabolism, attenuate hyperglycemia, dyslipidemia and insulin resistance, improve adipose tissue metabolism, and alleviate oxidative stress and stress-sensitive signaling pathways and inflammatory processes. Polyphenolic compounds can also prevent the development of long-term diabetes complications including cardiovascular disease, neuropathy, nephropathy and retinopathy. Further investigations as human clinical studies are needed to obtain the optimum dose and duration of supplementation with polyphenolic compounds in diabetic patients.

Keywords: Polyphenols Phenolic acids Flavonoids Stilbenes Lignans Type 2 diabetes Diabetes complications

INTRODUCTION

Type 2 diabetes is a complex metabolic disorder associated with developing insulin resistance, impaired insulin signaling and β-cell dysfunction, abnormal glucose and lipid metabolism, sub-clinical inflammation and increased oxidative stress; these metabolic disorders lead to long-term pathogenic conditions including micro- and macro-vascular complications, neuropathy, retinopathy, nephropathy, and a consequent decrease in quality of life and an increase in the rate of mortality [1, 2, 3]. Among the multiple risk factors underling the incidence and progression of type 2 diabetes, diet is the main modifiable factor. An increasing number of epidemiological investigations show that diet rich in foods with high-content of phytochemicals, high total antioxidant capacity and polyphenolic compounds may be related to lower risk of diabetes and predisposing factors [4, 5, 6, 7, 8, 9].

Based on the current understanding of pathophysiology of insulin resistance and type 2 diabetes, multiple pharmacological and non-pharmacological interventions have been developed with the aim of improving glycemic control and prevention of diabetes complications; in this area, recently the use of functional foods and their bioactive components have been considered as a new approach in the prevention and management of diabetes and its complications [10, 11, 12, 13].

Due to their biological properties, polyphenols may be appropriate nutraceuticals and supplementary treatments for various aspects of diabetes mellitus. Our aim here is to review the current evidences in relation to several potential efficacies of these bioactive components on type 2 diabetes mellitus and related metabolic disorders. We obtained relevant articles, including *in vitro*, animal models and human studies with appropriate design, as well as review articles with good quality, published between 1990 to 2013, through searches of the Medline and PubMed databases. We first describe a brief introduction on dietary polyphenols, food sources and properties, and then summarize the evidence from *in vitro,* animal models and clinical studies.

Dietary polyphenols: food sources, bioavailability and metabolism

Polyphenols are natural phytochemical compounds in plant-based foods, such as fruits, vegetables, whole grains, cereal, legumes, tea, coffee, wine and cocoa; more than 8000 polyphenolic compounds, including phenolic acids, flavonoids, stilbenes, lignans and polymeric lignans have been identified in whole plant foods [5]. These compounds are secondary metabolites of the plants that act as a defense against ultraviolet radiation, oxidants and pathogens [14].

Polyphenols may be classified into several categories based on the number of phenol rings and structural elements that bind these rings to one another [15]. Phenolic acids are approximately a third of the polyphenolic compounds in the diet and include two main classes hydroxybenzoic acid derivatives (protocatechuic acid, gallic acid, *p*-hydroxybenzoic acid) and hydroxycinnamic acid derivatives (caffeic acid, chlorogenic acid, coumaric acid, Ferulic acid, sinapic acid); berry fruits, kiwi, cherry, apple, pear, chicory and coffee are the foods with high content of these phenolic acids [16]. Flavonoids are the most abundant polyphenols in the human diet and more than 4000 types of these compounds have been identified. There are six subclasses of flavonoids including anthocyanins, flavonols, flavanols, flavanones, flavones and isoflavones; anthocyanins (cyanidin, pelargonidin, delphinidin, malvidin) are found in the berries family, red wine, red cabbage, cherry, black grape and strawberry. Flavonols, including quercetin, kampferol and myricetin, have been mainly detected in onion, curly kale, leeks, broccoli and blueberries. Isoflavones are other most important dietary flavonoids that include daidzein, genistein and glycitein; soybeans and soy products are the richest sources of these estrogen-like structure compounds. Lignans, diphenoilc components with phytoesterogenic activity, have been found in high concentrations in linseed and other grains and cereals. Stilbenes occur in the human diet in low quantities; resveratrol, one of the well studied compounds of these groups, is largely detected in grapes and red wine [5, 16, 17].

It is estimated that dietary intake of polyphenols is approximately 1 g/day [18, 19]. Bioavailability of these bioactive components is dependent on food preparation processes, gastrointestinal digestion, absorption and metabolism [20]. During the absorption pathway, dietary polyphenols must be hydrolyzed by the intestinal enzymes or colonic microflora, and then be conjugated in the intestinal cells and later in the liver by methylation, sulfation or glucuronidation [21]. Polyphenols consequently reach and accumulate in the target tissue and induce biological properties; the polyphenol derivates mainly excrete through bile and urine. Several studies showed rapid absorption of the polyphenolic compounds, such as procyanidins, quercetin and flavanols into plasma, with plasma concentrations peaking at 2 or 3 hours after ingestion [16].

Several biological activities and beneficial properties have been documented for dietary polyphenols, and some of the more well known ones include antioxidant, anti-allergic, anti-inflammatory, anti-viral and anti-microbial, anti-proliferative, anti-mutagenic, anti-carcinogenic, free radical scavenging, regulation of cell cycle arrest, apoptosis, and induction of antioxidant enzymes; more interestingly, dietary polyphenols could modulate some important cell signaling pathways such as nuclear factor kappa-B (NF-κB), activator protein-1 DNA binding (AP-1), extracellular signal-regulated protein kinase (ERK), phosphoinositide 3 (PI3) kinase/protein kinase B (Akt), mitogen-activated protein kinases (MAPK), and nuclear factor erythroid 2 related factor 2 (Nrf2) [22].

Anti-hyperglycemic effects of polyphenols with regard to carbohydrate metabolism, β-cell function and insulin resistance

Impaired carbohydrate metabolism and developing insulin resistance is the main metabolic disorder in non-insulin dependent diabetes mellitus leading to hyperglycemia. Altered digestion and absorption of dietary carbohydrate, depletion of glycogen storage, increased gluconeogenesis and over output hepatic glucose, β-cell dysfunction, insulin resistance of peripheral tissue and defect in insulin signaling pathways are more important causes of hyperglycemia [23]. Although the use of oral anti-diabetic drugs including α-glucosidase inhibitors, biguanides, meglitinides, sulfonylureas, thiazolidindiones or insulin therapies are common clinical options in management of type 2 diabetes and hyperglycemia, but traditionally used natural agents have been considered for a long period of time. Among the known natural bioactive components and phytochemicals, recently polyphenols are very popular because of their anti-hyperglycemic effects, safety and non side-effects. Potential efficacy of polyphenols on carbohydrate metabolism and glucose homeostasis has been well investigated in *in vitro*, animal models and some clinical trials [24].

In Figure 1 beneficial effects of polyphenols on management of blood glucose in diabetes are summarized. The hypoglycemic effects of polyphenols are mainly attributed to reduce intestinal absorption of dietary carbohydrate, modulation of the enzymes involved in glucose metabolism, improvement of β-cell function and insulin action, stimulation of insulin secretion, and the antioxidative and anti-inflammatory properties of these components [25, 26, 27].

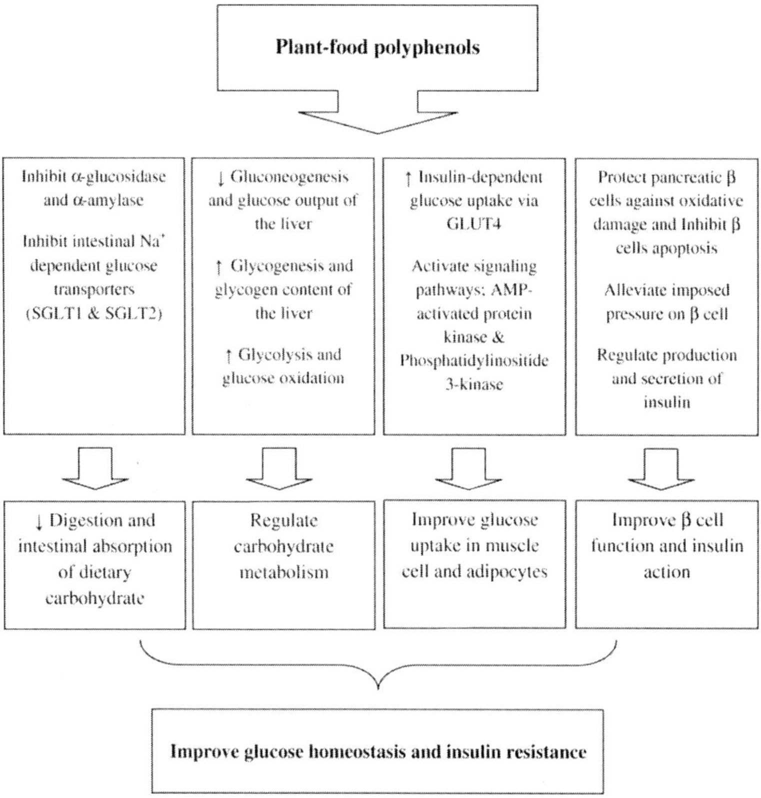

Figure 1. Beneficial effects of polyphenols on management of blood glucose in diabetes. The hypoglycemic effects of polyphenols are mainly attributed to reduce intestinal absorption of dietary carbohydrate, modulation of the enzymes involved in glucose metabolism, improvement of β-cell function and insulin action, and stimulation of insulin secretion.

One of the most well known properties of the polyphenols, especially flavonoids, phenolic acids and tannins, on carbohydrate metabolism is inhibition of α-glucosidase and α-amylase, the key enzymes responsible for digestion of dietary carbohydrates to glucose [26, 28]. Some polyphenols, including green tea catechins and epicatechins, chlorogenic acids, Ferulic acids, caffeic and tannic acids, quercetin and naringenin, could interact with absorption of glucose from intestine via inhibition of Na^+-dependent glucose transporters, SGLT1 and SGLT2

[29, 30]. Some investigations have shown that polyphenolic compounds are also able to regulate postprandial glycemia and inhibit the development of glucose intolerance by a facilitated insulin response and attenuated secretion of glucose-dependent insulinotropic polypeptide (GIP) and glucagon-like polypeptide-1 (GLP-1) [31, 32].

Some polyphenols are able to regulate the key pathways of carbohydrate metabolism and hepatic glucose homeostasis including glycolysis, glycogenesis and gluconeogenesis, usually impaired in diabetes. Ferulic acid, a hydroxycinnamic acid derivate, effectively suppresses blood glucose by elevating glucokinase activity and production of glycogen in the liver and increased plasma insulin levels in diabetic rats [33]. Supplementation of diabetic rats with hesperidin and naringin, two main citrus bioflavonoids, was accompanied with increased hepatic glucokinase activity and glycogen content, attenuated hepatic gluconeogenesis via decrease the activity of glucose-6-phosphatase and phosphoenolpyruvate carboxykinase (PEPCK), and subsequent improvement of glycemic control [34, 35]. Green tea polyphenols, mainly catechins and epicatechins have been shown to attenuate hyperglycemia and hepatic glucose output via downregulation the expression of liver glucokinase and upregulation of PEPCK [36]; in an *in vitro* study, epigallocatechin gallate (EGCG), one of the most abundant catechins in green tea, could activate AMP-activated protein kinase as a required pathway for the inhibition of gluconeogenic enzymes expression [37].

Dietary polyphenols also influence peripheral glucose uptake in both insulin sensitive and non-insulin sensitive tissues; one study showed that phenolic acids stimulated glucose uptake by comparable performance to metformin and thiazolodinedione, main common oral hypoglycemic drugs [38]. The results from the *in vitro* studies showed that some polyphenolic compounds such as quercetin, resveratrol and EGCG improved insulin-dependent glucose uptake in muscle cells and adipocytes by translocation of glucose transporter, GLUT4, to plasma membrane mainly through induction of the AMP-activated protein kinase (AMPK) pathway [39,40]. AMPK, an important sensor of cellular energy status, has a key role in metabolic control; activation of this pathway is considered as a new treatment for obesity, type 2 diabetes, metabolic syndrome and a main target for anti-diabetic drugs including metformin [41, 42]. Interestingly, effect of polyphenols in activation of AMPK has been reported 50-200 times more than metformin [43]. Some polyphenols also have potential to induce phosphatidylinositide 3-kinase (PI3k) as a key signaling pathway for up-regulation of glucose uptake [44].

Isoflavones, particularly genistein, have amazing effects on pancreatic β-cells; Liu et al reported that anti-diabetic effects of genistein are not associated with stimulation of insulin synthesis, expression of glucose tranporter-2 or glycolytic pathway, genistein acts as a novel agonist of cyclic AMP/protein kinas A signaling, an important physiological amplifier of glucose-induced insulin secretion by the pancreatic β-cells [45, 46]. Furthermore, Fu et al indicated that genistein could induce protein expression of cyclin D1, a major cell-cycle regulator of β-cell growth and subsequently improve islet β-cell proliferation, survival and mass [47].

Hyperglycemia-induced oxidative stress in pancreatic β-cells plays a pivotal role in the development of diabetes [48, 49]. Some of the polyphenolic compounds protect β-cells from hyperglycemia-induced and oxidative-induced damage; oral administration of phenolic-rich chestnut extract in STZ-induced diabetic rats had favorable effects on serum glucose and viability of β-cell through attenuation of oxidative stress, enhancing the natural antioxidant system, and inhibition of lipid peroxidation [50]. Another very known phenolic compound, resveratrol (3,4′,5-trihydroxystilbene) found in grapes, wine, grape juice, peanuts, and berries, improve glucose tolerance, attenuate β-cell loss, and reduce oxidative stress in pancreatic islet [51]. Resveratrol also alleviate chronic over stimulation induced-workload and impose pressure on the β-cells, and subsequently delay the degradation of pancreatic islets and progress of type 2 diabetes. This effect appears to be due to the diminished stimulatory effects of hyperglycemia in insulin secretion; some experimental and *in vitro* studies demonstrated that resveratrol has the potential to reduce insulin secretion through induction of metabolic changes in β-cells [51,52].

Some protective effects of polyphenols on β-cells are related to the ability to modulate key cellular signaling pathways; anthocyanins-rich Chinese bayberry extract showed protective effects for pancreatic β cells against oxidative damage through up-regulation of heme oxygenase-1, modulation of ERK1/2 and PI3K/Akt signaling pathway and inhibition of β cells apoptosis [39].

In summary, results of the studies acknowledge that plant polyphenols favorably affect several aspects of diabetes-induced metabolic disorders and modulate carbohydrate metabolism, glucose homeostasis, insulin secretion and insulin resistance.

Cardiovascular protective effects of polyphenols with regard to lipid metabolism, blood pressure, blood coagulation and vascular function

Progressive insulin resistance is mainly accompanied with pro-atherogenic cardiovascular risk profiles and consequently atherosclerotic coronary artery disease and other forms of cardiovascular disease are the major causes of mortality in type 2 diabetic patients [53]. Dyslipidemia, undesirable changes in vascular endothelial and smooth muscle cells, lipid peroxidation especially oxidized low-density lipoprotein particles, oxidative damage and increased inflammatory mediators including chemokines and cytokines, hyper-coagulation and platelet activation have been considered as the main metabolic abnormalities in diabetes mellitus leading to cardiovascular disease [54].

There is growing evidence suggesting that dietary intake of polyphenol-rich foods and supplementation with these bioactive components could have protective effects against diabetes-induced cardiovascular pathogenesis; the mechanisms involved in these properties mainly include regulation of lipid metabolism, attenuation of oxidative damage and scavenging of free radicals, improvement of the endothelial function and vascular tone, enhancement the production of vasodilating factors such as nitric oxide, and inhibition the synthesis of vasoconstrictors such as endothelin-1 in endothelial cells [55, 56, 57].

One of the most important favorable effects of polyphenols on cardiovascular system in diabetes probably is regulation of lipid and lipoprotein metabolism, and improvement of dyslipidemia. Based on research conducted in this area, polyphenolic compounds are capable of reducing digestion and absorption of dietary lipids. Oligomeric procyanidins, contained in apples had inhibitory effects on pancreatic lipase and triglyceride absorption [58]. Apple procyanidins also induce hypolipidemic effects by decreasing of apolipoprotein B synthesis and secretion, inhibition of cholesterol estrification and intestinal lipoprotein production [59]. The hypolipidemic effects of catechins and proanthcyanidins are related to inhibition of key enzymes in lipid biosynthesis pathways, reduce intestinal lipid absorption. Catechins also interact with proteins involved in cholesterol translocation from the enterocyte brush border (ATP-binding cassette proteins, multidrug resistance P-glycoprotein 1, B type1-scavenger receptors, Niemann Pick C-1 like 1 protein), change their function and effectively reduce cholesterol absorption [60]. Administration of tart cherries as medicinal food rich in anthocyanins was accompanied with decrease in hyperlipidemia, hyperinsulinemia, fatty liver and hepatic steatosis through enhanced hepatic PPARα and some target genes including acyl-coenzyme A oxidase [61].

Endothelial dysfunction, proliferation and migration of smooth muscle cells of the vessels are central events in the pathogenesis of diabetes-induced atherosclerosis. Some cardiovascular protective properties of polyphenols are attributed to modulatory effects on the vascular structure and function. Interestingly, some polyphenols inhibit the expression of major proangiogenic, prothrombotic and proatherosclerotic factors such as monocyte chemoattractant protein-1, vascular endothelial growth factor (VEGF) and matrix metalloproteinase-2 (MMP-2) in smooth muscle cells, by redox-sensitive and redox-insensitive mechanisms [62, 63, 64]. Oligomeric proanthcyanidins, found in red apple, cinnamon, cocoa, and grapes have the potential to protect vascular cell against diabetes-induced oxidative stress via increase in activity of superoxide, dismutase inhibition of NADPH oxidase and production of free radicals as well as decrease proliferation of smooth muscle cells [65]. Flanan-3-ols modulate platelet hyperactivity and aggregation, regulate coronary blood flow, reduce endothelial inflammatory cytokines and free radicals, increase production and bioavailability of nitric oxide, and consequently atherosclerosis development [66]. In human trials, consumption of high-polyphenol dark chocolate was accompanied with improvement of endothelial function in individuals with stage 1 hypertension, and attenuation acute transient hyperglycemia-induced endothelial dysfunction and oxidative stress in type 2 diabetic patients [67, 68]. Administration of other polyphenol-rich products such as grape seed extract, cranberry juice, grape and pomegranate juice also had a therapeutic role in decreasing cardiovascular risk factors in patients with type 2 diabetes and metabolic syndrome [69, 70].

Catechins, quercetin and anthocyanins have potent platelet-inhibitory properties and are considered as inhibitors of platelet cell signaling and thrombus formation [71]. As reviewed by Pascul-Tresa, bioactive anthocyanins including delphinidin-3-rotinoside, cyanidin-3-glucoside, cyanidin-3-rutinoside, malvidin-3-glucoside and intestinal metabolites such as dihydroferulic acid and 3- (hydroxyphenyl) propionic acid prevent platelet hyper-activation and aggregation through inhibition of peptides activating thrombin receptor [66].

Undoubtedly, one of the main protective properties of polyphenols in the development of cardiovascular dysfunction in diabetic condition is related to the ability of these bioactive components to prevent lipoproteins oxidation and production of advanced glycation end products. Dietary polyphenolic compounds also protect myocardial tissue against several undesirable changes and diabetic cardiomyopathy. Treatment of diabetic rat models with grape seed proanthcyanidins extracts effectively reduced the receptor of advanced glycation end products (RAGE), nuclear factor-kappaB (NF-kappaB), and transforming growth factor-β (TGF-β) gene expression in myocardial tissue [72].

Human studies have confirmed the benefits of polyphenols on the cardiovascular system; Rizza et al in a randomized cross-over clinical trial shown that oral administration (50 mg/d for 3 week) of hesperidin, a citrus flavonoids, increased flow mediated dilation and reduced circulating inflammatory biomarkers (hs-CRP, serum amyloid A protein, soluble E selectin), decreased adhesion of monocytes, expression of vascular cell adhesion moleculs-1 and generally improved vascular function in patients with metabolic syndrome [73]. Another cross-over trial conducted in postmenopausal type 2 diabetic patients, showed that supplementation with isoflavones from red clover (50 mg/day) after 4 weeks improved endothelial function and decrease systolic and diastolic blood pressure [74].

In summary, results of the studies confirm that polyphenolic compounds attenuate several cardiovascular risk factors in diabetes; dietary polyphenols modulate lipid metabolism and dyslipidemia, improve vascular function, decrease oxidative and inflammatory-induced vascular damage, and regulate blood pressure.

Antioxidative properties of polyphenols

One of the pathogenic mechanisms that explain the development and progression of micro and macro vascular complications in diabetes is oxidative stress; increased generation of free radicals and an impaired antioxidant defense system in diabetic conditions induces imbalance of the oxidant/antioxidant status [2, 75]. Inhibition of these oxidative processes could prevent the onset and development of long-term diabetic complications [76].

Most polyphenolic compounds and their active metabolites have been known as potent antioxidant phytochemicals due to their unique structure. As reviewed by Dembinska-Kiec, these compounds could scavenge free radicals, quench electronically excited compounds, reduce hydroperoxide formation, and attenuate production of reactive oxygen species (ROS) through modulation of several enzymes involved in the development of ROS including xanthine oxidase, cyclooxygenase, lipoxygenase, microsomal monooxygenase, NADH oxidase and mitochondrial succinoxidase [77]. Some experts believe that polyphenols beyond the direct antioxidant capacities in scavenging of free radicals mainly act by direct interactions with important cellular receptors or key signaling pathways, which may result in modification of the redox status of the cell and may trigger a series of redox-dependent reactions [78].

Plant polyphenols can enhance the endogenous antioxidative system, improve oxidant antioxidant balance, and effectively prevent oxidative damage; green tea catechins are the polyphenolic compounds most studied polyphenolic compounds in this area; these bioactive components decreased lipid peroxidation and increased plasma total antioxidant capacity; they also attenuated of stress-sensitive signaling pathways, prooxidant enzymes, and inducted of antioxidant enzymes including superoxide dismutase, catalase and glutathione peroxidase [79].

In summary, polyphenols effectively attenuate oxidative stress, promote endogenous antioxidant defense system, and modulate oxidant/antioxidant balance.

Effects of polyphenols on adipose tissue metabolism

Adipocyte dysfunction is strongly associated with the development of insulin resistance, sub-clinical inflammation, β cell impairment and type 2 diabetes [80]. Polyphenolic compounds have wonderful modulatory effects on many aspects of metabolic, endocrine and cellular signaling transduction of adipose tissue. Some polyphenols such as catechins increase β oxidation in adipocytes, down-regulate the enzymes and genes involved in lipogenesis including lipoprotein lipase, fatty acid synthase complex, peroxisome proliferator-activated receptor γ (PPARγ), CCAAT enhancer-binding protein-α, regulatory element-binding protein 1-c, fatty acid binding protein. Some polyphenols, up-regulate lipolysis pathways via induction of hormone sensitive lipase, adipose tissue lipase, increased gene expression of mitochondrial uncoupling protein 2 (UCP-2) and carnitin palmitoyl transferase-1 (CPT-1) in adipocytes [81, 82].

Anthocyanins, one group of phenolic compounds considered as modulators of adipose tissue metabolism, are bioactive components which improve adipocytes dysfunction and adipocytokines secretion in insulin resistance, increase β oxidation and decrease fat accumulation on adipocytes [83]. Cyanidin and cyanidin-3-glucoside have shown several therapeutic effects on adipocyte dysfunction through decrease in plasminogen activator inhibitor-1 and interleukin-6, induction of mitochondrial uncoupling proteins, acetyl CoA oxidase, perlipin and adiponectin gene expression [84].

Favorable effects of polyphenols in prevention of long-term diabetes complications

One of the most important properties of polyphenols recently identified is its preventive effect against long-term diabetes complications including retinopathy, nephropathy and neuropathy; based on research conducted in this area administration of anthocyanins, flavonoids and other polyphenolic compounds in diabetic conditions may facilitate new approaches for improving the quality of life in diabetic patients.

As reviewed by Ghosh et al, anthocyanins and anthocyanins-rich extracts have the potential to alleviate the developing pathways of some pathologic conditions related to diabetes; anthocyanins facilitate blood flow and prevent diabetes-induced microangiopathy, increase microvascular permeability, decrease leucocytes aggregation in vascular cell wall and improve capillary filtration of albumin [85]. Purple corn extract containing cyanidin 3-glucoside and cyanidin-3-(6″-malonylglucoside) attenuated hyperglycemia-induced mesangial cell proliferation and matrix accumulation, and inhibited over-expression intracellular cell adhesion molecule-1 and monocyte chemoattractant protein-1, as major features of diabetic mesangial fibrosis and glomerulosclerosis [86]. Recently there has been increasing interest in grape seed proanthcyanidin extracts as a natural treatment for some important diabetes complications; proanthcyanidin-rich grape seed extract inhibited the development of retinopathy, nephropathy and neurodegenerative damage in diabetic condition [87, 88].

Flavanols surprisingly have the potential to improve cognitive disorders and cholinergic dysfunction related to diabetes and other secondary consequence of changes in the nervous system induced by hyperglycemia and diabetes oxidative stress; administration of quercetin in diabetic rats improved mental function and memory via inhibition of acetylcholine esterase and attenuation of oxidative damage in nervous system [89].

Green tea catechins including epicatechin, epicatechin-3-gallat, and epigalocatechin gallat decreased the synthesis of thromboxane A2 (TXA2) and increased prostacyclin I2 (PGI2), modulate the impaired balance between these ecosanoids as accelerators of thrombogenesis in the renal tubules, leading consequently improved glomerular filtration and kidney function [90].

CONCLUSION

Type 2 diabetes, a clustering of metabolic disorder, is accompanied with other pathogenic conditions including sub-clinical inflammation and oxidative stress that subsequently leads to insulin resistance and long-term diabetes complications. The rising trend in the prevalence of diabetes complications suggests that current medical treatments for the management of diabetes are not sufficient and use of supplementary treatments, including functional foods and their nutraceuticals, could increase the effectiveness of diabetes management. Plant polyphenols including phenolic acids, flavonoids, stilbenes and lignans, based on *in vitro*studies, animal models and some clinical trials, have been proposed as effective supplements for diabetes management and prevention of its long-term complications. Further investigations using human clinical studies are needed to confirm the beneficial effects of polyphenolic compounds as supplementary treatments for diabetic patients.

ACKNOWLEDGMENTS

This study was funded by the Research Institute of Endocrine Sciences, Shahid Beheshti University of Medical Sciences, Tehran, Iran. The authors express to acknowledge the assistance given by Ms N.Shiva in language editing of the manuscript.

COMPETING INTERESTS

The authors declare that they have no competing interests.

AUTHORS' CONTRIBUTIONS

The study was designed and implemented by ZB and PM. The manuscript was prepared by ZB, PM, and FA. All authors read and approved the final manuscript.

REFERENCES

1. Santaguida PL, Balion C, Hunt D: Diagnosis, prognosis, and treatment of impaired glucose tolerance and impaired fasting glucose. *Evid Rep Technol Assess* 2008, 12: 1–11.

2. Evans JL, Goldfine ID, Maddux BA, Grodsky GM: Oxidative stress and stress-activated signaling pathways: a unifying hypothesis of type 2 diabetes. *Endocr Rev* 2002, 23: 599–622.

3. Spranger J, Kroke A, Möhlig M, Hoffmann K, Bergmann MM, Ristow M, *et al.*: Inflammatory cytokines and the risk to develop type 2 diabetes: results of the prospective population-based European Prospective Investigation into Cancer and Nutrition (EPIC)-Potsdam Study. *Diabetes* 2003, 52: 812–817.

4. Montonen J, Knekt P, Järvinen R, Reunanen A: Dietary antioxidant intake and risk of type 2 diabetes.*Diabetes Care* 2004, 27: 362–366.

5. Pandey KB, Rizvi SI: Plant polyphenols as dietary antioxidants in human health and disease. *Oxid Med Cell Longev* 2009, 2: 270–278.

6. Bahadoran Z, Golzarand M, Mirmiran P, Saadati N, Azizi F: The association of dietary phytochemical index and cardio-metabolic risk factors in adults: Tehran lipid and glucose study. *J Hum Nutr Diet*2013. In prin

7. Bahadoran Z, Golzarand M, Mirmiran P, Shiva N, Azizi F: Dietary total antioxidant capacity and the occurrence of metabolic syndrome and its components after a 3-year follow-up in adults: Tehran lipid and glucose study. *Nutr Metab (Lond)* 2012, 9: 70.

8. Mirmiran P, Bahadoran Z, Golzarand M, Shiva N, Azizi F: Association between dietary phytochemical index and 3-year changes in weight, waist circumference and body adiposity index in adults: Tehran lipid and glucose study. *Nutr Metab (Lond)* 2012, 9: 108.

9. Mirmiran P, Noori N, Zavareh MB, Azizi F: Fruit and vegetable consumption and risk factors for cardiovascular disease. *Metabolism* 2009, 58: 460–468.

10. Perera PK, Li Y: Functional herbal food ingredients used in type 2 diabetes mellitus. *Pharmacogn Rev*2012, 6: 37–45.

11. Bahadoran Z, Mirmiran P, Hosseinpanah F, Hedayati M, Hosseinpour-Niazi S, Azizi F: Broccoli sprouts reduce oxidative stress in type 2 diabetes: a randomized double-blind clinical trial. *Eur J Clin Nutr*2011, 65: 972–977.

12. Bahadoran Z, Mirmiran P, Hosseinpanah F, Asghari G, Rajab A, Azizi F: Broccoli sprouts Powder could improve serum triglyceride and oxidized LDL/LDL-cholesterol ratio in type 2

diabetic patients: a randomized double-blind placebo-controlled clinical trial. *Diabetes Res Clin Pract* 2012, 96: 348–354.

13. Bahadoran Z, Tohidi M, Nazeri P, Mehran M, Azizi F, Mirmiran P: Effect of broccoli sprouts on insulin resistance in type 2 diabetic patients: a randomized double-blind clinical trial. *Int J Food Sci Nutr*2012, 63: 767–771.

14. Beckman CH: Phenolic-storing cells: keys to programmed cell death and periderm formation in wilt disease resistance and in general defence responses in plants? *Physiol Mol Plant Pathol* 2000, 57:101–110.

15. Pietta P, Minoggio M, Bramati L: Plant polyphenols: structure, occurrence and bioactivity. *Stud Nat Pro Chem* 2003, 28: 257–312.

16. Manach C, Scalbert A, Morand C, Rémésy C, Jiménez L: Polyphenols: food sources and bioavailability.*Am J Clin Nutr* 2004, 79: 727–747.

17. Adlercreutz H: Lignans and human health. *Crit Rev Clin Lab Sci* 2007, 44: 483–525.

18. Chun OK, Chung SJ, Song WO: Estimated dietary flavonoid intake and major food sources of U.S. adults. *J Nutr* 2007, 137: 1244–1252.

19. Ovaskainen ML, Törrönen R, Koponen JM, Sinkko H, Hellström J, Reinivuo H, *et al.*: Dietary intake and major food sources of polyphenols in Finnish adults. *J Nutr* 2008, 138: 562–566.

20. Scalbert A, Williamson G: Dietary intake and bioavailability of polyphenols. *J Nutr* 2000, 130: 2073S-2085S.

21. Scalbert A, Morand C, Manach C, Rémésy C: Absorption and metabolism of polyphenols in the gut and impact on health. *Biomed Pharmacother* 2002, 56: 276–282.

22. Han X, Loa T: Dietary polyphenols and their biological significance. *Int J Mol Sci* 2007, 8: 950–988.

23. Dinneen S, Gerich J, Rizza R: Carbohydrate metabolism in non-insulin-dependent diabetes mellitus. *N Engl J Med* 1992, 327: 707–713.

24. Hanhineva K, Törrönen R, Bondia-Pons I, Pekkinen J, Kolehmainen M, Mykkänen H, *et al.*: Impact of dietary

polyphenols on carbohydrate metabolism. *Int J Mol Sci* 2010, 11: 1365–1402.

25. Iwai K, Kim MY, Onodera A, Matsue H: Alpha-glucosidase inhibitory and antihyperglycemic effects of polyphenols in the fruit of Viburnum dilatatum Thunb. *Agric Food Chem* 2006, 54: 4588–4592.

26. Iwai K: Antidiabetic and antioxidant effects of polyphenols in brown alga Ecklonia stolonifera in genetically diabetic KK-A(y) mice. *Plant Foods Hum Nutr* 2008, 63: 163–169.

27. Cabrera C, Artacho R, Giménez R: Beneficial effects of green tea-a review. *J Am Coll Nutr* 2006, 25: 79–99.

28. Tadera K, Minami Y, Takamatsu K, Matsuoka T: Inhibition of alpha-glucosidase and alpha-amylase by flavonoids. *J Nutr Sci Vitaminol (Tokyo)* 2006, 52: 149–153.

29. Kobayashi Y, Suzuki M, Satsu H, Arai S, Hara Y, Suzuki K, *et al.*: Green tea polyphenols inhibit the sodium-dependent glucose transporter of intestinal epithelial cells by a competitive mechanism. *J Agric Food Chem* 2000, 48: 5618–5623.

30. Johnston K, Sharp P, Clifford M, Morgan L: Dietary polyphenols decrease glucose uptake by human intestinal Caco-2 cells. *FEBS Lett* 2005, 579: 1653–1657.

31. Johnston KL, Clifford MN, Morgan LM: Coffee acutely modifies gastrointestinal hormone secretion and glucose tolerance in humans: glycemic effects of chlorogenic acid and caffeine. *Am J Clin Nutr*2003, 78: 728–733.

32. Dao TM, Waget A, Klopp P, Serino M, Vachoux C, Pechere L, *et al.*: Resveratrol increases glucose induced GLP-1 secretion in mice: a mechanism which contributes to the glycemic control. *PLoS One*2011, 6: e20700.

33. Jung EH, Kim SR, Hwang IK, Ha TY: Hypoglycemic effects of a phenolic acid fraction of rice bran and ferulic acid in C57BL/KsJ-db/db mice. *J Agric Food Chem* 2007, 55: 9800–9804.

34. Jung UJ, Lee MK, Jeong KS, Choi MS: The hypoglycemic effects of hesperidin and naringin are partly mediated by hepatic glucose-regulating enzymes in C57BL/KsJ-db/db mice. *J Nutr* 2004, 134: 2499–2503.

35. Jung UJ, Lee MK, Park YB, Kang MA, Choi MS: Effect of citrus flavonoids on lipid metabolism and glucose-regulating enzyme

mRNA levels in type-2 diabetic mice. *Int J Biochem Cell Biol* 2006, 38:1134–1145.

36. Waltner-Law ME, Wang XL, Law BK, Hall RK, Nawano M, Granner DK: Epigallocatechin gallate, a constituent of green tea, represses hepatic glucose production. *J Biol Chem* 2002, 277: 34933–34940.

37. Collins QF, Liu HY, Pi J, Liu Z, Quon MJ, Cao W: Epigallocatechin-3-gallate (EGCG), a green tea polyphenol, suppresses hepatic gluconeogenesis through 5′-AMP-activated protein kinase. *J Biol Chem* 2007, 282: 30143–30149.

38. Prabhakar PK, Doble M: Synergistic effect of phytochemicals in combination with hypoglycemic drugs on glucose uptake in myotubes. *Phytomedicine* 2009, 16: 1119–1126.

39. Zhang B, Kang M, Xie Q, Xu B, Sun C, Chen K, Wu Y: Anthocyanins from Chinese bayberry extract protect β cells from oxidative stress-mediated injury via HO-1 upregulation. *J Agric Food Chem* 2011,59: 537–545.

40. Park CE, Kim MJ, Lee JH, Min BI, Bae H, Choe W, *et al.*: Resveratrol stimulates glucose transport in C2C12 myotubes by activating AMP-activated protein kinase. *Mol Med* 2007, 39: 222–229.

41. Towler MC, Hardie DG: AMP-activated protein kinase in metabolic control and insulin signaling. *Circ Res* 2007, 100: 328–341.

42. Zhou G, Myers R, Li Y, Chen Y, Shen X, Fenyk-Melody J, *et al.*: Role of AMP-activated protein kinase in mechanism of metformin action. *J Clin Invest* 2001, 108: 1167–1174.

43. Zang M, Xu S, Maitland-Toolan KA, Zuccollo A, Hou X, Jiang B, *et al.*: Polyphenols stimulate AMP-activated protein kinase, lower lipids, and inhibit accelerated atherosclerosis in diabetic LDL receptor-deficient mice. *Diabetes* 2006, 55: 2180–2191.

44. Kumar R, Balaji S, Uma TS, Sehgal PK: Fruit extracts of Momordica charantia potentiate glucose uptake and up-regulate Glut-4, PPAR gamma and PI3K. *J Ethnopharmacol* 2009, 126: 533–537.

45. Fu Z, Liu D: Long-term exposure to genistein improves insulin secretory function of pancreatic beta-cells. *Eur J Pharmacol* 2009, 616: 321–327.

46. Liu D, Zhen W, Yang Z, Carter JD, Si H, Reynolds KA: Genistein acutely stimulates insulin secretion in pancreatic beta-cells through a cAMP-dependent protein kinase pathway. *Diabetes* 2006, 55: 1043–1050.

47. Fu Z, Zhang W, Zhen W, Lum H, Nadler J, Bassaganya-Riera J: Genistein induces pancreatic beta-cell proliferation through activation of multiple signaling pathways and prevents insulin-deficient diabetes in mice. *Endocrinology* 2010, 151: 3026–3037.

48. Kajimoto Y, Kaneto H: Role of oxidative stress in pancreatic beta-cell dysfunction. *Ann NY Acad Sci*2004, 1011: 168–176.

49. Drews G, Krippeit-Drews P, Düfer M: Oxidative stress and beta-cell dysfunction. *Pflugers Arch* 2010,460: 703–718.

50. Yin P, Zhao S, Chen S, Liu J, Shi L, Wang X, Liu Y, Ma C: Hypoglycemic and hypolipidemic effects of polyphenols from burs of Castanea mollissima Blume. *Molecules* 2011, 16: 9764–9774.

51. Szkudelski T, Szkudelska K: Anti-diabetic effects of resveratrol. *Ann NY Acad Sci* 2011, 1215: 34–39.

52. Szkudelski T: Resveratrol inhibits insulin secretion from rat pancreatic islets. *Eur J Pharmacol* 2006,552: 176–181.

53. Kalofoutis C, Piperi C, Kalofoutis A, Harris F, Phoenix D, Singh J: Type II diabetes mellitus and cardiovascular risk factors: Current therapeutic approaches. *Exp Clin Cardiol* 2007, 12: 17–28.

54. Thomas JE, Foody JM: The pathophysiology of cardiovascular disease in diabetes mellitus and the future of therapy. *J Cardiometab Syndr* 2007, 2: 108–113.

55. Lecour S, Lamont KT: Natural polyphenols and cardioprotection. *Mini Rev Med Chem* 2011, 11: 1191–1199.

56. Schini-Kerth VB, Auger C, Etienne-Selloum N, Chataigneau T: Polyphenol-induced endothelium-dependent relaxations role of NO and EDHF. *Adv Pharmacol* 2010, 60: 133–175.

57. Stoclet JC, Chataigneau T, Ndiaye M, Oak MH, El Bedoui J, Chataigneau M, *et al.*: Vascular protection by dietary polyphenols. *Eur J Pharmacol* 2004, 500: 299–313.

58. Sugiyama H, Akazome Y, Shoji T, Yamaguchi A, Yasue M, Kanda T, *et al.*: Oligomeric procyanidins in apple polyphenol are main

active components for inhibition of pancreatic lipase and triglyceride absorption. *J Agric Food Chem* 2007, 55: 4604–4609.

59. Vidal R, Hernandez-Vallejo S, Pauquai T, Texier O, Rousset M, Chambaz J, *et al*.: Apple procyanidins decrease cholesterol esterification and lipoprotein secretion in Caco-2/TC7 enterocytes. *J Lipid Res*2005, 46: 258–268.

60. Koo SI, Noh SK: Green tea as inhibitor of the intestinal absorption of lipids: potential mechanism for its lipid-lowering effect. *J Nutr Biochem* 2007, 18: 179–183.

61. Seymour EM, Singer AA, Kirakosyan A, Urcuyo-Llanes DE, Kaufman PB, Bolling SF: Altered hyperlipidemia, hepatic steatosis, and hepatic peroxisome proliferator-activated receptors in rats with intake of tart cherry. *J Med Food* 2008, 11: 252–259.

62. Oak MH, Chataigneau M, Keravis T, Chataigneau T, Beretz A, Andriantsitohaina R, *et al*.: Red wine polyphenolic compounds inhibit vascular endothelial growth factor expression in vascular smooth muscle cells by preventing the activation of the p38 mitogen-activated protein kinase pathway.*Arterioscler Thromb Vasc Biol* 2003, 23: 1001–1007.

63. Oak MH, El Bedoui J, Schini-Kerth VB: Antiangiogenic properties of natural polyphenols from red wine and green tea. *J Nutr Biochem* 2005, 16: 1–8.

64. Ndiaye M, Chataigneau T, Chataigneau M, Schini-Kerth VB: Red wine polyphenols induce EDHF-mediated relaxations in porcine coronary arteries through the redox-sensitive activation of the PI3-kinase/Akt pathway. *Br J Pharmacol* 2004, 142: 1131–1136.

65. Wang L, Zhu LH, Jiang H, Tang QZ, Yan L, Wang D, *et al*.: Grape seed proanthocyanidins attenuate vascular smooth muscle cell proliferation via blocking phosphatidylinositol 3-kinase-dependent signaling pathways. *J Cell Physiol* 2010, 223: 713–726.

66. de Pascual-Teresa S, Moreno DA, García-Viguera C: Flavanols and anthocyanins in cardiovascular health: a review of current evidence. *Int J Mol Sci* 2010, 11: 1679–1703.

67. Nogueira Lde P, Knibel MP, Torres MR, Nogueira Neto JF, Sanjuliani AF: Consumption of high-polyphenol dark chocolate improves endothelial function in individuals with stage 1

hypertension and excess body weight. *Int J Hypertens* 2012, 2012: 147321.

68. Mellor DD, Madden LA, Smith KA, Kilpatrick ES, Atkin SL: High-polyphenol chocolate reduces endothelial dysfunction and oxidative stress during acute transient hyperglycaemia in Type 2 diabetes: a pilot randomized controlled trial. *Diabet Med* 2012, 30: 478–483.

69. Kar P, Laight D, Rooprai HK, Shaw KM, Cummings M: Effects of grape seed extract in Type 2 diabetic subjects at high cardiovascular risk: a double blind randomized placebo controlled trial examining metabolic markers, vascular tone, inflammation, oxidative stress and insulin sensitivity. *Diabet Med*2009, 26: 526–531.

70. Shidfar F, Heydari I, Hajimiresmaiel SJ, Hosseini S, Shidfar S, Amiri F: The effects of cranberry juice on serum glucose, apoB, apoA-I, Lp(a), and Paraoxonase-1 activity in type 2 diabetic male patients. *J Res Med Sci* 2012, 17: 355–360.

71. Hubbard GP, Wolffram S, Lovegrove JA, Gibbins JM: Ingestion of quercetin inhibits platelet aggregation and essential components of the collagen-stimulated platelet activation pathway in humans. *J Thromb Haemost* 2004, 2: 2138–2145.

72. Cheng M, Gao HQ, Xu L, Li BY, Zhang H, Li XH: Cardioprotective effects of grape seed proanthocyanidins extracts in streptozocin induced diabetic rats. *J Cardiovasc Pharmacol* 2007, 50:503–509.PubMedGoogle Scholar

73. Rizza S, Muniyappa R, Iantorno M, Kim JA, Chen H, Pullikotil P, *et al.*: Citrus polyphenol hesperidin stimulates production of nitric oxide in endothelial cells while improving endothelial function and reducing inflammatory markers in patients with metabolic syndrome. *J Clin Endocrinol Metab* 2011,96: E782-E792.

74. Howes JB, Tran D, Brillante D, Howes LG: Effects of dietary supplementation with isoflavones from red clover on ambulatory blood pressure and endothelial function in postmenopausal type 2 diabetes.*Diabetes Obes Metab* 2003, 5: 325–332.

75. Goycheva V, Gadjeva BP: Oxidative stress and its complications in diabetes mellitus. *Trakia J of Sci*2006, 4: 1–8

76. Pérez-Matute P, Zulet MA, Martínez JA: Reactive species and diabetes: counteracting oxidative stress to improve health. *Curr Opin Pharmacol* 2009, 9: 771–779.

77. Dembinska-Kiec A, Mykkänen O, Kiec-Wilk B, Mykkänen H: Antioxidant phytochemicals against type 2 diabetes. *Br J Nutr* 2008, 99: ES109-ES117.

78. Scalbert A, Johnson IT, Saltmarsh M: Polyphenols: antioxidants and beyond. *Am J Clin Nutr* 2005, 81:215S-217S.

79. Crespy V, Williamson G: A review of the health effects of green tea catechins in in vivo animal models. *J Nutr* 2004, 134: 3431S-3440S.

80. Guilherme A, Virbasius JV, Puri V, Czech MP: Adipocyte dysfunctions linking obesity to insulin resistance and type 2 diabetes. *Nat Rev Mol Cell Biol* 2008, 9: 367–377.

81. Nakazato K, Song H, Waga T: Effects of dietary apple polyphenol on adipose tissues weights in Wistar rats. *Exp Anim* 2006, 55: 383–389. 10.1538/expanim.55.383

82. Osada K, Suzuki T, Kawakami Y, Senda M, Kasai A, Sami M, *et al.*: Dose-dependent hypocholesterolemic actions of dietary apple polyphenol in rats fed cholesterol. *Lipids* 2006, 41: 133–139.

83. Tsuda T, Horio F, Uchida K, Aoki H, Osawa T: Dietary cyanidin 3-O-beta-D-glucoside-rich purple corn color prevents obesity and ameliorates hyperglycemia in mice. *J Nutr* 2003, 133: 2125–2130.

84. Tsuda T, Ueno Y, Yoshikawa T, Kojo H, Osawa T: Microarray profiling of gene expression in human adipocytes in response to anthocyanins. *Biochem Pharmacol* 2006, 71: 1184–1197.

85. Ghosh D, Konishi T: Anthocyanins and anthocyanin-rich extracts: role in diabetes and eye function. *Asia Pac J Clin Nutr* 2007, 16: 200–208.

86. Li J, Lim SS, Lee JY, Kim JK, Kang SW, Kim JL, *et al.*: Purple corn anthocyanins dampened high-glucose-induced mesangial fibrosis and inflammation: possible renoprotective role in diabetic nephropathy. *J Nutr Biochem* 2012, 23: 320–331.

87. Li BY, Cheng M, Gao HQ, Ma YB, Xu L, Li XH, *et al.*: Back-regulation of six oxidative stress proteins with grape seed proanthocyanidin extracts in rat diabetic nephropathy. *J Cell Biochem* 2008, 104: 668–679.

88. Cui XP, Li BY, Gao HQ, Wei N, Wang WL, Lu M: Effects of grape seed proanthocyanidin extracts on peripheral nerves in

streptozocin-induced diabetic rats. *J Nutr Sci Vitaminol (Tokyo)* 2008, 54: 321–328.

89. Bhutada P, Mundhada Y, Bansod K, Bhutada C, Tawari S, Dixit P, *et al.*: Ameliorative effect of quercetin on memory dysfunction in streptozotocin-induced diabetic rats. *Neurobiol Learn Mem* 2010, 94: 293–302.

90. Rhee SJ, Choi JH, Park MR: Green tea catechin improves microsomal phospholipase A2 activity and the arachidonic acid cascade system in the kidney of diabetic rats. *Asia Pac J Clin Nutr* 2002, 11: 226–231.

10

FROM FUNCTIONAL FOOD TO MEDICINAL PRODUCT: SYSTEMATIC APPROACH IN ANALYSIS OF POLYPHENOLICS FROM PROPOLIS AND WINE

Marica Medić-Šarić*[1], Vesna Rastija[2], Mirza Bojić[1] and Željan Maleš[3]

[1]Department of Medicinal Chemistry, Faculty of Pharmacy and Biochemistry, University of Zagreb, A. Kovačića 1, 10000 Zagreb, Croatia,

[2]Faculty of Agriculture, Josip Juraj Strossmayer University of Osijek, Trg Sv. Trojstva 3, 31000 Osijek, Croatia

[3]Department of Pharmaceutical Botany, Faculty of Pharmacy and Biochemistry, University of Zagreb, Schrottova 39, 10000 Zagreb, Croatia

ABSTRACT

In the last decade we have been working on standardization of propolis extract and determination of active constituents of wine those are rich in polyphenolics and have nutritional as well as therapeutic value. Here we are summarizing our results and providing overview on systematic approach how to analyse natural products rich in flavonoids and phenolic acids.

Chromatographic methods (thin layer chromatography and high performance liquid chromatography) were used for identification, quantification, and characterization of individual flavonoid or phenolic acid. Total content of active constituents and antioxidant activity were determined by spectrophotometry. Pharmacokinetic parameters were determined by high performance liquid chromatography and using appropriate software. Quantitative structure-activity relationship study of antioxidant activity was conducted, as well as assessment of prolonged propolis supplementation on antioxidative status of organism.

Thin layer chromatography-densitometry has been proven as quick and reliable method for standard analysis of propolis and wine; the best mobile phase being chloroform – methanol – formic acid (98–100%) in ratio 44 : 3.5 : 2.5 (*v/v*). Higher number of polyphenolics was determined by high performance liquid chromatography; 15 compared to 9 by thin layer chromatography. Interactions *in situ* with acetylsalicylic acid were detected with most of polyphenolics analysed. Plasma protein binding and blood-barrier penetration was greatest for flavone. The interactions with human serum albumin have been grater than 95% for all flavonoids analysed. The prolonged propolis consumption increased superoxide dismutase activity.

The necessity of standardization of natural products and their registration as functional nutraceuticals demand easy, quick and inexpensive methods of analysis. In this work we provided overview of analytical part for polyphenolics that could be used as data for possible registration of final products either as functional food or medicinal product.

This feature introduces the readers to the authors' research through a concise overview of the selected topic. Reference to important work from others in the field is included.

BACKGROUND

The main causes of death in western countries are cardiovascular diseases and cancer. Over 50 percent of the population has some kind of chronic condition (high blood pressure, high cholesterol, arthritis, diabetes, asthma, osteoporosis...), so the goal of the many researches in the last decades is improving the quality of life. Much of the interested was transfered to homeopathy, alternative, and folk medicine, evincing polyphenols as one of the main nutraceuticals [1].

The most abundant sources of polyphenols, mainly flavonoids and phenolic acids, are propolis and wine. Flavonoids and phenolic acids have antibacterial, antifungal, antiviral, antineoplastic, hepatoprotective, immunomodulating, and antiinflammatory properties. Their use has been proven beneficial in allergies, asthma, diabetes, hypertension, micro bleeding, etc. Much of these pharmacological effects can be associated with antioxidant activity. Hence, antioxidant activity is the most studied property of polyphenols [2].

In the last decade, we were working on several projects with the aim of developing standardized extracts of propolis and determination of active constituents of wine, transferring knowledge from the laboratory to everyday-practice for the purpose of analyzing natural products. To accomplish this we used rather simple, reliable, and quick spectrophotometric and liquid chromatography methods for analysis of polyphenols, the results of which are reviewed here. These were used to suggest mixtures of propolis that will provide the best final product.

In this review we wanted to systematize the approach in analysis of polyphenols rich samples providing mostly unpublished data (Published data is marked as reference). Some basic concepts of optimization of chromatographic system, chromatographic parameters describing pharmacokinetic and quantitative structure-activity relationship are described. The use of liquid chromatography for different objectives is thoroughly illustrated: identification, quantification, characterization; ADME study (Absorption, Distribution, Metabolism, Excretion) and interactions. To demonstrate *in vivo* antioxidant effects of polyphenols from propolis preliminary clinical trial of prolongated propolis is presented.

Flavonoids and Phenolic Acids. Propolis and Wine

Flavonoids and phenolic acids are plant polyphenols characterized by having one or more phenolic hydroxyl groups or carboxylic group in phenolic acids. The major classes of polyphenols are phenolic acids (hydroxycinnamic and hydroxybenzoic acids), flavonoids, anthocyanins, and tannins (Figure 1) [2, 3].

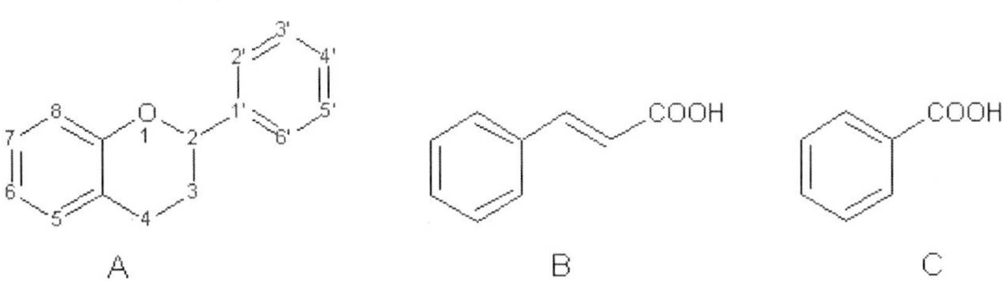

Figure 1. Basic structures of flavonoids (A) and phenolic acids (B-cinnamic acid, C-benzoic acid).

Propolis is a resinous substance collected by honeybees (*Apis mellifera*, L.) from a variety of plant sources. Its chemical composition is very complex and varies with geographic origin, depending on the local flora and phenology of the source plants. The benefits of effects of propolis on human health were recognized thousand of years ago. It has wide range of biological activities including antibacterial, antiviral, antiinflammatory, and antioxidative [4]. To illustrate the regions where our propolis samples originate, the map of Croatia is provided on Figure 2.

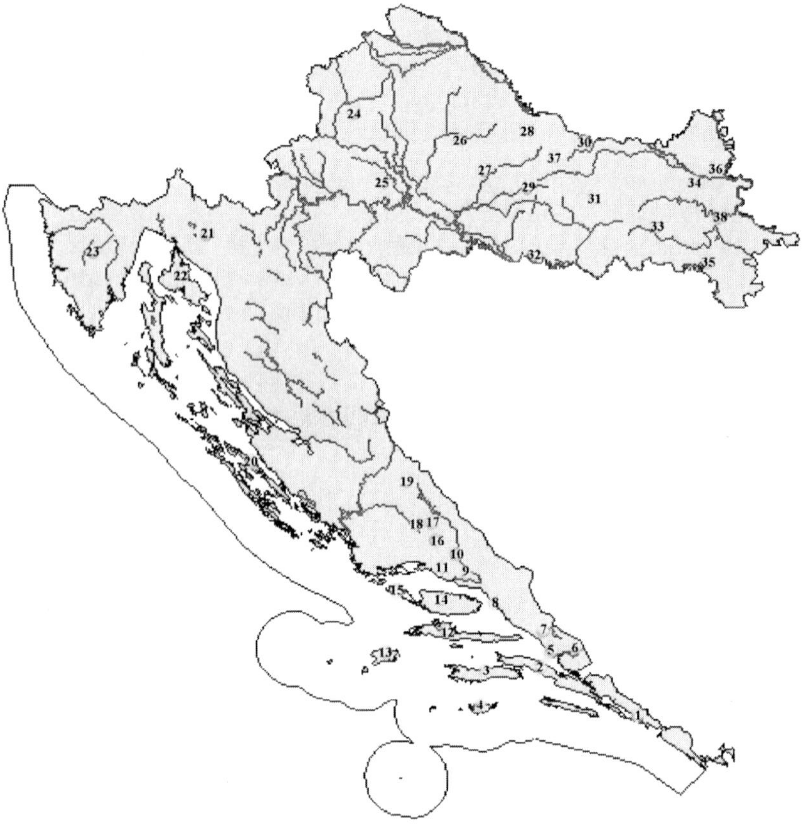

Figure 2. The map of Croatia. Areas of origin of propolis samples (marked by numbers).

Wine is an alcoholic beverage that contains a large amount of different polyphenols extracted from grapes during the processes of vinification. These molecules are responsible for color, acerbity, flavor, and antioxidant properties of wine [5].

Optimization of Chromatographic Systems [6]

The purpose of optimization of chromatographic systems is to find the one that shows the greatest difference in identification characteristics between substances e.g. retention factor (R_F) value in thin layer chromatography.

To accomplish this numerical taxonomy methods were used. Taxonomic entities are polyphenols and their numerical characteristic is R_F value. Matrix of resemblance of R_F values is analyzed to find the mobile phase in which the resemblance is the lowest and separation of analyzed substances is optimal. In short, the matrix of N substances and t mobile phases is reduced using different algorithms to form a cluster of similar mobile phases, the procedure is repeated until the final cluster including all mobile phases is formed and the results are presented in form of dendrogram.

Complementary mathematical methods are used. If the R_F values are distributed into groups of width E, in R_F units, then in group k n_k R_F values are present, and the average information content is described by Shannon equation:

$$I(X) = -\sum_k \frac{n_k}{n} \, ld \, \frac{n_k}{n}, \quad (1)$$

with the assumption that substances with the R_F value in the same group can not be identified. The higher the average information content is, the better results of separation for mobile phase are. To positively identify two substances difference between R_F values has to be greater than E(usually 0.05). Discriminating power (DP) is used as a measure of the effectiveness of chromatographic systems. The DP of a chromatographic system is the probability of separating two flavonoids (or phenolic acids) selected at random from a specific substance population. Two flavonoids (or phenolic acids) are chromatographically similar if the differences in their identification values do not exceed the error factor E. In case of mixture of eluents DP is defined as probability that two randomly selected substances can be distinguished by one mobile phase. Mathematically it can be expressed by the following equation:

$$DP_k = 1 - \frac{2M}{N(N-1)}, \quad (2)$$

where k is the number of mobile phases, N number of substances analyzed and M the total number of matching pairs. The average number of similar substances T, for each mobile phase, is defined by expression:

$$T = 1 + \frac{N-1}{1-DP_k}. \quad (3)$$

The highest DP and the smallest T value are attributed to the most appropriate combination of eluents.

This procedure of optimization has been used in the analysis of numerous plant samples:*Zizyphus jujuba* Mill., *Chamomilla recutita* (L.) Rauschert, *Rosmarini folium, Guiera senegalensis*J.F.GMEL., *Rhamni cathartici fructus, Lavandulae flos, Sambuci flos, Helleborus atrorubens*Waldst. et Kit. etc. [7, 8, 9, 10, 11, 12, 13, 14].

Chromatographic Parameters Describing Pharmacokinetics of Polyphenols [15]

As our samples are consumed orally absorption and distribution of polyphenols are of interest. Absorption through the gastrointestinal tract (GIT) membrane, plasma protein binding and the penetration through blood brain barrier (BBB) was studied using *in silico* approaches and liquid chromatography.

In reverse phase thin layer chromatography (RP-TLC), the chromatographic parameter R_M is used to describe the lipophilicity of a substance:

$$R_M = \log\frac{b-a}{a} = \log\frac{1-R_F}{R_F}. \quad (4)$$

It represents a logarithm of ratio of spot distance from the front and from the start. The higher the value of R_F, chromatographic parameter is lower and the substance is more polar. As $R_M$depends on the percentage of the organic modifier in mobile phase, R_{Mw} value with 0% of organic modifier is used and can be extrapolated using the equation:

$$R_M = R_{Mw} + b\varphi, \quad (5)$$

where b is the coefficient of the slope and Φ is the concentration of the organic modifier.

In reverse phase high performance liquid chromatography (RP-HPLC) $\log k$ is used as a measurement of distribution between hydrophobic (stationary) and hydrophilic (mobile) phase:

$$\log k = \log\frac{c_{stationary}}{c_{mobile}} = \log\frac{t_R - t_0}{t_0}. \quad (6)$$

The values of log k are compared at a 0% concentration of organic modifier based on the equation:

$$\log k = \log k_w + b\varphi. \tag{7}$$

As mucosa membranes are modified with phospholipids that are changed under physiological pH due to interaction, absorption and distribution of polyphenols can be changed, too. To predict this interaction immobilized artificial membrane (IAM) columns are used (Figure 3). The measurement of these interactions as well as for RP-HPLC is log k_{wIAM}.

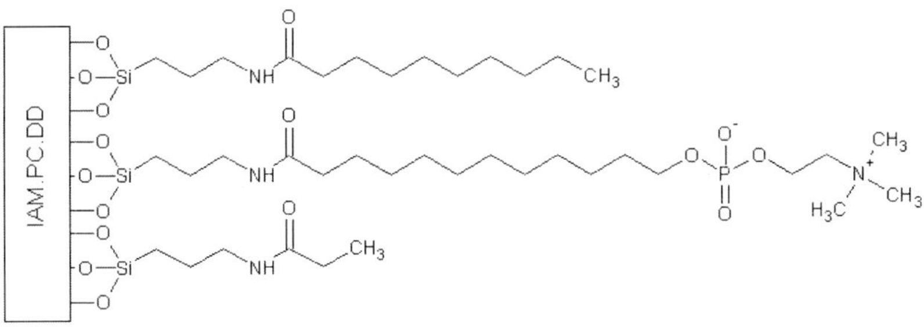

Figure 3. The structure of stationary phase of immobilized artificial membrane – phosphatidylcholine – drug-discovery column (IAM.PC.DD).

To assess the binding of polyphenols to the plasma protein columns containing human serum albumin (HSA) and alfa1-glycoprotein acid are used. The percentage of polyphenol bounded to HSA is calculated using the equation:

$$\%HSA = 100\frac{c_{stationary}}{c_{stationary}+c_{mobile}} = 100\frac{k}{k+1}. \tag{8}$$

If the polyphenol shows a binding of over 95% it can potentially interact with other drugs of high affinity to HSA as the concentration of active (free) drug can increase significantly (e.g. 5% to 8% is increase of 60% in active form of drug).

Quantitative Structure-Activity Relationship [16]

Quantitative Structure-Activity Relationship (QSAR) represents the analysis in which the structure of molecules is quantitatively correlated to biological activity. QSAR is now an irreplaceable technique in the rational design of drugs. The main postulate of QSAR is: biological activity is the consequence of chemical structure. To characterize the structure, different topological indices and three-dimensional (3D) descriptors are used. The most common topological indices are described in Table 1.

Table 1. The most commonly used topological indices.

Index	Expression for calculation	Observation
Wiener index	$W(G)=\frac{1}{2}\sum_{i,j} D_{i,j}$	D_{ij} represents off-diagonal elements of matrix which stands for the shortest distance in term on number of bonds between atom *i* and *j*
Valence connectivity index	$\chi^{v}(G)=\sum_{i,j}\frac{1}{\sqrt{v_i v_j}}$	v_i and v_j are weights (valence delta values) of vertices *i* and *j* making up edge in vertex weighted graph *G*
Balaban index	$J(G)=\frac{E}{\mu+1}\sum_{edges}\frac{1}{\sqrt{ds_i ds_j}}$	the average distance sum connectivity; where *E* is the number of edges, μ is cyclomatic number of *G* and ds_i is a distance sum
Information-theoretic index	$I(G)=-\sum_{i}\frac{2N_i}{N(N-1)}\log_2\frac{2N_i}{N(N-1)}$	modified Shannon's equation where *n* is the number of different sets of elements, N_i is the number of elements in the *i*-th set of elements and the sum is over all sets of elements
Shultz index	$MTI=\sum_{i} e_i$	molecular topological index (MTI) is based on adjacency matrix (*A*), the distance matrix (*D*) and the valency matrix (*v*); the of elements e_i of the row matrix *v* [*A*+*D*] gives Shultz index

Besides QSAR, evolution in rational design has been achieved by using software for assessing physicochemical properties and parameters of bioavailability.

REVIEW

Thin Layer Chromatography

Thin layer chromatography of standard solutions of flavonoids and phenolic acids was performed on silicagel plates 60 F_{254} using different mobile phases (Table 2) and was visualized under short and long ultraviolet (UV) light after spraying with 1% $AlCl_3$. The optimization was done using program KT1 [17]. Eleven mobile phases, for separation of flavonoids and phenolic acids were analyzed. The most suitable mobile phases were number 7 (*n*-hexane : ethyl acetate : acetic acid (glac.) = 31 : 14 : 5 *v/v*) and number 11 (chloroform : methanol : formic acid = 44 : 3.5 : 2.5 *v/v*), as shown by dendrogram (Figure 4) and confirmed by values of discriminating power and the average information content (Table 3) [17]. Using mobile phases 11 and 7 we succeeded to identify up to 9 polyphenols in samples of Croatian propolis.

Table 2. The mobile phases studied.

No	Solvents	Proportions (*v*/*v*)
1	toluene – ethyl acetate – formic acid (98–100%)	36 : 12 : 5
2	cyclohexane – ethyl acetate – formic acid (98–100%)	30 : 15 : 5
3	toluene – ethyl acetate – glacial acetic acid	36 : 12 : 5
4	cyclohexane – ethyl acetate – glacial acetic acid	31 : 14 : 5
5	*n*-hexane – ethyl acetate – formic acid (98–100%)	31 : 14 : 5
6	toluene – acetone – formic acid (98–100%)	38 : 10 : 5
7	*n*-hexane-ethyl acetate – glacial acetic acid	31 : 14 : 5
8	petroleum ether (40–70°C) – ethyl acetate – formic acid (98–100%)	30 : 15 : 5
9	carbon tetrachloride – acetone – formic acid (98–100%)	35 : 10 : 5
10	*n*-hexane – ethyl acetate – glacial acetic acid	30 : 20 : 1.5
11	chloroform – methanol – formic acid (98–100%)	44 : 3.5 : 2. 5

Table 3. *DP* and *I* output date for error factor $E = 0.03$ for each mobile phase.

Mobile phase	*DP*	*I* (bit)
1	0.8538	3.221
2	0.7836	2.735
3	0.8655	3.076
4	0.8947	3.616
5	0.8187	2.860
6	0.8480	3.011
7	**0.9298**	**3.682**
8	0.7895	3.050
9	0.9240	3.511
10	0.9181	3.471
11	**0.9415**	**3.827**

Analysis of flavonoids and phenolic acids in propolis was performed by two-dimensional thin layer chromatography (2D-TLC) using optimized chromatographic systems and detection and quantification was done using CAMAG Reprostar 3 densitometer with CAMAG VideoScan TLC/HPTLC evaluation software. The absorbance was recorded at 254 and 366 nm, the later being the wavelength of quantification [18]. Since propolis is a rather complex mixture for simple TLC, 2D-TLC analysis of propolis samples previously optimized chromatographic systems were used. Plate and densitograms of standard solution of caffeic acid and propolis sample from Peruča are presented in Figure 5.

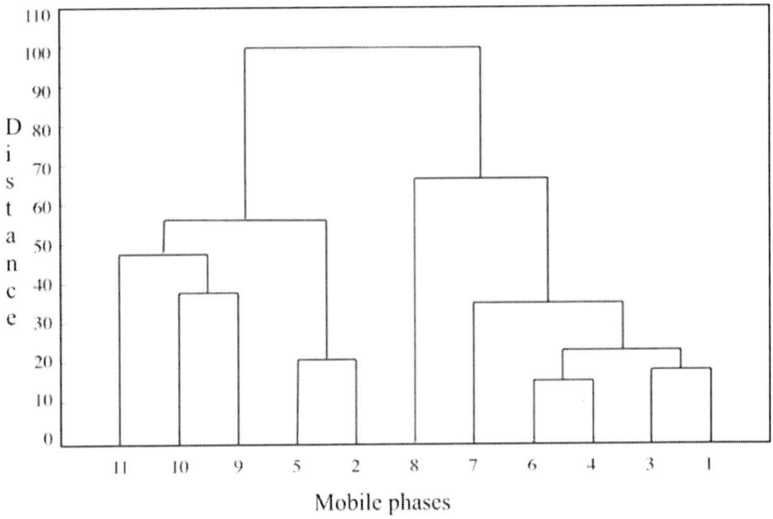

Figure 4. Dendrogram for eleven TLC mobile phases used fot determination of polyphenols in samples of Croatian propolis.

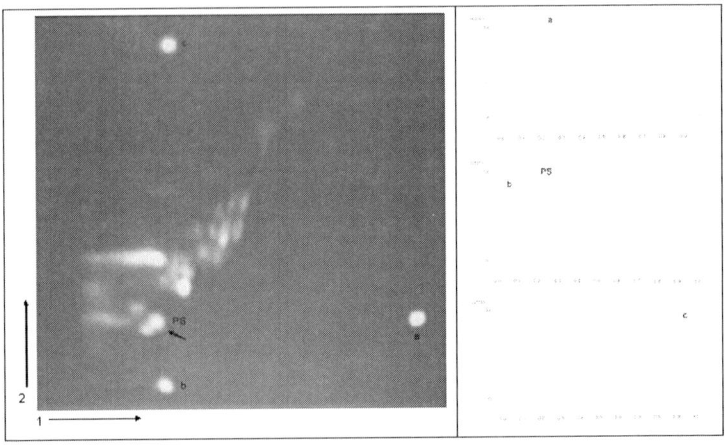

Figure 5. 2D-TLC of caffeic acid in propolis sample from Peruča and standards of caffeic acid. The plate was first developed in the direction 1 then 2 using mobile phase 1 (n-hexane : ethyl acetate : glacial acetic acid = 31 : 14 : 5 *v/v*) and mobile phase 2 (chloroform : methanol : formic acid = 44 : 3.5 : 2.5*v/v*). Bands were visualized under short and long wave UV light and under long wave UV light after spraying with 1% $AlCl_3$ ethanol solution. Concetration obtained from chromatograms: a = m_{max} = 2.50 µg, b = m_{min} = 0.83 µg, c = m_{mid} = 1.67 µg, PS = $m_{propolis\ sample}$ = 2.91 µg [18].

2D-TLC was shown to be a suitable method for quantitative determination of flavonoids and phenolic acids in Croatian propolis samples. The linear relationship between absorbance and mass of standard was established:

$$A = 9706.6 + 4487.0m;\ r = 0.98 \tag{9}$$

The presence of coumaric and cinnamic acids could not be established, as these compounds do not form fluorescent complexes with $AlCl_3$.

For the quantification purpose high performance thin layer chromatography (HPTLC) under previously optimized conditions was used. Seven polyphenols (Figure 6) have been quantified and the method was validated for a routine control of propolis tinctures [19]. HPTLC method was used for quantification and the results of validation are shown in Table 4. HPTLC method was applied to 7 propolis samples and results are shown in Table 5.

Table 4.. Results of validation of HPTLC method [19].

Validation data	Value
linearity	r > 0.99
precision	
repeatability of the sample application and intra-day precision	RSD < 3.8%
repeatability of peak-area measurement	RSD < 2.4%
accuracy	RSD < 6.5%
limit of detection	PME 7.5 ng/band IFA 7.5 ng/band CA 60 ng/band
limit of quantification	PME 22.5 ng/band IFA 22.5 ng/band CA 180 ng/band
robustness	
inter-day precision and stability of standard solutions	RSD < 5% (two days)
stability on the plate	RSD < 3.4% (up to 2 hours)*
effect of temperature	RSD < 4.6% (20/26°C)
selectivity	absorption spectra matching > 0.99

*only caffeic acid degraded up to 9.4% in 120 minutes, but as the analysis lasts less, this was not of great significance; CA: caffeic acid; IFA: isoferulic acid; PME: pinocembrin-7-methylether; RSD: relative standard deviation.

Table 5. Phenolic acid and flavonoid content (expressed as mean of mass concentration in mg/mL) of the Croatian propolis samples analyzed [19].

propolis sample\polyphenolic	*p*-coumaric acid	caffeic acid	chrysin	tectochrysin	pinocembrin	pinocembrin-7-methyl ether	isoferulic acid
Veliki Zdenci	0.3223+1.32	0.1204+0.99	-	-	-	-	-
Sisak	0.1331+8.22	0.2675+0.22	0.1423+4.09	0.0845+2.90	-	-	-
Labin	0.1464+3.82	0.3000+0.74	0.3987+3.30	-	-	-	-
Čisla (Omiš)	0.2047+2.09	0.4123+0.51	0.1247+1.84	-	-	0.0593+7.36	-
Pelješac	-	0.4196+0.38	0.4896+1.46	0.6775+1.45	0.8454+2.13	0.7452+0.84	0.5068+0.59
Metković	0.2968+1.04	0.3538+0.79	0.5616+2.62	1.1816+0.81	0.6725+1.54	1.1621+0.85	0.4376+2.42
Mixture of propolis	0.1908+2.14	0.3398+0.92	0.6237+4.47	0.4179+1.71	1.1465+3.24	0.2305+5.49	0.4109+4.54

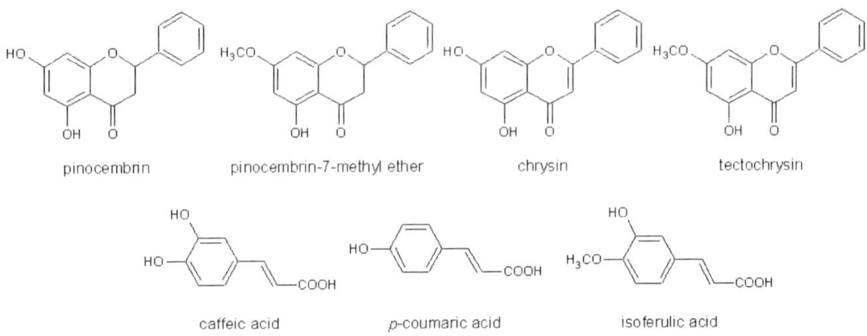

Figure 6. Structures of flavonoids and phenolic acids quantified in propolis tinctures.

For the investigation of ADME for flavonoids reversed-phase thin layer chromatography was used. Chromatography was performed on RP-18F$_{254s}$ plates with binary mobile phase prepared from methanol and phosphate buffer. The pH was at least 2 units lower than pK_a value of phenolics, and organic modifier was varied from 30 to 80% in 5% increments. ADME data was calculated using the following programs: CLOGP, KowWin, Molinspiration, MolSoft, XLOGP, Osiris, VEGA ZZ, DRAGON, ChemSilico, ALOGPS, Interactive Analysis, SPARC [20]. Regular retention behaviour was observed for all the polyphenols investigated – a liner decrease of retention with increased concentration of organic modifier of mobile phase, with standard deviation of less than 0.1. To compare values of retention of polyphenols R_{Mw} values were extrapolated to 100% buffer in mobile phase by using the equation:

$$R_M = R_{Mw} + b\varphi, \quad (10)$$

where Φ is the concentration of organic modifier. R_{Mw} values of flavonoids were in the range 2.309–3.580 and phenolic acids 1.318–2.176. The correlation between R_{Mw} and Φ_0 ($R_M = 0$) was established:

$$R_{Mw} = 4.1854(\pm 0.2238) - 0.0569(\pm 0.0079)\varphi_0,$$
$$n = 30, r = 0.941, s = 0.226, F = 216. \quad (11)$$

It is evident that R_{Mw} and Φ_0 are well correlated but are not identical. This is the case with isomers sakuranetin and isosakuranetin that have the same chromatographic lipophilicity R_{Mw}= 3.111, but different Φ_0, 19.61 and 20.22 respectively.

Most of the used programs are "blind" to this difference occurring between structural isomers, and for MLOGP even different classes of flavonoids could not be distinguished: galangin (flavonol) and apigenin (flavone).

Besides lipophilicity, that is the main determinant for ADME, using ChemSilico software plasma protein binding, blood-brain barrier penetration and human absorption were predicted (Table6).

Table 6. Results obtained using ChemSilico software [20].

ADME data	Results
plasma protein binding	
- flavonoids	85.41% (myricetin) – 95.65% (flavone)
- phenolic acids	70.22% (sinapic acid) – 85.99% (cinnamic acid)
blood-brain barrier penetration	negative except flavon and flavanone
human absorption	significant

BBB penetration was positive only for flavone and flavanone, as these do not have hydroxyl groups. Human absorption was the lowest for myricetin (58%).

Surprisingly, correlation of R_{Mw} and calculated log P values was rather poor, and the best correlations were found between Φ_0 and XLOGP values for flavonols, and human intestinal absorption calculated by ChemSilico and chromatographic RMw (for flavanones) and Φ_0 (for phenolic acids) values.

Based on the procedure developed by Ramić *et al.* [21] chemical interactions were studied using the optimized chromatographic system for polyphenols. Interactions of 19 polyphenols and over-the-counter (OTC) analgesic (acetylsalicylic acid, paracetamol, diclofenac, ibuprofen and ketoprofen) and vitamins (C and E) were examined. Interactions were detected between acetylsalicylic acid and acacetin, galangin, chrysin, pinocembrin and cinnamic acid; ibuprofen and flavone, ketoprofen and pinocembrin, vitamin C and myricetin, morin and quercetin; and vitamin E with flavanone. Example of chromatogram obtained is shown on Figure 7.

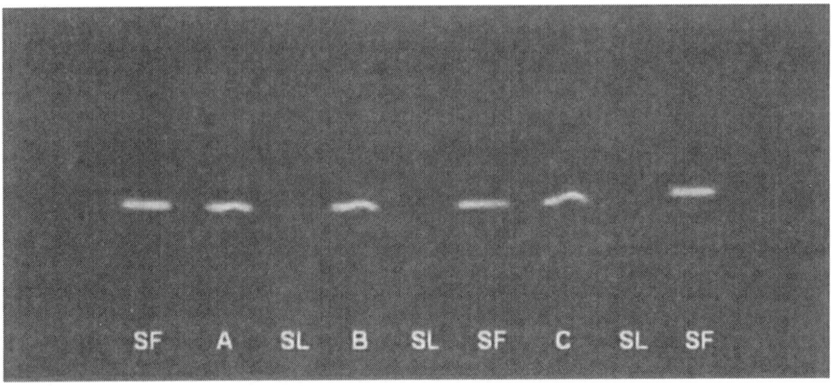

Figure 7. Chromatogram of interaction of flavonoid pinocembrin and ketoprofen. Interaction of flavonoid pinocembrin and ketoprofen obtained under long wave UV light. SF – standard of flavonoid (0.33 mg/mL), A, B, C – interaction lines of pinocembrin and ketoprofen in concentration 0.5, 1.0 and 1.5 mg/mL respectively, SL – standard of ketoprofen in the same concentration as in A, B and C.

These chemical interactions cannot be replaced *in vivo* analysis, but rather be used as basis for further research of phenolics in biological systems.

Band-blot test was used to evaluate antioxidant activity of propolis samples compared to standard mixture of caffeic acid, galangin and pinocembrin using stable free radicals: 2,2'-azino-bis(3-ethylbenzothiazoline-6-sulphonic acid) ($ABTS^{\cdot+}$) and the 2,2-diphenyl-1-picryl-hydrazyl ($DPPH^{\cdot}$) [22]. Band-blot test was performed instead of original dot-blot test using the stable free radical of $DPPH^{\cdot}$. The reason for replacing dots with bands is equal to the distribution of samples in a line instead of over-concentrated centre of spot that can not be easily quantified. Antioxidant efficacy (AOE) was expressed as the slope of the dose-response curve of decrease in $DPPH^{\cdot}$ radical absorbance was used. The chromatogram for standard mixture is shown on Figure 8. Band-blot test has proven a rather quick method for assessing antioxidant activity of a great number propolis samples as the only application of samples and visualization after spraying was done, taking less than 10 minutes.

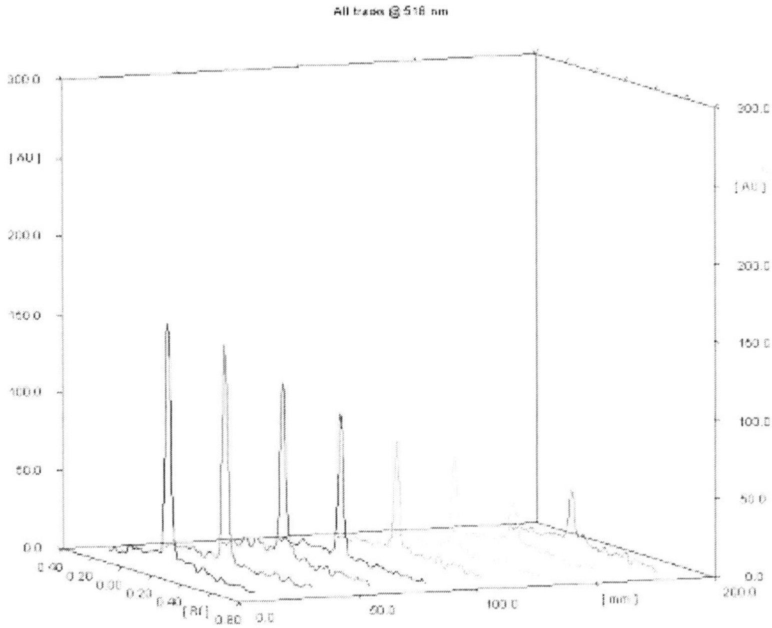

Figure 8. Band-blot test of polyphenols present in propolis using the stable free radical DPPH·. Chromatogram obtained after spraying the layer (applied polyphenol standard mixture bands in the range from 45 (track 1) to 10 μg/mL (track 8)) with 0.3 mM solution of DPPH· radical. *AOE* of standard mixture is 1.89 ($H = 1.89c + 22.856$, $r^2 = 0.974$) [22].

For wine samples the same procedure of optimization was used to select the most appropriate mobile phase (benzene : ethyl acetate : formic acid = 30 : 15 : 5 *v/v*). Six phenolic compounds were indetified in the tested samples. The plates are shown on Figure 9[23]. TLC quantification of polyphenols in wine was performed using CAMAG system. The substances were identified on basis of R_F values and UV spectra. Densitometric quantitative analysis of gallic acid in wine extract is presented on Figure 10, as an example.

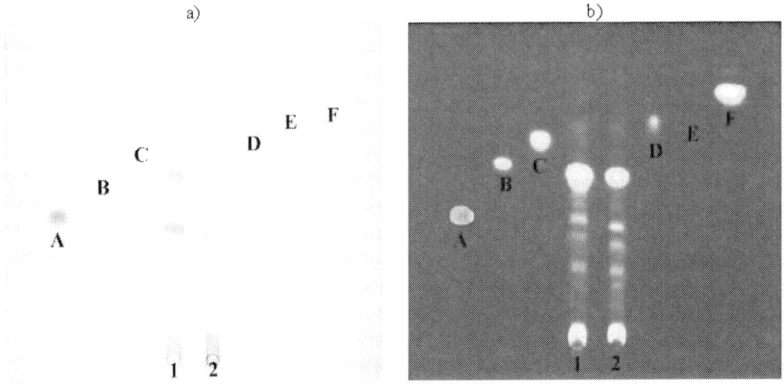

Figure 9. Chromatograms of extracts of red wines "Merlot" (1) and "Frankovka" (2) by use of mobile phase benzene : ethyl acetate : formic acid = 30 + 15 + 5 *v* / *v* / *v*. a) recorded under UV light λ = 254 nm; b) recorded under UV light λ = 366 nm, after spraying with 1% ethanol solution of $AlCl_3$. The standard substances used: A – gallic acid, B – caffeic acid, C – apigenin, D – kaempferol, E – *p*-coumaric acid, F – naringenin [23].

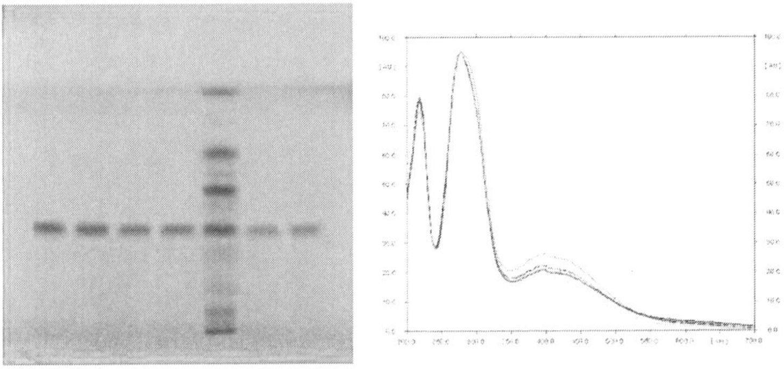

Figure 10. TLC identification and quantification of gallic acid. Photograph of the chromatographic plate recorded at UV light λ = 254 nm, for the purpose of quantification of gallic acid in the sample of wine, with the spectrum of marked peaks obtained using CAMAG densitometer.

High Performance Liquid Chromatography

HPLC analysis of propolis was conducted on Agilent 1100 using X-bridge C18 column. Binary mobile phase of eluents A (10 mM ammonium-formiate in water) and B (10 mM ammonium-formiate in methanol) both of pH = 7 (adjusted with formic acid) was used with the gradient stated in Table 7[22]. Flow rate was 0.5 mL/min at room temperature. 21 standards of polyphenols were used; their identification was based on retention time and UV spectrum, and quantification was done at 270 nm.

Table 7. Gradient of mobile phases used for HPLC analysis of propolis.

time (min)									
mobile phase	0	15	25	30	40	50	60	75	80
%A	90	50	50	40	40	10	10	90	90
%B	10	50	50	60	60	90	90	10	10

Reverse phase HPLC was used for the lipophilicity/hydrophobicity of flavonoids and phenolic acids. Mobile phase A was 2% acetic acid in water and B 2% acetic acid in methanol. Gradient method started with 95% of mobile phase A and 5% of mobile phase B that was linearly increased to 100% during 20/60 minutes [24]. As shown on chromatogram, phenolic acids as more polar substances were first eluted from the column, followed by more hydrophilic and lipophilic flavonoids. HPLC results were used to identify flavonoids and phenolic acids present in propolis samples, to quantify the content of polyphenols, to explain the antioxidant activity *in vitro* and *in vivo* as well as they were used for calculations of pharmacokinetic parameters [22].

For the IAM-HPLC analysis IAM.PC.DD 2 column was used. Mobile phase was phosphate buffer modified with different volumes of methanol. For the HSA-HPLC analysis Chiral HSA column and gradient of phosphate and 2-propanol were used. IAM-HPLC analysis showed that ionization of polyphenolic under physiological pH was influencing the retention of the substance due to ion-ion interaction. The strongest interactions were in the group of flavonoids (kaempferide log k_{wIAM} = 3.581) and lower for phenolic acids (log k_{wIAM} = 1.35–1.68).

From the results of HSA-HPLC analysis it has to be noticed that all the flavonoids have percentage of bonded fraction grater than 95%, which can have repercussions to the interactions with drugs. Binding to HSA was higher for myricetin (%HSA = 99.8) from the group of flavonoids and the lowest for caffeic acid (%HSA = 81.8) from the phenolic acids analyzed, both having the greatest number of hydroxyl groups. Enantiomers could have been differentiated using this method, as expected. This is the case with flavanons shown on Figure11.

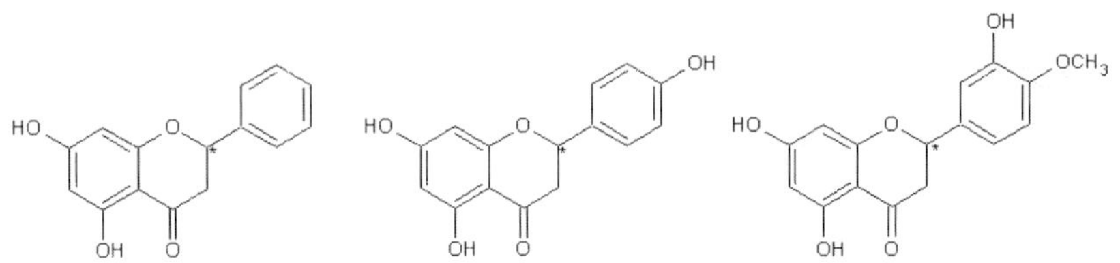

pinocembrin (Δ%HSA=4.7) naringenin (Δ%HSA=0.5) hesperetin (Δ%HSA=0.6)

Figure 11. Structure and differences in HSA binding of enantiomers.

HPLC analysis of wine was conducted on Agilent 1100 using Zorbax StableBond C18 column [5]. Binary mobile phase of eluents A (phosphoric acid (c = 0.02 M, pH = 3.0 adjusted with triethylamin) : methanol = 90 : 10 *v/v*) and B (phosphoric acid (c = 0.02 M, pH = 3.0 adjusted with triethylamin) : methanol = 10 : 90 *v/v*) was used with the gradient stated in Table 8. Flow rate was 1 mL/min at 35°C. 15 standards of polyphenols were used; their identification was based on retention time and UV spectrum, and quantification was done at 280 nm. HPLC analysis of samples of wine has shown discrepancy in results compared to TLC. This has been described in literature [25, 26] and can be explained by lower limit of detection and possibility of overleaping the peaks in HPLC. To illustrate this comparative results for Pelješac sample are shown in Table9. Chromatogram of wine samples from Croatia obtained by HPLC analysis is shown on Figure12.

Table 8. Gradient of mobile phases used for HPLC analysis of wine.

time (min)			
mobile phase	0	25	30
%A	85	15	5
%B	15	85	95

Legend: *only caffeic acid degraded up to 9.4% in 120 minutes, but as the analysis lasts less, this was not of great significance; CA: caffeic acid; IFA: isoferulic acid; PME: pinocembrin-7-methylether; RSD: relative standard deviation.

Table 9. Comparison of the results obtained by HPLC and TLC analysis for Pelješac sample.

	gentisic acid	gallic acid	cinnamic acid	o-coumaric acid	m-coumaric acid	p-coumaric acid	caffeic acid	ferulic acid	chlorogenic acid	catehin	quercetin	kaempferol	myricetin	quercitrin	apigenin	naringenin	trans-resveratrol
HPLC	na	8.4	na	-	-	-	5.0	0.7	-	4.1	4.1	0.4	-	-	-	-	0.8
TLC	48.23	8.92	36.56	na	-	-	3.50	0.93	na	na	5.06	-	na	na	-	-	na

Results expressed as mean of mass concentration in mg/L (na – not analyzed, - – not identified)

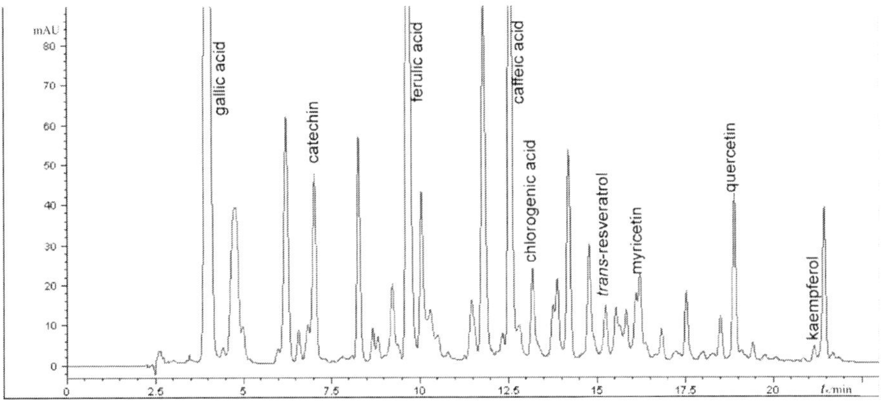

Figure 12. HPLC chromatogram of wine sample Postup registered at 280 nm.

SPECTROPHOTOMETRY

The Folin-Ciocalteu method was used for quantification of total polyphenols according to the method described by Slinkard and Singleton [27]. The method is based on the reduction of MoO^{4+} to MoO^{3+} that is detected by color change from yellow to blue; measured at 765 nm. The results were expressed as equivalents of gallic acid from the calibration curve.

The results for determination of total polyphenols, according to the Folin-Ciocalteu method have shown that white wines (malvazija (*malv*), Traminac (*tram*), Pelješac (*pelj*)) have a lower content of polyphenols [5]. Red wine contains more polyphenols than white wine. This may be ascribing to the fact that making of white wine requires the removal of the skins after the grapes are crushed. Wines containing higher contents of polyphenols are those from the south of Croatia (Plavac(*plav*), Postup (*post*), Dingač (*ding*)) (Figure 13). These findings have been confirmed by TLC analysis.

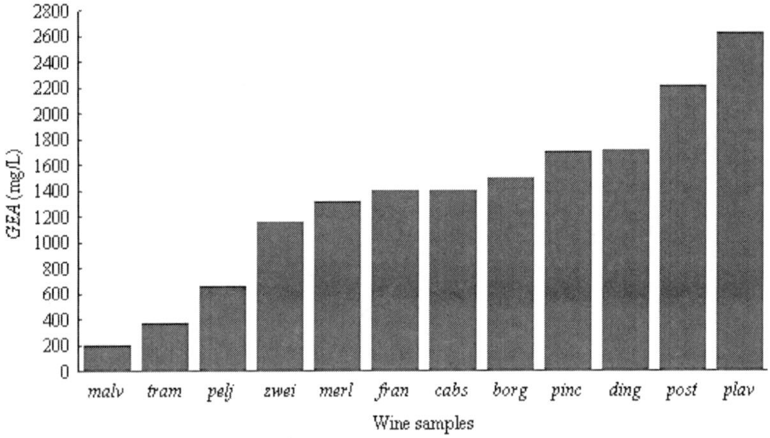

Figure 13. Total polyphenols in wine samples as equivalents of gallic acid (GAE, mg/L) [5]. Codes for wine samples: *malv* – Malvazija; *tram* – Traminac; *pelj* – Pelješac; *zwei* – Zweigelt; *merl* – Merlot; *fran* – Frankovka; *cabs* – Cabernet Sauvignon; *borg* – Borgonja; *pinc* – Pinot crni; *ding* – Dingač; *post* – Postup; *plav* – Plavac.

Free stable radicals $DPPH^{\cdot}$ and $ABTS^{\cdot+}$ were used to assess the antioxidant activity. The method is based on lost of violet/blue color of radicals in presence of substance capable to accept free electron. Discoloration was measured on spectrophotometer at 518 and 730 nm respectively [22]. The spectrophotomety assays, using stable free radicals to assess the antioxidant activities have proven reliable and precise. As most of the suggested procedures could not differentiate similar samples, kinetics of different concentrations of propolis samples has been studied and antioxidant efficiency was introduced (AOE). $DPPH^{\cdot}$ radical was more stable than $ABTS^{\cdot+}$ and results of the $DPPH^{\cdot}$ assay showed better reproducibility. Based on the content of flavonoids and phenolic acids identified and quantified by HPLC analysis we obtained the following correlation:

$$AOE_{DPPH} = 0.5637 + 0.0285c_{phenolic\ acids} + 0.0063c_{flavonoids},$$
$$n = 5, r = 0.878, s = 0.4713, F = 3.3623. \quad (12)$$

Quantitative Structure-Activity Relationship

Experimental data used for QSAR analysis was taken from the literature. Wiener index, connectivity index, Balaban index, Balaban-type indices from atomic number, mass, van der Waals, electronegativity and polarizability weighted distance matrix, information-theoretic index, Shultz index, together with molecular weight, n-octanol/water partition coefficient, van der Waals volume, molar refractivity and polar surface area of polyphenols were calculated using TAM [28], HyperChem 8.0 Evaluation software, PCLIENT, Dragon 3.0. Four groups of 3D descriptors were used: geometrical, GETAWAY (Geometry, Topology and Atom Weights Assembly), 3D-MoRSE and RDF (Radial Distribution Function). Linear, polynomial and multiple linear regression analysis was conducted using Statistica 6.0 [16].

Statistically significant QSAR models for lipid peroxidation inhibiting effects of flavonoids were obtained by polynomial and multiple regression using lipophilicity, Balaban index, Balaban-type index and 3D GETAWAY descriptor. The reason for selecting the 3D descriptors was the possibility of discriminating stereoisomers, like catechin and epicatechin (Figure 14).

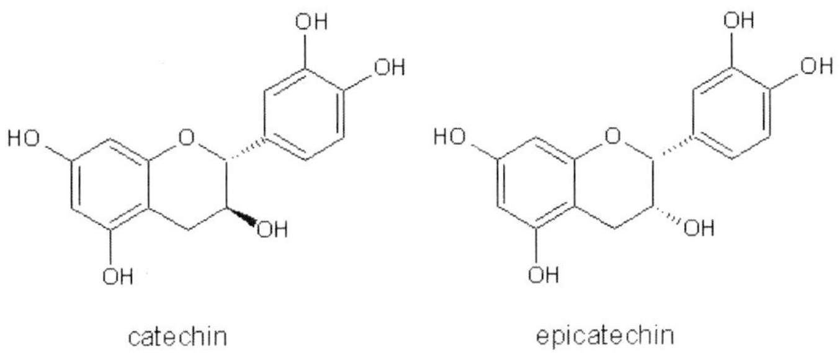

Figure 14. Structures of catechin and epicatechin.

The best model that includes 3D descriptor $H_7(p)$ in combination with Balaban-type index from mass-weighted distance matrix (J_m) was chosen by the best-subset regression:

$$IC_{50} = 320.3(\pm 247.9) + 17.46(\pm 1.92)J_m + 19.63(\pm 2.59)H_7(p),$$
$$n = 8, r^2 = 0.95, S = 7.87, F = 47.66. \quad (13)$$

$H_7(p)$ is an autocorrelation descriptor calculated for 3D-spatial molecular geometry based on lag (topological distance) and weighted by atomic polarizabilities. This descriptor belongs to the group of H-GETAWAY descriptors that have been calculated from the molecular influence matrix H. These descriptors are sensitive to significant conformational changes and to the bond lengths that account for atom types and bond multiplicity.

This QSAR investigation of wine polyphenols could be extended to a larger number of substances, including anthocyanins and dimeric procyanidins as the most common polyphenols in wine.

Clinical Trial [29]

An *in vivo* study has been conducted on 47 healthy women and men in order to investigate whether daily intake of powdered propolis extract during 30 days has any influence on antioxidative status based on the following blood parameters: activity of superoxide dismutase, glutathione peroxidase and catalase, concentration of plasma malondialdehyde, total cholesterol, low- and high-density lipoprotein cholesterol, triglycerides, glucose, uric acid, ferritin and transferrin, together with routine red blood cell parameters.

This was the first reporting of the effects of prolonged propolis supplementation on redox-status of human organism. The benefit of propolis use was only shown in male population demonstrating reduction in free-radical-induced lipid peroxidation as well as increase in activity of superoxide dismutase. A 23.2% decrease in malonaldehyde (degradation product of peroxidation of polyunsaturated fatty acids) concentration and a 20.9% increase in superoxide dismutase activity (first and most important line of antioxidant enzyme defense) were observed (Figure 15).

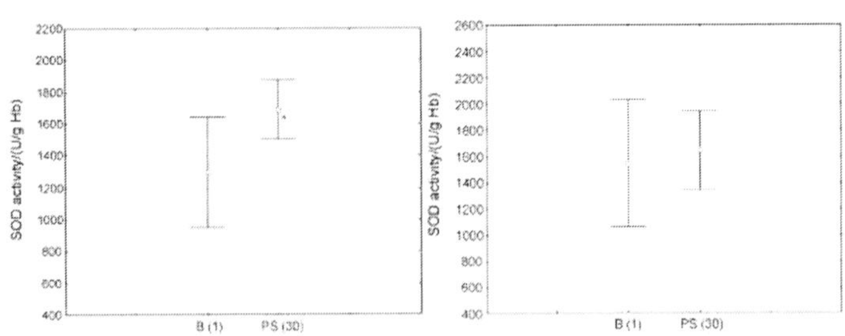

Figure 15. Antioxidant activity of propolis *in vivo*. Activity of superoxide-dismutase (SOD) (U/g Hb) during the study: a) in the men test group and b) in the women test group. Data are expressed as means ± S.D.; B (1) represents the baseline on the 15th day prior to the study and PS (30) represents propolis supplementation on the 30th day. The symbol (*) denotes statistically significant change [29].

Absence of the same results in women was probably due to uncoordinated menstrual cycles. Hence, estrogens are powerful antioxidants, modulators of antioxidant enzyme expression and levels of lipid peroxidase and lipoproteins.

Summary and conclusion

In the last decade interest on nutraceuticals and natural medicinal products is constantly growing. The market is full of antioxidant formulations of wide variety of sources. For the registration of nutraceutical as natural medicinal product analytical procedures have to be developed, product has to be standardized and their functionality and beneficial effects have to be demonstrated. The goal of our studies was standardization of Croatian propolis extracts as a rich sample of flavonoids and phenolic – active components to which pharmacological (antioxidant) activity is attributed. Parallel research on wine samples was done, as wine represents another sample rich in polyphenolics that has been used as constituents e.g. iron wine, tonics.

Identification and quantification of flavonoids and phenolic acids

Although the methods for identification and quantification of propolis samples using HPLC combined with mass spectrometry (MS) and nuclear magnetic resonance (NMR) have been developed and alternative was provided in capillary electrophoresis coupled with MS, these are rather expensive, not readily available and inappropriate for routine analysis [30, 31]. Thus we have decided for TLC method combined with HPLC-diode array detection (DAD) method. Out of 11 mobile phases available from literature based on numerical taxonomy chloroform : methanol : formic acid in volume ratio 44 : 3.5 : 2.5 was selected as the most appropriate for TLC identification of 9 polyphenols [17]. Better separation for identification was achieved using 2D-TLC chromatography, although for quantification we decided for high performance TLC plates using which clear identification and quantification of 7 polyphenols (namely: *p*-coumaric acid, caffeic acid, chrysin, tectochrysin, pinocembrine-7-methyl ether, isoferulic acid) was performed [18, 19]. Major limiting factor of TLC is length of the plate, so for better separation HPLC was used.

Total content of polyphenols was determined using Folin-Ciocalteu method. As we have done identification using liquid chromatography we did not separately analyze total content of phenolic acids and flavonoids which can be done using well known procedures described in Ph. Eur. and Christ and Müller, respectively [32, 33].

Pharmacokinetic (ADME) parameters of flavonoids and phenolic acids

Passive transport through membranes is mainly determined by the lipophilicity of the substance. The most commonly used experimental value of lipophilicity is chromatographic parameter R_M. This parameter was determined by TLC as well by HPLC and to assess lipophilicity within the group of polyphenolics. As this parameter cannot distinguish isomers, additional parameter Φ_0 was used differentiating sakuranetin and isosakuranetin.

Using ChemSilico software plasma protein binding of flavonoids was found rather high (85–96%) compared to phenolic acids (70–86%). High values of flavonoid binding are in accordance to the experimental date e.g. for quercetin (99%) [34]. Passage through blood-brain barrier was negative which is expected for compounds having acidic phenolic and carboxylic groups. Absorption was mainly greater than 60%, but this has to be taken with dose of doubt, as experimental data is contradictory [35].

Chemical interaction with most commonly used non-steroidal anti-inflammatory drugs (NSAID) and vitamins where characterized on TLC plate. The interactions were most common with acetylsalicylic acid. At the moment this has no practical value as further *in vivo* studies have to demonstrate applicability of this model [21].

Interactions of polyphenolics with artificial membranes were probably based on ion-ion and passive diffusion as interaction showed greater partition coefficient for flavonoids than phenolic acids. Binding on HSA-column was higher compared to ChemSilico predictions and more in accordance to experimental data obtained *in vivo*.

Antioxidant activity of flavonoids and phenolic acids

Antioxidant activity of polyphenolics is well known. To assay the antioxidant activity different methods are used: electron paramagnetic resonance (EPR) spectroscopy, chemiluminescence, enzyme assays... Most often used and readily available is spectrophotometric method using stable free radicals. $DPPH^{\cdot}$ and $ABTS^{\cdot+}$ were used for spectrophotometry as well TLC *in situ* for analysis of total antioxidant capacity of propolis. The most active propolis comes from coastal Croatia [22].

QSAR analysis of polyphenolics based on Trolox test date from literature pointed out that antioxidant activity of polyphenols as hydrogen donating free radical scavengers, is closely related to their chemical structure, especially with the number and arrangement of free hydroxyl groups of polyphenol skeleton [16].

In vivo study of propolis prolonged used showed beneficial in male population demonstrating reduction in free-radical-induced lipid peroxidation as well as increase in activity of superoxide dismutase. Production of malonaldehyde (degradation product of peroxidation of polyunsaturated fatty acids) reduced and activity of superoxide dismutase (first and most important line of antioxidant enzyme defense) was increased [29].

Antioxidant supplements are flooding the market. Asking pharmacist for a new product – extract of the plant coming from exotic country, will usually end with the answer "its antioxidant and thus good for your health". The necessity of standardization natural antioxidant products made us write this minireview-providing basis for standardization of natural antioxidant products rich in polyphenols using simple and readily available techniques based on our research on propolis and wine.

ACKNOWLEDGEMENTS

This work was supported by the Ministry of Science, Education and Sports of the Republic of Croatia (projects No. 006-0061117-1237 – MMŠ and 006-0061117-1239 – ŽM). The authors wish to thank all the associates involved in these as well as antecedent projects.

COMPETING INTERESTS

The authors declare that they have no competing interests.

AUTHORS' CONTRIBUTIONS

All authors contributed equally to this work, read and approved the final manuscript.

REFERENCES

1. Bradamante V, Lacković Z: Oxidative stress and efficiency of antioxidants. 2001, Zagreb: Medicinska naklada
2. Havsteen B: Flavonoids, a class of natural products of high pharmacological potency. Biochem Pharmacol. 1983, 7: 1141-1148.
3. Smirnoff N: Antioxidants and reactive oxygen species in plants. 2005, Oxford: Blackwell Publishing
4. Castalado S, Capasso F: Propolis, an old remedy used in modern medicine. Fitoterapia. 2002, 73 (Suppl 1): S1-S6.
5. Rastija V, Medić-Šarić M: Polyphenolic composition of Croatian wines with different geographical origins. Food Chem. 2009, 115: 54-60.
6. Kaštelan-Macan M, Medić-Šarić M, Turina S: Planar chromatography. 2006, Zagreb: Faculty of Pharmacy and Biochemistry
7. Medić-Šarić M, Maleš Ž, Stanić G, Šarić S: Evaluation and selection of optimal solvent and solvent combinations in thin-layer chromatography of flavonoids and of phenolic acids of *Zizyphus jujuba* Mill. Croat Chem Acta. 1996, 69: 1265-1274.
8. Medić-Šarić M, Stanić G, Maleš Ž, Šarić S: Application of numerical methods to thin-layer chromatographic investigation of the main components of chamomile (*Chamomilla recutita* (L.) Rauschert) essential oil. J Chromatogr A. 1997, 776: 355-360.
9. Medić-Šarić M, Maleš Ž: Application of numerical methods to the TLC analysis of flavonoids and phenolic acids of *Rosmarini folium*. J Planar Chromatogr. 1997, 10: 182-187.
10. Maleš Ž, Medić-Šarić M, Bucar F: Flavonoids of *Guiera senegalensis* J.F.GMEL. – thin-layer chromatography and numerical methods. Croat Chem Acta. 1998, 71: 69-79.
11. Medić-Šarić M, Maleš Ž, Šarić S, Debeljak Ž: Use of information theory and numerical taxonomy methods for evaluating the quality of thin-layer chromatographic separations of flavonoids and phenolic acids of *Rhamni cathartici fructus*. J Liq Chrom & Rel Technol. 1999, 22: 83-103.

12. Medić-Šarić M, Maleš Ž: Selection of an optimal set of solvents in thin-layer chromatography of flavonoids and phenolic acids of *Lavandulae flos*. Pharmazie. 1999, 54: 362-364.

13. Maleš Ž, Medić-Šarić M: Investigation of the flavonoids and phenolic acids of *Sambuci flos* by thin-layer chromatography. J Planar Chromatogr. 1999, 12: 345-349.

14. Maleš Ž, Medić-Šarić M: Optimization of flavonoids and phenolic acids of *Helleborus atrorubens* Waldst. et Kit. J Pharm Biomed Anal. 2001, 24: 353-359.

15. Waterbeemd van de H, Hans Lennernäs H, Per Artursson P: Drug Bioavailability: Estimation of Solubility, Permeability, Absorption and Bioavailability. 2003, Weinheim: Wiley-VCH

16. Rastija V, Medić-Šarić M: QSAR Study of antioxidant activity of wine polyphenols. Eur J Med Chem. 2009, 44: 400-408.

17. Jasprica I, Smolčić-Bubalo A, Mornar A, Medić-Šarić M: Investigation of the flavonoids in Croatian propolis by thin-layer chromatography. J Planar Chromatogr. 2004, 17: 95-101.

18. Medić-Šarić M, Jasprica I, Mornar A, Smolčić-Bubalo A, Golja P: Quantitative analysis of flavonoids and phenolic acids in propolis by two-dimensional thin layer chromatography. J Planar Chromatogr. 2004, 17: 459-463.

19. Cvek J, Medić-Šarić M, Jasprica I, Mornar A: High-performance thin-layer chromatographic analysis of the phenolic acid and flavonoid content of Croatian propolis samples. J Planar Chromatogr. 2007, 20: 429-435.

20. Mornar A, Medić-Šarić M, Jasprica I: ADME data for polyphenols characterized by reversed-phase thin-layer chromatography. J Planar Chromatogr. 2006, 19: 409-417.

21. Ramić A, Medić-Šarić M, Turina S, Jasprica I: TLC detection of chemical interaction of vitamins A and D with drugs. J Planar Chromatogr. 2006, 19: 27-31.

22. Jasprica I, Bojić M, Mornar A, Bešić E, Bućan K, Medić-Šarić M: Evaluation of antioxidant activity of Croatian propolis samples using DPPH and $ABTS^+$ stable free radical assays. Molecules. 2007, 12: 1006-1021.

23. Rastija V, Mornar A, Jasprica I, Srečnik G, Medić-Šarić M: Analysis of phenolic components in croatian red wine by thin-layer chromatography. J Planar Chromatogr. 2004, 17: 26-31.

24. Medić-Šarić M, Mornar A, Jasprica I: Lipophilicity of flavonoids and phenolic acids determined by shake-flask and high performance liquid chromatography methods. Proceedings of the 6th AFMC International Medicinal Chemistry Symposium: 8–11 July 2007; Istambul. 2007, Barcelona: Prous science, 133-133

25. Shi R, Schwedt G: HPLC and TLC analysis of phenolic compounds in wine. Deut Labensm-Rundsch. 1995, 1: 14-17.

26. de Rijke E, Out P, Niessen WMA, Ariese F, Gooijer C, Brinkman UATh: Analytical separation and detection methods for flavonoids. J Chromatogr A. 2006, 1112: 31-36.

27. Slinkard K, Singleton VL: Total phenol analysis: automation and comparison with manual methods. Am J Enol Vitic. 1977, 28: 49-55.

28. Vedrina M, Marković S, Medić-Šarić M, Trinajstić N: TAM: a program for the calculation of topological indices in QSPR and QSAR studies. Computers Chem. 1997, 21: 355-361.

29. Jasprica I, Mornar A, Debeljak Ž, Smolčić-Bubalo A, Medić-Šarić M, Mayer Lj, Romić Ž, Bućan K, Balog T, Sobočanec S, Šverko V: *In vivo* study of propolis supplementation effects on antioxidative status and red blood cells. J Ethnopharmacol. 2007, 110: 548-554.

30. Cuesta-Rubio O, Piccinelli AL, Fernandez MC, Hernandez IM, Rosado A, Rastrelli L: Chemical characterization of Cuban propolis by HPLC-PDA, HPLC-MS, and NMR: the brown, red, and yellow Cuban varieties of propolis. J Agric Food Chem. 2007, 55: 7502-7509.

31. Gomez-Romero M, Arraez-Roman D, Moreno-Torres R, Garcia-Salas P, Segura-Carretero A, Fernandez-Gutierrez A: Antioxidant compounds of propolis determined by capillary electrophoresis-mass spectrometry. J Sep Sci. 2007, 30: 595-603.

32. Council of Europe: European Pharmacopoeia. Strasbourg. 2007

33. Christ B, Müller KH: Zur serienmäßigen bestimmung des gehaltes an flavonol derivaten in drogen. Arch Pharm. 1960, 293: 1033-1042.

34. Hollman PC, Katan MB: Absorption, metabolism and health effects of dietary flavonoids in man. Biomed Pharmacother. 1997, 51: 305-310.

35. Walle T: Absorption and metabolism of flavonoids. Free Radic Biol Med. 2004, 36: 829-837.

11

NUTRACEUTICAL EFFECTS OF TABLE GREEN OLIVES: A PILOT STUDY WITH NOCELLARA DEL BELICE OLIVES

Giulia Accardi[1], Anna Aiello[1] , Valeria Gargano

[1]Sezione di Patologia generale del Dipartimento di Biopatologiae Biotecnologie Mediche (DIBIMED), Università di Palermo, Corso Tukory 211, 90134 Palermo, Italy

ABSTRACT

Background

The aim of this study was to analyse the nutraceutical properties of table green olives *Nocellara del Belice*, a traditional Mediterranean food. The Mediterranean Diet has as key elements olives and extra virgin olive oil, common to all Mediterranean countries. Olive oil is the main source of fat and can modulate oxidative stress and inflammation, whereas little is known about the role of olives. Moreover, emerging evidences underline the association between gut microbiota and food as the basis of many phenomena that affect health and delay or avoid the onset of some age-related chronic diseases.

Methods

In order to show if table green olives have nutraceutical properties and/or probiotic effect, we performed a nutritional intervention, administering to 25 healthy subjects (mean age 38,3), 12 table green olives/day for 30 days. We carried out anthropometric, biochemical, oxidative stress and cytokines analyses at the beginning of the study and at the end. Moreover, we also collected fecal samples to investigate about the possible variation of concentration of*Lactobacilli*, after the olives consumption.

Result

Our results showed a significant variation of one molecule related to oxidative stress, malondialdehyde, confirming that *Nocellara del Belice* green olives could have an anti-oxidant effect. In addition, the level of interleukin-6 decreased significantly, demonstrating how this food could be able to modulate the inflammatory response. Moreover, it is noteworthy the reduction of fat mass with an increase of muscle mass, suggesting a possible effect on long time assumption of table olives on body mass variation. No statistically significant differences were observed in the amount of *Lactobacilli*, although a trend towards an increased concentration of them at the end of the intervention could be related to the nutraceutical effects of olives.

Conclusion

These preliminary results suggest a possible nutraceutical effect of daily consumption of green table olives *Nocellara del Belice*. To best of our knowledge, this is the first study performed to assess nutraceutical properties of this food. Of course, it is necessary to verify the data in a larger sample of individuals to confirm their role as nutraceuticals.

Keywords: Table green olives Mediterranean Diet Nutraceuticals Dietary intervention Oxidative stress Inflammatory status

BACKGROUND

Nowadays, ageing process and the related diseases constitute one of the bigger challenges in Western countries. The general increase of lifespan does not go, hand in hand, with the increase of healthy lifespan, the so-called "healthspan". This constitutes a worldwide problem, in particular due to age-related chronic diseases [1].

It is well known that the pathogenesis of age-related diseases is characterized by a low-grade inflammation. In particular, the visceral adipose tissue is a source of inflammatory mediators produced by adipocytes and infiltrating monocytes [2].

Abdominal obesity with dyslipidaemia, elevated blood pressure and impaired glucose tolerance characterizes metabolic syndrome (MS) that predisposes to the onset of age-related diseases. As many studies demonstrate, a dietary Mediterranean regimen can positively influence these parameters. Large intervention trials showed, in fact, that Mediterranean Diet (MedDiet) could prevent and or delay the onset of age-related diseases with a great implication in the health social system [3, 4, 5, 6, 7].

The traditional MedDiet is a common dietary pattern, adopted by inhabitants of countries within Mediterranean basin where the olive tree, *Olea europaea*, is widely cultivated for the production of table olives and oil. They are the essential components of the MedDiet with a very significant economic value. Besides of the economical contribution to national economies, these are important in terms of nutritional value. Extra virgin olive oil (EVOO) has been claimed to play a key role in the prevention of age-related diseases and in the attainment of longevity. This is due to the high levels of monounsaturated fatty acids, likely responsible for the decreased low density lipoprotein levels, and phenolic compounds claimed to play a role as antioxidants and anti-inflammatories [6, 8, 9].

Foods with bioactive molecules can be considered "nutraceuticals", defined as "Naturally derived bioactive compounds that are found in foods, dietary supplements and herbal products, and have health promoting, disease preventing, or medicinal properties". The term was coined in 1989 by Stephen De Felice and was born from the conjunction between nutrition and pharmaceutics [10].

As reported in a recent review, table olives are extremely rich sources of polyphenols, especially oleuropein and hydroxytyrosol, comprising 1–3 % of the fresh pulp weight. Despite the high levels of hydroxytyrosol in both table olives and EVOO, in humans its bioavailability was proved only in oil. Accordingly, to the best of our knowledge, there are no human studies on health effects of table olives [11]. However, the amount of polyphenols is strongly influenced by the variety and the geographical origin. *Greek Koroneiki* have a very high level of them, while the polypenol content of the *Spanish Arbequina* is low and that of *Sicilian Nocellara* is medium-high [12]. So, a possible anti-inflammatory and anti-oxidant effect of these Sicilian olives is conceivable.

The development of strategies aimed at counterbalancing the frailty in the elderly is a major challenge for the medicine of 21st century [1]. As recently reviewed, ageing affects the gut microbiota composition and its influence in immune response. Age-related gut microbiota changes are associated with immunosenescence and inflamm-ageing. Hence, the gut ecosystem shows the potential to become a promising target for strategies able to contribute to the health status of elderly. In this context, the consumption of pro/prebiotics may be useful in both prevention and treatment of age-related pathophysiological conditions, favouring the attainment of longevity [13].

Probiotics are defined as "Live microorganisms which when administered in adequate amounts confer a health benefit on the host". *Lactobacilli* (*L.*) and *Bifidobacteria* are the most commonly used bacterial probiotics [14]. Nutritional supplementation in aged people might help to maintain good immune-inflammatory responses by re-equilibrating the gut microbiota.

Fermentation is one of the oldest methods to preserve olives. It has applied worldwide for thousands of years. The microbiota of olives during fermentation, that varies somewhat from*cultivar* to *cultivar*, has been recently reviewed, showing that *L.* are the major constituents of*Nocellara del Belice* olives microbiota [15, 16]. So, a possible probiotic-like effect of these olives is feasible.

The aim of this pilot study was to evaluate the effect of green table olives *Nocellara del Belice* on clinical and biological parameters of healthy individuals at baseline (T0) and after the assumption of 12 olives/day for 30 days (T1) (this amount was chosen to assure the administration of $2x10^7$ *L.*/die, see below).

RESULTS AND DISCUSSION

Hematochemical tests

At the end of the intervention, all hematochemical parameters did not experienced variations, with the exception of alkaline phosphatase that significantly increased (Table 1).

However, the increased values were in normal range. This means that a regular consumption of 12 green olives/day for 30 days does not have a detrimental effect on liver and kidney function and on lipid values.

Table 1. The Table shows the arithmetic average values at T0 and T1, the p-value and the variation in percentage (+ indicates an increase of the variable at T1; - a decrease at T1)

Variable	T0 ± SD	T1 ± SD	p-value	%
Alkaline phosphate (IU/L)	49.95 ± 13.26	53.73 ± 16.81	0.022	+7.57
Fat mass%	29.70 ± 7.92	28 ± 7.24	0.004	−5.72
Muscle mass %	66.97 ± 7.62	68.36 ± 6.85	0.003	+2.09
IL-6 (FI)	31.52 ± 29.37	20.89 ± 11.93	0.027	−33.73
MDA (μmol/L)	2.72 ± 0.64	2.33 ± 0.49	0.005	−14.24
Weight (Kg)	70.44 ± 14.07	69.93 ± 13.77	0.08	−0.72
BMI (Kg/m^2)	24.37 ± 4.19	24.24 ± 4.16	0.22	−0.53

T0 baseline, *T1* the end of the nutritional intervention (30 days), *BMI* Body Mass Index, *IL-6* interleukin-6, *IF* indirect fluorescence, *MDA* malondialdehyde, *SD* standard deviation

Anthropometric measurements

At T1, in analysed subjects the fat mass significantly decreased together to an increase of muscle mass (Table 1). The possible explanation could be linked to the capacity of conjugated linoleic acid (CLA) to reduce the body fat levels [17]. This molecule is present both in EVOO and table olives, and can also be produced during their digestion. In experimental models, acting as signalling mediators, CLAs inhibit lipogenesis, increase fat oxidation, and reduce adipocytes size [18, 19].

Cytokines analyses

The serological analysis of the levels of the main pro and anti-inflammatory cytokines was conducted. Although it was not possible to evaluate the absolute concentration of interleukin (IL)-6 because it is too low, a significant variation was measured in the indirect fluorescence (IF). In fact, its levels significantly decreased at the end of the dietary intervention (Table 1).

IL-6 is a pleiotropic cytokine capable of regulating proliferation, differentiation and activity in a variety of cell types. In particular, it plays a pivotal role in acute phase responses and in the balancing of the pro and anti-inflammatory pathways. It is involved in impaired lipid metabolism and in the production of triglycerides. Moreover, it decreases lipoprotein lipase activity and monomeric lipoprotein lipase levels in plasma which contributes to increased macrophage uptake of lipids [20]. This datum suggests that a regular consumption of green olives can have anti-inflammatory effects linked to polyphenols, known to have anti-inflammatory properties [6].

Oxidative stress analyses

At the end of intervention, the values of malondialdehyde (MDA) significantly decreased (Table 1), while paraoxonase (PON) plasma levels and reduced glutathione in the red blood cells were not changed (data not shown). MDA is the main product of the polyunsaturated fatty acids peroxidation and is an important index of oxidative stress [21]. So, its reduction should be linked to the increased assumption of mono-unsatured oleic acid by olives.

Microbiological analyses on feces

The amount of *L.*/g of feces was quantified before and after the intervention. No statistically significant differences were observed, although a trend towards an increased amount of *L.* was highlighted in some subjects at T1 (data not shown). Thus, we can speculate that a more durable dietary intervention and a bigger sample of people could give more interesting results.

CONCLUSIONS

The traditional MedDiet is a common dietary pattern that identify a lifestyle and a culture. It was proven that it contributes to better health and quality of life. Concerning its healthy effects, low content of animal protein and low glycaemic index may directly modulate the insulin/insulin-like growth factor-1 and the mammalian target of rapamycin pathways, known to be involved in ageing, age-related diseases and longevity. In addition to the influence on nutrient sensing pathways, many single components of MedDiet are known to have positive effects on health, reducing inflammation, oxidative stress and other important risk factors of age-related diseases [6].

This pilot study demonstrates an anti-inflammatory and anti-oxidant effect of daily consumption of green table olives *Nocellara del Belice*. Moreover, it is noteworthy the reduction of fat mass with an increase of muscle mass. Although no statistically significant probiotic effect was observed, the positive trend related to *L.* amount at T1 could represent a starting point for further studies.

It is to note that the study presents limitations. One is strictly related to the intrinsic complexity of human as study model and to the inter/intra-individual variability. These features are more evident in ageing than in younger people. This is the reason why we chose middle age people. So, our choice represented the second limitation of the study because we did not analyze the effects of the intervention in elderly. Thirdly, it is necessary to verify these data in a larger sample of individuals to confirm the role of table green olives as nutraceutical foods. Also the duration of the intervention could be inadequate. In fact, we developed a short-term dietary regimen (30 days). This is a good choice in terms of compliance to the study because the more is the time of intervention the more is the drop out effect. But, a long-term dietary intervention could be stronger in terms of variation of analyzed parameters (e.g., *L.* amount in feces).

However, these new knowledges give an important achievement for the food and farming industry, especially in Sicily, where the olives represent a great potential resource. No approved healthy property and claim exist for them. Therefore, adding such a common product to the class of nutraceuticals could represent a big deal.

In the era of many expansive and mysterious longevity elixirs, the olives could represent a traditional, cheap and accessible to everyone "healthy food".

METHODS

Study design

The trial consisted in the assumption of 12 olives/day for 30 days. They belonging to the variety*Nocellara del Belice*, were processed in salt solution without any chemical additives.

See Fig. 1 for the flow chart of the study design.

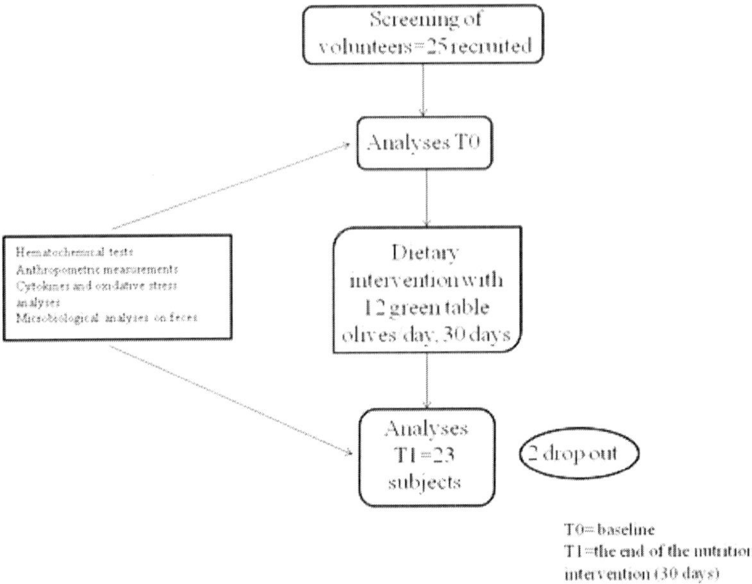

Figure 1. The figure shows the flow chart of the study design

Study population

Twenty-five randomized volunteers (mean age 38,3), both men and women, were recruited from April 2015 to July 2015. The subjects included were: healthy, with age between 18 and 65 years and Caucasian. The exclusion criteria provided: a history of the absence of pathologies (obesity, MS); a history of use of any pre or probiotics as dietary supplements within 3 months prior to the study; a history of treatment with statins or similar and with lyposoluble drugs; the onset of gastrointestinal disorders or the use of antibiotics during the nutritional intervention. No restriction related to sex was considered. Two subjects dropped out of the trial. All participants signed an informed consent before the enrolment. To respect the privacy, everyone was identified with an alphanumeric code. Height and weight were measured wearing light clothes and barefoot. The body composition was registered using specific hardware and software. Body mass index was calculated as weight (in kilos) over height squared (in square metre) (Table 1). Dietary habits were assessed through a food frequency questionnaire, officially validate by the EPIC study. Blood tests, oxidative stress and cytokines analyses were carried out for all subjects at T0 and T1. Molecular analyses were conducted on *L.* DNA obtained from fecal samples to measure the variation of its amount. A database was created to insert all participants' data and to handle the collected information.

Hematochemical tests

The recruited people underwent to venipuncture at T0 and at T1. Blood samples were collected in specific blood collection tubes containing ethylenediaminetetraacetic acid (EDTA) for plasma analyses and in serum tubes with no additives. Plasma and sera were separated from whole blood by low-speed centrifugation at 2,500 rpm for 15′ at 4 °C. After separation, the samples were stored at −80 °C for further tests. We also obtained gruel of red blood cells from blood collected in tubes with EDTA through three washes with physiological solution (centrifugation at 2,500 rpm for 15′ at 4 °C).

Evaluation of parameters of oxidative stress

These analyses were conducted in collaboration with the University of Sassari. Thiobarbituric acid reactive substances (TBARS) were determined according to the method described by Esterbauer and Cheeseman [22]. TBARS methodology measures MDA and other aldehydes produced by lipid peroxidation induced by hydroxyl free radicals. For the measurements, plasma was mixed with 10 % trichloroacetic acid and 0.67 % thiobarbituric acid and heated at 95 °C in thermoblock heater for 25′. TBARS were determined by measuring the absorbance at 535 nm. A calibration curve was obtained using standard MDA and each curve point was subjected to the same treatment as that of the samples.

PON activity was determined by measuring the increase in absorbance at 412 nm (formation of 4-nitrophenol), using paraoxon (O, O diethyl-O-p-nitrophenyl phosphate) as a substrate [22]. The enzyme activity was calculated by using the molar extinction coefficient of 17,100 $M^{-1}cm^{-1}$and one unit of PON activity was defined as 1 nanomole of 4-nitrophenol formed per minute. For red blood cell glutathione quantification, 200 µl (µL) of thawed packed cells were lysed by adding 600 µL of cold water and keeping the samples at 4 °C for 15′. 200 µL of lysed samples were deproteinized by adding 200 µL acetonitrile and centrifuged at 2,000 × g for 5′. Samples were then derivatized by mixing 100 µL of supernatant with 100 µL of sodium phosphate buffer (60 µmol (mmol)/L, pH 12.5), and 25 µL of 5-Iodoacetamidofluorescein (4.1 mmol/L). After vortex mixing, samples were incubated for 15′ at room temperature. Derivatized samples were diluted 100-fold in water and analysed by capillary electrophoresis with laser induced fluorescence detection [23].

Pro and anti-inflammatory cytokines analyses

These analyses were conducted using Luminex assays, coupled to Bio-Plex Manager software.

Data obtained have been checked by technical department and quality control parameters. Values of the standard curve were compared to the values provided by the manufacturer of the kits used and must not exceed a CV of 15 %. All of above parameters were applied on, at least, the 90 % of the standard curve values.

Microbiological and molecular analyses of *Lactobacilli*

In order to quantify the amount of *L.* in each olive, 1 g of pulp was suspended in phosphate-buffered saline solution (1 mL), homogenized for 2′ at maximum speed, and then serially diluted. Decimal dilutions were plated and incubated on *de Man, Rogosa and Sharpe* at 30 °C for 48 h to observe the *L.* growth. The colonies' count was performed in triplicate and the *L.* DNA was extracted from them to perform molecular analyses. Moroever, colony suspension were used as a template for Real Time PCR. The primers and probes used to detect *L. species* (*spp*) were based on 16S rRNA gene sequences retrieved from the NCBI databases (Table 2). The amplification reactions were carried out in a total volume of 25 ml containing 1X SSoFast Probe mix (BIORAD), primers (each at 200 nM concentration), 100 nM TaqMan MGB probe, 60 ng purified target DNA. Amplification (1 cycle of 5′ at 95 °C, 45 cycles of 15″ at 95 °C and 1 cycle of 1′ at 60 °C) and detection were carried out on a CFX Real Time system (BIORAD).

Table 2. Primer and probe sequences for analyses of *L. spp* in Real Time PCR

	Oligonucleotide sequence 5′-3′
Primer Forward	GAGGCAGCAGTAGGGAATCTTC
Primer Reverse	GGCCAGTTACTACCTCTATCCTTCTTC
Probe	FAM-ATGGAGCAACGCCGC-QUENCER

Fluorescent probe was labeled at 5′ end with the reporter dye 6-carboxyfluorescein and at 3′ end with a quencher dye. A negative and a positive control were included on the reaction plate.

In order to perform the quantification of *L.* in each feces sample, the QIAamp DNA Stool Minikit (Qiagen) was used to extract DNA from an appropriate amount of frozen stool sample, according to the manufacturer's instructions. The Real Time PCR was performed as previous described and the cycle threshold of each sample was compared to a standard curve made by diluting genomic DNA (10-fold serial dilution) from cultures of known concentrations of *L.*(10^6 CFU/ml).

Statistical analyses

The paired comparisons were performed with the Student's *t*-test or the Wilcoxon signed rank test, according to the normality of samples. Statistical analyses were performed with the IDE RStudio for the R (version 3.2.2) software [24, 25].

ACKNOWLEDGMENTS

This work was supported by PON DIMESA (Programma Operativo Nazionale Ricerca e Competitività 2007/2013 - Progetto "DI.ME.Sa." PON02_00451_3361785. Valorisation of typical products of the Mediterranean diet and their nutraceutical use to improve health) to CC. GA is a Post Doc at DiBiMed. AA and CMG are students of the PhD course directed by CC.

We are grateful to Dr. Nicola Locorotondo for his continuous enthusiastic support.

COMPETING INTERESTS

The authors declare that they have no competing interest.

AUTHORS' CONTRIBUTION

GA, AA, VG, and CC* conceived and designed the study; GA, AA, CMG, VG, SM, SC, GV, AZ, CC* and CC** performed or supervised experiments. MZ executed statistical analysis. GA, AA, VG, CC*, and CC** analyzed and interpreted data; GA and AA drafted the paper. GC, CC* and CC** made critical revisions to the draft. All authors read and approved the final manuscript. CC*: Calogero Caruso. CC**: Ciriaco Carru

REFERENCES

1. Longo VD, Antebi A, Bartke A, Barzilai N, Brown-Borg HM, Caruso C, Curiel TJ, de Cabo R, Franceschi C, Gems D, Ingram DK, Johnson TE, Kennedy BK, Kenyon C, Klein S, Kopchick JJ, Lepperdinger G, Madeo F, Mirisola MG, Mitchell JR, Passarino G, Rudolph KL, Sedivy JM, Shadel GS, Sinclair DA, Spindler SR, Suh Y, Vijg J, Vinciguerra M, Fontana L. Interventions to Slow Aging in Humans: Are We Ready? Aging Cell. 2015;14:497–510.

2. Balistreri CR, Caruso C, Candore G. The role of adipose tissue and adipokines in obesity-related inflammatory diseases. Mediators Inflamm. 2010.

3. Estruch R, Martínez-González MA, Corella D, Salas-Salvadó J, Ruiz-Gutiérrez V, Covas MI, Fiol M, Gómez-Gracia E, López-Sabater MC, Vinyoles E, Arós F, Conde M, Lahoz C, Lapetra J, Sáez G, Ros E; PREDIMED Study Investigators. Effects of a Mediterranean-style diet on cardiovascular risk factors: a randomized trial. Ann Intern Med. 2006;145:1–11.

4. Fitó M, Guxens M, Corella D, Sáez G, Estruch R, de la Torre R, Francés F, Cabezas C, López-Sabater Mdel C, Marrugat J, García-Arellano A, Arós F, Ruiz-Gutierrez V, Ros E, Salas-Salvadó J, Fiol M, Solá R, Covas MI; PREDIMED Study Investigators. Effect of a traditional Mediterranean diet on lipoprotein oxidation: a randomized controlled trial. Arch Intern Med. 2007;167:1195–203.

5. Casas R, Sacanella E, Estruch R. The immune protective effect of the Mediterranean diet against chronic low-grade inflammatory diseases. Endocr Metab Immune Disord Drug Targets. 2014;14:245–54.

6. Vasto S, Buscemi S, Barera A, Di Carlo M, Accardi G, Caruso C. Mediterranean diet and healthy ageing: a Sicilian perspective. Gerontology. 2014;60:508–18.

7. Kastorini CM, Milionis HJ, Esposito K, Giugliano D, Goudevenos JA, Panagiotakos DB. The effect of Mediterranean diet on metabolic syndrome and its components: a meta-analysis of 50

studies and 534,906 individuals. J Am Coll Cardiol. 2011;57:1299–313.

8. Uylaşer V, Yildiz G. The historical development and nutritional importance of olive and olive oil constituted an important part of the Mediterranean diet. Crit Rev Food Sci Nutr. 2014;54:1092–101.

9. Vasto S, Rizzo C, Caruso C. Centenarians and diet: what they eat in the Western part of Sicily. Immun Ageing. 2012;9:10.

10. DeFelice SL. FIM, Rationale and Proposed Guidelines for the Nutraceutical Research & Education Act NREA, Foundation for Innovation in Medicine. 2002.http://www.fimdefelice.org/archives/arc.researchact.htm l archact.html. Accessed 10 Nov 2002.

11. Hoffman R, Gerber M. Food Processing and the Mediterranean Diet. Nutrients. 2015;7:7925–64.

12. Aiello A, Guccione GD, Accardi G, Caruso C. What olive oil for healthy ageing? Maturitas. 2015;80:117–8.

13. Biagi E, Candela M, Turroni S, Garagnani P, Franceschi C, Brigidi P. Ageing and gut microbes: perspectives for health maintenance and longevity. Pharmacol Res. 2013;69:11–20.

14. Lefevre M, Racedo SM, Ripert G, Housez B, Cazaubiel M, Maudet C, Jüsten P, Marteau P, Urdaci MC. Probiotic strain Bacillus subtilis CU1 stimulates immune system of elderly during common infectious disease period: a randomized, double-blind placebo-controlled study. Immun Ageing. 2015;12:24.

15. Heperkan D. Microbiota of table olive fermentations and criteria of selection for their use as starters. Front Microbiol. 2013;4:143.

16. Aponte M, Ventorino V, Blaiotta G, Volpe G, Farina V, Avellone G, Lanza CM, Moschetti G. Study of green Sicilian table olive fermentations through microbiological, chemical and sensory analyses. Food Microbiol. 2010;27:162–70.

17. Lehnen TE, da Silva MR, Camacho A, Marcadenti A, Lehnen AM. A review on effects of conjugated linoleic fatty acid (CLA) upon body composition and energetic metabolism. J Int Soc Sports Nutr. 2015;12:36.

18. Fazzari M, Trostchansky A, Schopfer FJ, Salvatore SR, Sánchez-Calvo B, Vitturi D, Valderrama R, Barroso JB, Radi R, Freeman

BA, Rubbo H. Olives and olive oil are sources of electrophilic fatty acid nitroalkenes. PLoS One. 2014;14(9):e84884.

19. Wang Y, Jones PJ. Dietary conjugated linoleic acid and body composition. Am J Clin Nutr. 2004;6 Suppl 79:1153S–8S.

20. Ershler WB, Keller ET. Age-associated increased interleukin-6 gene expression, late-life diseases, and frailty. Annu Rev Med. 2000;51:245–70.

21. Czerska M, Mikołajewska K, Zieliński M, Gromadzińska J, Wąsowicz W. Today's oxidative stress markers. Med Pr. 2015;66:393–405.

22. Gan KN, Smolen A, Eckerson HW, La Du BN. Purification of human serum paraoxonase/arylesterase. Evidence for one esterase catalyzing both activities. Drug Metab Dispos. 1991;19:100–6.

23. Zinellu A, Sotgia S, Usai MF, Chessa R, Deiana L, Carru C. Thiol redox status evaluation in red blood cells by capillary electrophoresis-laser induced fluorescence detection. Electrophoresis. 2005;26:1963–8.

24. RStudio Team. RStudio: Integrated Development for R. Boston, MA: RStudio, Inc.; 2015.http://www.rstudio.com/.

25. R Core Team. R. A language and environment for statistical computing. Vienna, Austria: R Foundation for Statistical Computing; 2015. https://www.R-project.org/.

INDEX